Positive Approaches to Dementia Care

They're lucky here Lord,
   They each have a wardrobe and a dressing table,
   and the large dormitory is divided so that
      there is some privacy when they go to bed,
      there is space to keep clothes, a few photographs,
      some books, a box of chocolates:
      yes they're lucky here, not like some of the others:
         the first day Mrs Lawrie went to the
         Old Folk's Home they emptied out her handbag
         to make sure there were no valuables in it –
         nobody had ever touched her handbag before;
         Carrie lay in a bedroom with nine others,
         one tatty bedside locker each, and a jam jar
         with flowers in it to share between them,
         a transistor crackled somewhere,
         but nobody was listening,
         they stared at each other,
         stared, and said nothing;
         they let Vi have her canary and kept it
         in the living-room,
         but she couldn't keep books by her bedside,
         and she loved books;
         Bill used to sit with his buttons undone,
         he was beyond pride and caring
         and nobody seemed to mind,
            clothes were something to shamble in and out of,
            morning and evening.

Lord, those who care for the aged do a job I couldn't do,
   give them the strength and kindness,
      patience and cheerfulness
      to do it;
   and may those who organize the care of the elderly,
   government, local councils, hospital boards,
   voluntary agencies, trustees —
   may all of them create conditions in which
   people can grow old with dignity,
   enjoy the life that remains to them,
   and die, cradled in love.

(Reprinted from 'The old folk's home' by
Michael Walker, with the permission of the
publishers, Arthur James Ltd.)

Positive Approaches to Dementia Care

Una P. Holden BA FBPsS
Consultant Clinical Psychologist,
Freelance, and providing clinical input to NHS East Cumbria, UK

Robert T. Woods MA MSc FBPsS
Senior Lecturer in Psychology,
University College, London, UK

THIRD EDITION

UNIVERSITY OF WOLVERHAMPTON
LIBRARY

Acc No. 2010753

CLASS 618. 976'

CONTROL 044304970x

DATE 26. JUN 1996

SITE BUR

89 HOL

CHURCHILL LIVINGSTONE
EDINBURGH HONG KONG LONDON MELBOURNE NEW YORK AND TOKYO 1995

CHURCHILL LIVINGSTONE
Medical Division of Pearson Professional Limited

Distributed in the United States of America by Churchill
Livingstone, 650 Avenue of the Americas, New York,
N.Y. 10011, and by associated companies, branches and
representatives throughout the world.

First edition (*Reality Orientation—Psychological Approaches to
the Confused Elderly*) 1982
Second edition (*Reality Orientation—Psychological Approaches
to the Confused Elderly*) 1988
Third edition 1995

ISBN 0-443-04970-X

British Library Cataloguing in Publication Data
A catalogue record for this book is available from the British
Library.

Library of Congress Cataloging in Publication Data
A catalog record for this book is available from the Library
of Congress.

For Churchill Livingstone:

Editorial director: Mary Law
Project editor: Valerie Bain
Copy editor: Jane Ward
Project manager: Valerie Burgess
Project controller: Nicola Haig/Pat Miller
Sales promotion executive: Maria O'Connor
Design direction: Judith Wright

The
publisher's
policy is to use
**paper manufactured
from sustainable forests**

Produced through Longman Malaysia

Contents

Preface to the third edition

This revised edition enjoys a completely new title (formerly *Reality Orientation*), and is indeed almost a completely new book. Over 15 years have now passed since we first began working on a book to describe the theory and practice of psychological approaches with older people suffering from a dementia, with the aim of convincing those working in this field that something could be done to help older 'confused' people. Our initial work with Reality Orientation (RO), as the first positive approach, has broadened into other areas and intervention programmes. There have been considerable advances in the understanding of normal ageing, research on degenerative conditions and outstanding developments in care settings with regard to awareness of needs, changes in institutional environments and a greater understanding of the individual older person. The RO banner is no longer able to encompass the range of material we wish to cover. Previous editions of the book were not simply about RO, of course; but a variety of approaches are now sufficiently developed to enable this edition to more clearly treat RO as one of many, rather than first of a few, ways of working with people with dementia.

Positive Approaches to Dementia Care refers to attitudes as well as active interventions. Far too frequently, older people are lumped together as though they are clones and are perceived as dependent, demanding and deteriorated; a problem for the family and the state. This stigmatisation of ageing results in discrimination and depersonalisation. The individual is lost in this false, negative perception and his or her skills,

experiences and wisdom are lost to the community. *Positive Approaches to Dementia Care* requires others to look again; to see and employ such retained abilities in order to allow the older individual the opportunity to continue to function as he or she would wish and to contribute to society's well-being; and, in the case of a degenerative condition, making it possible for the person to continue to care for him or herself as far as possible, again employing retained abilities in order to do so.

In the UK, as elsewhere, dramatic changes in systems of care are underway. Far-reaching changes in both health and community care have enormous implications for the care of people with a dementia. Greater emphasis on care in the community, together with a massive growth in the number of providers offering continuing care has made the need even more critical for all staff to be provided with as much information, skill and knowledge regarding dementia care as possible. This dispersal of care, whilst welcome in some respects, requires good training opportunities, and inter-disciplinary contact through team work if the advances that have been achieved are not to be lost in the chaos of re-organisation.

In order to make way for the new material in this edition, including over 150 additional references, we have in the text referred where appropriate to other sources for specific topics, recognising the welcome availability of an increasing number of books and articles on specific aspects of care for older people. Details of many of the earlier studies are no longer described ·

here; however, reviews of the earlier work are available and are cited in the text. The intention is to provide a handbook that will enable care staff and their managers to use a variety of interventions for the different individuals in their care.

Once again our families have proved patient and supportive, and we are grateful for their understanding. We continue to be appreciative of the many letters received from the UK, and far beyond, asking for further information or advice – we remain only too pleased to respond and welcome comments and useful suggestions.

Please send any correspondence to:

Una Holden-Cosgrove,
Ironmacannie Mill,
Balmaclellan,
Castle Douglas,
Kirkcudbrightshire,
DG7 3QS,
UK

Bob Woods,
Sub Department of
Clinical Health
Psychology,
University College
London,
Gower Street,
London WC1E 6BT,
UK

London 1995

PART 1

Positive approaches: theory and research

1

Introduction

Old age is for life what the evening is for the day. So one may call the evening the old age of the day and old age the evening of life.

Aristotle

Although the evening of life has arrived for elderly people, it does not follow that old age is something to be feared, dreaded and regarded with distaste. Glorious sunsets only occur in the evening, which is also the time when the problems and pressures of the day are eased with relaxation and peace. Many older people *are* unhappy, but many more are not. A number of factors are involved in determining a person's reaction to advancing years—social, economic, health, personality and so on. Generalisations about 'the elderly' should then be made cautiously.

This book concerns itself primarily with a section of the elderly population often described with such terms as 'confused', 'senile' and 'demented'. These people could be said to be ageing abnormally; they form—as we shall see below—a minority of elderly people. However, those working with them day-by-day may lose sight of what constitutes 'normal ageing', of what the evening of life can be. To provide a context for the abnormal, some psychological findings on normal ageing will be briefly discussed. Fuller reviews are provided by Woods & Britton (1985), Stuart-Hamilton (1994) and Stokes (1992) with in-depth coverage to be found in the *Handbook of the Psychology of Aging* edited by Birren & Schaie (1990).

NORMAL AGEING

Intellect

In the past, intellectual ability was thought to reach a peak in early adulthood. A decline in functioning from this time on accelerated as the seventh and eighth decades were reached. This view is reflected in standardisation data for commonly used intelligence tests (see Woods & Britton 1985, p. 25). It adds support to the general belief that most elderly people suffer from impaired intellect.

This simple notion of progressive decline throughout the adult years is now accepted to be totally misleading. In fact, age-related decline has been overestimated for a number of reasons.

Cross-sectional differences

The early studies that showed progressive deterioration were cross-sectional in nature. Results of, say, groups of 20, 30, 40, 50, 60 and 70-year-olds would be compared on a particular measure. The problem here is that the groups differ in many ways apart from age per se. Educational opportunities in 1920 and 1970, for example, were considerably different and may have restricted the education and intellectual development of today's 70-year-olds.

Differences in nutrition, culture, environment and medical care in the early years of life could also significantly disadvantage the older groups. At the time of assessment, differences between age groups in physical health, economic status and social contact could be present—all of which could have some impact on intellectual test performance. Intelligence tests often seem to be designed for younger people; the older person may be less motivated and less competitive and so would not perform as well as a younger person. The 80-year-old in a wheelchair may fail to see the relevance—to take an extreme example from Wechsler's Adult Intelligence Scale—of what one should do if lost in a forest in the daytime!

In a series of large-scale studies in the USA, Schaie and his colleagues (1990) have confirmed that when these factors are taken into account, and the emphasis placed more on changes with age rather than differences between age groups at one point in time, decline is only apparent in groups in their 60s and 70s. In these age groups there are large individual differences, with a number showing improvements in function, while others do show a decline, often related to poor health, sensory loss or other factors (Rabbitt 1988, Holland & Rabbitt 1991).

Differential relationship of age with various aspects of intelligence

In a number of studies, it has been noted that some aspects of intellectual performance show decline at an earlier age than others. In particular, tests with a large speed component show deterioration most rapidly; tests of verbal knowledge, however, may well show improvements into the 70s (Rabbitt 1988). These findings have been repeated by many researchers, who have related this to the notion of 'fluid' and 'crystallised' intelligence. Fluid intelligence is involved in adapting to novel situations, grasping new ideas, reasoning rapidly and so on. Crystallised intelligence reflects the person's acquired knowledge or accumulated wisdom. Fluid intelligence, then, is seen as declining more rapidly with age, while crystallised intelligence may well increase. More recent models emphasise a greater variability between individuals in the pattern of retained abilities, with increasing evidence of maintained function and even continued development of ability in areas of particular interest/ significance to the individual (Rybash et al 1986). For example, Schaie (1990) shows that, over a 7-year period, 90% of individuals initially aged 74 maintained or improved performance on at least two out of the five areas of cognitive function assessed; the areas retained differed greatly between individuals, however. These variations lead to considerable overlap between younger and older people; on most tests, some older people will perform better than a number of those who are 40 or 50 years their junior.

Memory and learning

The old adage that 'you can't teach an old dog

new tricks' reflects the stereotypical view of elderly people's memory and learning ability. They are thought of as living in the past, with excellent recall for years gone by, but inability to recall the events of the previous day!

Research evidence, however, provides similar findings to those regarding intellectual ability, with the memory loss that has been described being relatively small. Older people tend to be more variable in their performance, and a large overlap remains with the performances of younger people. Normal elderly people are able to learn and remember new things; the conditions under which learning and recall take place are much more important, however. For example, they are particularly impaired by fast rates of presentation of information and differentially helped by retrieval cues. A study in Australia showing that a group of 65–85-year-olds were able to learn German for the first time as proficiently as 16-year-olds (Naylor & Harwood 1975) affirms the capabilities of normal elderly people to learn in situations which are of importance to them.

There is increasing evidence that with special training programmes memory function can be enhanced in older people; for example, Schaie & Willis (1986) report a re-training programme with elderly subjects who had showed decline over a 14-year period; skills were improved, with almost half regaining their previous level of ability. There have been suggestions that lifestyle, such as a stimulating environment (Huppert 1988), may enhance the maintenance of function, and that factors such as anxiety, mild depression and low expectations from others may be relevant (Rabbitt 1988, Yesavage et al 1982). Older people may also underestimate their own ability, and this can become a self-fulfilling prophecy.

Personality and adjustment

Personality, defined as the person's usual ways of responding across a range of situations, tends to show continuity across the adult years into later life (Costa & McCrae 1978). However, it must be recognised that older people often face situations they have never encountered pre-

viously. Current older people have opportunities for leisure and travel that previous generations could not have imagined. The post-work phase of life, the so-called third age, has become increasingly significant, with older people having considerable political and economic influence. The expectations of successive cohorts of older people are shaped by their earlier experiences, and it seems likely that older people in the future may expect more from 'old age' than their predecessors.

The spectre of illness, frailty and death cannot, of course, be avoided. Although the aim of medical science may be to reduce what might be described as the fourth age to a minimum, many older people will face a period where their health becomes a real constraint rather than an inconvenience. The ways in which the person is able to bring to bear the coping strategies learned earlier in life to handle disability, pain, loss of function and control will play a key role in determining his adjustment in the final part of his lifespan. A flexible, compensatory stance is likely to be most helpful in adapting to enforced changes and unwelcome circumstances, finding ways around obstacles and seeking out new ways of reaching a goal.

In this period of life, the person will often need to develop a sense of priorities; there simply is not enough energy—physical or mental—to do everything. Routines may come to the fore, as an effective energy-saving strategy rather than a reflection of rigidity. Personality and intellect are interdependent domains, although often written about separately. The accumulated knowledge of life, of how people function, of relationships, and of the ways of the world may find application in the older person's wisdom and maturity, which may shine through the person's own difficulties in a sense of peace. Others may have reached this stage with too many of their own tensions and conflicts unresolved and be unable to deal with their inner turmoil or feelings of anxiety, anger or rejection. Therefore, late life may present the older person with a set of challenges, the adjustment to which will be largely determined by the resources the person brings with him.

Conclusions on normal ageing

In this extremely brief review, three major areas of psychological functioning have been considered. It has been suggested that changes do occur, but that these are usually relatively small. The diversity of older people must be stressed; normal ageing can be rich and full; it can be empty and sad. The whole range exists and cannot be constrained into any stereotype or image, whether blissful or miserable.

The importance of other factors relating to poor performance should be noted. Physical health is particularly important; Holland & Rabbitt (1991) review its relationship to impaired cognitive functioning in elderly people, but it also constrains the opportunities the person has to live life to the full and so is also relevant to personal adjustment. It could, indeed, be argued that many apparently age-related changes may be brought about by the increased incidence of ill-health in the elderly. This serves as a reminder, also, that the passage of time itself does not bring about any changes in functioning. It is other processes—of disease, environment or whatever—also varying in time, that actually lead to changes in behaviour.

Losses of various types are experienced by most people as they age. Sensory losses, reduced physical speed and power, loss of physical health, loss of hair, loss of loved ones, loss of status and so on. The remarkable feature of elderly people from a psychological perspective is their ability to cope in the face of losses and adversity. Most elderly people are able to show good psychological function and adjustment, especially in those areas of life which they see as important and relevant.

DEMENTIA

Recent years have seen dramatic changes in our understanding of dementia, which have required definitions of dementia and diagnostic guidelines to be re-examined. Dementia is a clinical state with many different causes and characterised by loss of previous cognitive and social abilities. The variety of disease processes under-lying the disability is one of the factors leading to considerable variability in clinical presentation. The identification of new causes and disease processes—such as Lewy body dementia, frontal dementia and Prion diseases—means that previous work on, for example, the prevalence or clinical features of Alzheimer's disease has to be re-evaluated (Burns 1993). The pattern of dysfunction and the impact on daily living and social behaviour vary greatly. Dementia itself is then a blanket category that can never be considered as an adequate description or explanation of a person's condition.

The dementias should be distinguished from delirium. Here the patient is not alert and shows clouding of consciousness. It usually arises from an acute illness: infection, drug intoxication, the effects of surgery and so on. The major treatment approach to delirium is, naturally enough, to treat the underlying cause. Many doctors use the term 'acute confusional state' in place of delirium. The condition may occur with younger people during a fever or coming round from an anaesthetic: not knowing where they are or what is happening to them; seeing things that are not there and becoming disturbed and restless, perhaps. In older people, the signs may be less dramatic and, if the underlying cause is not dealt with, it may persist, often resulting in misunderstanding and perhaps misdiagnosis as a degenerative condition (see Byrne 1987).

The traditional distinction of dementias into 'senile' and 'pre-senile', according to the age of onset (with 65 the usual arbitrary dividing line) has little to commend it. The major form of dementia in both middle-aged and older patients is Alzheimer's disease; at postmortem, Alzheimer's disease appears to occur in about half the population of elderly people with dementia. It is associated with particular brain changes—including plaques and neurofibrillary tangles—which can only be seen under the microscope at postmortem. The frequency of plaques and tangles has been found to correlate with deterioration in intellectual and behavioural function (Blessed et al 1968, Wilcock & Esiri 1982). It should be noted that small numbers of plaques and tangles are often found in postmortem studies of the brains of normal older people. Larger numbers seem to be required before any impairment occurs. The pathological research is reviewed by Burns (1993). Studies have also indicated deficits in certain chemical substances in the brains of sufferers of Alzheimer's disease. This reduction in the amount of certain neurotransmitters has led to hopes of pharmacological therapy, by replacing the missing substances. In practice, this has proved difficult to achieve so far. There are some encouraging signs of progress (e.g. Wilcock 1984, Little et al 1985, Eagger et al 1991), but as yet there is no proven medical treatment for Alzheimer's disease; the first step is likely to be a drug which slows down the rate of decline for a period in a proportion of people with Alzheimer's disease.

The second major form of dementia traditionally identified is multi-infarct (or arteriosclerotic) dementia. This results from, in effect, a number of small strokes damaging brain tissue. Its progressive decline is usually described as sudden and stepwise, in contrast to the gradual, steady decline of Alzheimer's disease. There may even be a period of improvement if the interval between strokelets is long enough. Multi-infarct dementia occurs more commonly in people with other cardiovascular problems (e.g. high blood pressure).

Medical assessment of patients with dementia has as its primary aim the exclusion of the potentially treatable causes for the person's condition and of treatable dementias (Cummings 1984). These—with the exception of depression, discussed below—are, regrettably, rarely identified in older people in practice.

Recently, it has become clear that within what has been thought of as Alzheimer's disease there may be a number of distinct conditions that have in common some of the characteristic brain changes of Alzheimer's disease, but in other ways are quite different. A good example of this is Lewy body disease, which may, in fact, be the second most common form of dementia after Alzheimer's disease (Perry et al 1990). Patients with this disorder are more likely to suffer from hallucinations and other disturbances, to fluctuate cognitively and to be particularly sensitive to the side-effects of neuroleptic medication, i.e. major tranquillisers (Perry & Perry 1993). Similarly, there may be several forms of dementia related to vascular (blood supply) problems, which are currently thought of simply as multi-infarct dementias (Peisah et al 1993). Genetic studies suggest that there are forms of Alzheimer's disease that are inherited (in a very few families), with others not showing the same genetic fingerprint. Distinguishing types of dementia while the person is still alive is problematic, as so much depends on the specific changes occurring in the brain, which can only be confirmed under a powerful microscope at postmortem. The various brain scans being used at present cannot reliably distinguish them, nor is the pattern of impairment of function sufficiently specific in each to make diagnosis of the exact condition reliable during the person's life. When seen over a period of time, and when the disorder goes beyond a mild impairment, the diagnosis that a dementia is present is reasonably accurate, even if the exact disorder cannot be identified with certainty.

Whatever the type of dementia, memory difficulties are usually prominent among the first indications that something is wrong. Typically, new learning ability will be particularly impaired. Well-established habits and memories from the past are usually retained—initially at least. Those affected may forget an appointment, or arrive on the wrong day. They may become lost in unfamiliar surroundings or reach the shops and forget what they had intended to buy. The person loses the ability to grasp complex ideas, and reasoning becomes less abstract. Self-neglect may occur, and, as the condition progresses, the person may lose the ability to look after such personal needs as washing, dressing, toileting and even eating.

Perhaps partly as a result of there being a number of different conditions, and partly the random element of where exactly damage occurs, the pattern of dysfunction varies from person to person. Some may have particular difficulties in speech, or in tasks like dressing and other practical skills requiring hand–eye coordination. The rate of deterioration is also variable, although the progressive nature of the disease may be an important feature in distinguishing these conditions from static damage to a specific area of the brain. The rate of deterioration often seems slower when the condition begins in the 80s, rather than when the person is 60. As a group, their life expectancy is much reduced (particularly for younger sufferers), but the total time course is extremely variable (Burns & Lewis 1993). Personality changes do sometimes occur, and the person may lose a sense of what is socially acceptable. Relatives are very distressed to see patients begin to swear crudely for the first time in their lives, for example. Retention of personality traits—pleasant and unpleasant—is more frequently encountered than this distressing reversal of personality. Some patients retain an excellent social facade and are able to engage in small talk despite severe deterioration.

Sufferers from these conditions are often said to lack insight into what is happening to them, as it is the very organ of insight that is dysfunctional. Certainly, very few sufferers have awareness of their condition in the sense of being able to name it. In our experience, however, many people do have some level of awareness, particularly when the condition is less advanced. It is not unusual for a sufferer to show signs of anxiety and depression, perhaps in response to the repeated failures being experienced. Some patients admit loss of memory or show awareness of disintegration. One severely impaired lady, for example, responded 'my brain has gone' to an enquiry about her health. Through a miasma of rambling, confused talk that was difficult to comprehend, this comment had a poignant clarity. The sufferers who do deny their problems, perhaps to the extent of accusing neighbours of stealing a purse that they have mislaid, may be seen as defending themselves from an awesome reality. Despair, anxiety, self-blame and anger are all reactions seen in unimpaired people in the face of severe stress. It may well be that by giving more attention to the processes by which the dementing person is attempting to cope with what is happening to him or her, differences in behaviour between different sufferers could be better understood (e.g. Cohen et al 1984). The so-called 'happily dementing' person may have found his or her own way of facing the threat to his or her identity that dementia poses, in acceptance and resignation to the disability involved.

Careful evaluation and investigations to exclude other possible causes of the presenting picture are important in every case. In the early stages of these disorders, some diagnostic problems do arise. Most people would probably have to admit to episodes of forgetfulness. Thankfully, a saucepan boiled dry or a missed appointment do not in themselves mean some form of dementia is present! A history of progressive decline is a more serious indication.

Some older people who are depressed show some memory problems and other cognitive difficulties. This has been described as 'depressive pseudo-dementia' (Sahakian 1991). In many cases these deficits improve to some extent following the depression being appropriately treated. A diagnosis made while the person remains depressed is likely to be unreliable. Certain psychological tests are claimed to be able to discriminate well between groups of patients suffering from depression and dementia (e.g. Roth et al 1986). However, there are still patients who remain diagnostic puzzles over a period of months or even years. Diagnostic tests are usually standardised on groups of people with clear-cut depression and dementia. These are the patients who rarely need to be assessed in this way in practice!

The nature and cause of cognitive impairment in depression remain unclear (Sahakian 1991). Deficits are likely to be less consistent, more task specific and may be, in part, related to depressed people's reluctance to 'guess' when not completely certain of their answer, and their inability to produce sustained motivation and effort in demanding tasks (Woods & Britton 1985). Depression can then lead to diagnostic errors, unless a 'wait and see' approach is adopted. If depression is present, it should be treated; time will tell whether the person also has a progressive cognitive impairment. In studies such as Portalska & Bernstein (1988) and Ryan (1994) it is depression which leads to many errors in diagnosis at the initial assessment. These mistakes, which usually became evident in the course of time, illustrate the pitfalls of relying on assessment at a single point in time only.

It often seems to be assumed that depression and dementing disorders are mutually exclusive; of course they are not. They are both common disorders in older people. Both could occur together simply by chance, even if depression were not a predictable reaction to the experience of the early stages of a dementing disorder (see Miller & Morris 1993, p. 63–64).

Most elderly people do not and will not experience a dementing process. The EURODEM group results from a collaborative European project using stringent criteria indicate that the present norm for an overall rate of dementia in those over 65 years is between 4% and 7% (Hofman et al 1991). A good updated account of prevalence and incidence is provided by Jagger & Lindesay (1993). The number of people in the UK over 65 is now levelling off, having risen greatly in previous decades, but the number of 'old old' people (i.e. over 80) continues to increase. This latter age group is more prone to a dementing disorder; studies indicate around a fifth of over 80s have a dementia (Livingston & Hinchliffe 1993), but the condition tends not to be so severe as in younger old people.

Whilst people with dementia form a minority of elderly people, they are a sizeable, visible group. They make great demands upon health and social services. Although many are accommodated in hospitals, and residential and nursing homes, in the UK approximately three-quarters of dementia sufferers will be in the community: living alone or with relatives or friends. Families play a large part in supporting them (Bergmann et al 1978) and the strain on the family can be considerable (Gilleard 1984c, Morris et al 1988). Many severely disabled people with these conditions are supported by families, neighbours and social services. There has been a great deal of research on services, the care-giving role and education/training programmes to aid the care-

giver to cope (Morris & Morris 1993, Gilleard 1992, Brodaty 1992). Moriarty & Levin (1993) discuss dementia within the context of the community care arrangements in the UK and stress the need to ensure the continuation of a range of services and a team approach that can meet the full potential extent of the individual's needs.

Psychosocial factors, such as life events, isolation, bereavement, social class and personality have not been shown to have any significance in causing dementias (Gilhooly 1984). It is possible that factors such as diet and exercise, which contribute to better cardiovascular function, would also be preventative factors in relation to multi-infarct dementia. In some cases, a bereavement, change of house or other upheaval brings the dementia to the attention of family members living away from the person, or to doctors and social workers. Usually close examination reveals, for example, that the spouse who died was doing a great deal to compensate for the person's deficits, which were developing before the bereavement. Similarly, the change of house removes a number of environmental props that were helping to sustain the person's failing function.

Dementia is then a blanket term for a number of conditions involving progressive decline in intellect, skills and memory, which affect a large minority of elderly people. Diagnosis needs to be carefully made to exclude any treatable conditions and to ensure that depression is appropriately treated. There are currently no medical treatments available for the most common dementias. These conditions place great strain on families, hospitals, residential care and community services. Of all the problems experienced by elderly people, it has the most distressing impact for all concerned. Its study has been particularly hampered by the assumption that it is an inevitable part of old age, that nothing can be done to alleviate its impact or modify its course. In recent years, this attitude has begun to change and Alzheimer's disease, particularly, is now attracting considerably more attention. More resources for research and care are becoming available and interest is growing rapidly. This trend must continue, for the sake of the sufferers, their families and indeed for all our futures.

A POSITIVE APPROACH

Attitudes towards the elderly in Western society have often in the past been discriminatory, rejecting and negative. Those attributes that elderly people do have have been discounted in a society where speed, innovation and physical attributes are placed on a pedestal. Wisdom, experience and a sense of perspective are not valued as much as in certain other cultures, where to be an elder is an aspiration—rather than a fear—of the young.

If healthy elderly people have received a raw deal, how much more have mentally and physically disabled elderly suffered? In terms of facilities, medical geriatric and psychogeriatric units have often been housed in the oldest buildings, quite unsuitable for the purpose. Such hospitals may be in splendid isolation, many miles from relatives, friends and familiar surroundings. The grounds may be glorious, but few go out and enjoy them. Visitors—often equally elderly—find that the journey restricts visits severely.

The role of the staff has been seen as custodial rather than restorative or treatment-orientated. Morale, typically, has been low; recruitment of staff difficult. Extra payments for working on geriatric wards in the UK have been considered necessary. Nurses would be deliberately moved from geriatric wards after a certain time. The expectation was that the work must be unpleasant, tiresome and depressing. Anyone expressing a desire to work in this field was viewed with surprise and bewilderment, as if no one in possession of their senses would choose to do so.

In recent years, the growth in the old old population that has been and is taking place has grasped the attention of those at every level of health, social and voluntary services. Fresh approaches are being pursued, and more resources directed towards the ageing population. Custodial care concepts have been replaced by 'community care' as the sheer number of disabled elderly people being supported by relatives, friends and other social supports outside institutions has been realised. However, there are fears that the previous hospital provision is being replaced by nursing home environments, some just as institutional, with little monitoring, back-up or attention to the special needs of people with dementia. There are more positive approaches filtering through institutions catering for the elderly, there is more readiness to review traditional practices; the concern is that pressures of finance and the fragmentation of services resulting from the effective transfer of long-term care for people with dementia from the NHS to the independent sector will halt this progress and reverse some of what has been achieved.

Attitudes have by no means changed completely. There is perhaps now greater diversity; some are fully in tune with a positive, person-centred approach; in others there is resistance to change. New ideas often need more resources that are not forthcoming. The elderly are still perceived generally as an unattractive group with whom to work; problems of recruitment in this field occur in a variety of professions: doctors, psychiatrists, nurses, social workers, etc. Our own profession of clinical psychology has shown an enormous increase in the last 15 years of the number working at least part of the time with the elderly. Yet this area remains unattractive for most trainees coming into clinical psychology, until they experience the potential scope for positive psychological approaches at first hand.

This book focuses on positive approaches to working with elderly people disabled by a dementia. We are not advocating a particular set of techniques that all those working in this field should carry out on all their clients. Rather, we are commending a much more broadly based means of working with these people. It begins with basic attitudes, values and principles concerning the worth, humanity and dignity of those suffering from dementia. Any positive methods not based on such values and attitudes may do more harm than good. They must be the starting point for good practice in this area. Then there are techniques for helping communication, maintaining and developing skills and abilities and for tackling common areas of difficulty. Our experience is that the various positive approaches can complement, rather than compete with, each other. Our scheme has roots in reminiscence therapy, reality orientation, validation therapy, learning theory, the social psychology of group interaction and communication, individual programme planning and the nursing process. We emphasise the importance of seeing each elderly person as an individual and as a 'whole person' with psychological, social and emotional needs in addition to the physical needs which have been the main focus in the past, perhaps because they are in many ways easier to meet.

We hope readers will take from this book an integrated, individualised, value-based means of working and communicating with elderly people with dementia. We commend this approach not simply because of any benefits that may accrue in terms of quality of life for the elderly people concerned, but also because of the increased morale often noted among those using such methods. This may then bring further benefits for the elderly person in relationship with the helper.

Part 2 of the book gives practical guidance as to how to put this philosophy and some of the techniques into practice. The remainder of Part 1 focuses on specific approaches, giving the background on strategies contributing to our overall scheme. There is still a need for further development; there is always scope for fresh insights, better research studies, more inspired theorising and greater experience. No approach should be static or incapable of further development and revision. The challenges of working positively with people afflicted by what can be such severe and disabling conditions are immense. They need to be tackled with determination, flexibility and persistence.

2

An overview of positive approaches

INTRODUCTION

Psychological approaches to working with people with dementia have taken many forms and have been described in a variety of ways over a number of years. Several reviews of the earlier reports have appeared (e.g. Miller 1977, Woods & Britton 1977, 1985), and a number of other sources provide simple outlines of a variety of approaches (e.g. Stokes & Goudie 1990). There is considerable overlap and much common ground; our grouping of approaches, though arbitrary, should help to draw together the now extensive literature. Discussion of reality orientation (RO) is reserved for Chapter 3, in view of the greater amount of research interest it has attracted.

It must be appreciated that there is a wide variation in the type and degree of dementia and impairment of function from individual to individual. The special needs and strengths of the individual are the prime consideration; an approach applicable to one person with dementia may not be appropriate for another. Different approaches may be indicated at different points, as the person's condition changes. In this and the succeeding chapter we are seeking to give the reader a sense of the range of positive approaches available in dementia care and of the evidence for their effectiveness.

STIMULATION AND ACTIVITY PROGRAMMES

Sensory deprivation, stimulation and activity

Cameron (1941) demonstrated elegantly that the often observed increase in confusion and wandering at night in elderly people was related not to the effects of fatigue but simply to the effects of reduced sensory input, by showing that such confusion occurred in a darkened room during daytime. Elderly people may experience reduced sensory input for several reasons: first, by virtue of normal deterioration in sensory acuity: sight can show loss, as can sensitivity of hearing and touch. Secondly, some of the environments in which older people live—in institutional care or isolated in the community—can be monotonous and lacking in sensory stimulation. Thirdly, there are instances where the person 'chooses' to withdraw and reject stimulation, refusing to respond to the environment or react to it, perhaps as a means of coping with a large, unfamiliar institution.

These considerations suggest that sensory deprivation can increase confusion in elderly people and that many elderly people are deprived of sensory stimulation. Early studies (Corso 1967) clearly demonstrated that even young people suffered from confusion when deprived of sensory stimulation for a period of time. It should be noted that sensory deprivation results as much from monotony as from lack of stimulation. The constant playing of the radio or non-stop TV lead to a lack of response even to items the person would otherwise have found interesting. The person shuts her eyes to escape from the continuous background noise and joins the others who are already dozing... It is *change* in sensory input that is stimulating.

Whether based on this rationale or simply on the notion that activity is a 'good thing', there were a number of studies offering a range of social, physical and psychological stimulation (including occupational therapy, domestic and recreational activities) that reported positive effects (see Woods & Britton 1977). Such activities have become a widely accepted aspect of good practice,

are offered in many care settings and are the subject of various resource books and guides (see Appendix 3). The focus of attention has now shifted to more detailed consideration of different types of stimulation or activity, and to ways of increasing the response of people with dementia—including those most severely impaired—to activity and stimulation.

For example, much more specific forms of stimulation were used by Norberg et al (1986). They evaluated the effects of music, touch and objects expected to stimulate the person's senses of taste, touch and smell (e.g. fur, hay, bread, camphor). Two severely impaired patients with dementia, who showed little, if any, verbal communication, were carefully observed whilst receiving the various forms of stimulation. The results indicated a definite positive response to music, but no differences in reaction to different objects or to touch were detected. In similar vein, Gaebler & Hemsley (1991) identified a response to music in the majority of a group of six patients, whose dementia was very advanced and with whom verbal communication was impossible. These studies are particularly important in that they focused on patients who would normally be excluded from evaluative studies and they developed means by which the response to environmental stimulation of patients with extremely limited communicative skills could be reliably monitored. Very detailed, careful observation is required to build up a consistent, measurable pattern of response from the movements of the person's head, body, limbs and face, which to the untrained eye appear random and without purpose.

An evaluation of the effects of music on a less impaired group of 'Alzheimer patients' is reported by Lord & Garner (1993). Groups of 20 nursing home residents were given 'Big band' music from the 1920s and 1930s, puzzle exercises or the 'standard' recreational activities of drawing and painting and TV over a 6-month period in daily half-hour recreational sessions. The evaluation clearly favoured the music group; their recall of personal information was better, and their mood and social interaction also showed improvement compared with the other two groups. 'The subjects in the music therapy sessions always smiled, laughed, sang, danced and whistled while listening to the music.' The other groups did not elicit the same degree of anticipation, enjoyment and pleasure and were less effective as triggers of social interaction. Bright (1992) describes further the implementation and value of music therapy in dementia.

Two other sources of stimulation that perhaps approach the almost universal appeal of music are pets and children. An innovative programme bringing school-age children into hospitals and homes to get to know and work with older people (including a number with dementia) has been described by Langford (1993); the increase in interaction and activity prompted by the (carefully planned and prepared) presence of the children is remarkable. The children place the older person in a position of knowledge and experience; the older person is allowed to relax and play again without concern about appearing childish. Many will have observed a dramatic effect when younger children (and babies) are brought to visit; overlearned parenting responses re-emerge. Such stimulation needs careful handling—the attraction wears off rapidly when the children are too noisy and lively, or run around out of control. Several evaluative studies of the impact of pets have been reported. For example, Elliott & Milne (1991) and Haughie et al (1992) evaluated the impact of a visitor with a dog on a psychiatric hospital ward where most patients had a diagnosis of dementia. In both studies, interaction levels increased markedly when the dog and visitor were present. In the latter study, to control for novelty, photographs of the dog and visitor were also used as stimuli; they were associated with a smaller, but still significant, increase in interaction. Nursing staff rated a number of aspects of the patients' behaviour—including mobility and dependency—as improved during the sessions when the dog was present. The improvements were not maintained on days subsequent to the visits of the dog. The presence of a stimulus is needed to elicit the higher level of interaction and other changes.

A recent development that appears more immediately related to the concept of sensory deprivation is 'Snoezelen', an approach originating in Holland which seeks to increase the amount of sensory stimulation through changing coloured lights and visual effects, relaxing armchairs and cushions, pleasant smells and even a vibrating cushion and a soap bubble machine! The word 'Snoezelen' is a contraction of two Dutch words, meaning 'sniffing and dozing'. A positive evaluation has appeared (Benson 1994) that suggests increased relaxation, improved mood and decreased agitation during Snoezelen sessions, although with little carry over beyond the session. This article also suggests that conventional relaxation techniques—gentle music and one-to-one encouragement of slow deep breathing—were equally effective in calming patients with dementia. Methods of providing tactile stimulation, hand/foot massage, aromatherapy, etc, are also suggested as relaxing, enjoyable activities (e.g. West & Brockman 1994). Further support for the usefulness of relaxation techniques with this population is provided by Welden & Yesavage (1982). Twenty-four matched pairs of patients with dementia attended either a relaxation training group or a current affairs discussion group for an hour three times a week over a 3-month period. Relaxation instructions included progressive muscle relaxation and a self-hypnosis technique. Subjects attending relaxation sessions showed improvement on ratings of behavioural function compared with the control group. In addition, just over 40% of those taught relaxation techniques no longer required sleeping medication; none of the control group was able to discontinue.

Physical exercise

Most activity programmes have included some form of physical exercise, although there is, at times, a reluctance to encourage the involvement of older, frailer people. Can aged muscles and weakened stamina stand the strain of such exercise? Bassey (1985) reviewed and examined the literature on the effects of exercise on physical health and well-being in older people, and concluded that they can take the 'strain' and that there was sufficient evidence to show that inactivity is the major weakening factor. Improvements may be slower and smaller but contribute greatly to independent living and to circulation. She states that exercise may be of *more* value to the aged than the young. Blumenthal et al (1989) reported a number of physical benefits from 4 months of aerobic exercises in a group of older people, compared with a waiting-list control group and a group taking part in yoga and flexibility sessions.

Can physical exercise make a difference to older people with dementia? Morgan (1991) reviews several studies (mainly from the 1970s) with a bearing on this question. There have been some indications of limited benefits on aspects of cognitive function (e.g. Molloy et al 1988), but overall the studies have not been well controlled, so any benefits cannot be linked with certainty to the physical exercise component of the total treatment package. Also, there has been a tendency to use institutionalisation rather than a diagnosis of dementia as the criterion for inclusion in the study.

Physical activity as studied has been highly structured: light bending and stretching exercises whilst sitting in a chair, throwing a ball, knocking down skittles, brisk walking, rhythmical movements, movement to music, etc, all demanding task attention. Several manuals and audiotapes are available to assist care-workers in planning such programmes (e.g. Fisher (1994) *Creative Movement for Older Adults* and Strickland & Hill (1992) *Gentle Exercises for the Elderly*, both Winslow Press).

There is, therefore, evidence that physical exercise can produce changes of a physical nature in older people in general, with much weaker evidence that cognitive function in people with dementia might be enhanced. Physical exercise may be important in that it is one of the simplest forms of activity for this population. Future studies should also explore its impact on sleep patterns; Morgan (1987) suggests that 'activities which result in both mental and physical stimulation have implications for improved sleep quality'. Holden (1991) recommends that some physical exercise should be performed during the daytime or early evening, with late evenings offering quieter activities in preparation for sleep.

CHANGES IN THE ENVIRONMENT

Introduction

This group of approaches is based on the underlying idea that the elderly person will respond to her environment, which can be manipulated to produce and maintain positive changes in the person's functioning. The environment is thought to have a particularly influential role with older people with dementia; Lawton's model of 'environmental docility' (see Parmelee & Lawton 1990) suggests that the lower the person's level of competence, the more behaviour is determined by the environment. The person becomes less able to act on, adapt and shape the environment for themselves, or to use internal strategies to compensate for environmental deficiencies.

Clearly there is here an overlap with the previous section, where a stimulating environment was the therapeutic tool, and the next section, where behavioural methods largely based on environmental manipulation (together with a reinforcement system) will be discussed. Reality orientation (RO) also has effects on the person's overall environment through 24 hour RO. In this section, those studies not subsumed under the other approaches will be discussed. It is quite conceivable that all these approaches owe whatever effectiveness they possess to processes they have in common. A priority for future research should be the finer analysis of the mechanisms of change.

Physical changes in the environment

This includes attempts to bring about changes by design, by structural alteration or by rearrangement in some way of the physical environment. This tends to be particularly relevant in residential or daycare settings; in the person's own home in the community the emphasis is more on retaining all that is familiar to the person, only making changes where absolutely necessary, e.g. to reduce risk of harm to the person.

In a review of innovations in long-stay care for people with dementia, Carr & Marshall (1993) highlight the trend towards units specialising in the care of people with dementia; in many instances these are planned to be small and local to the area from which the residents come and to be more domestic in scale and style than the long-stay hospital units they often replace. Residents are much more likely to have their own rooms in such units. Single rooms represent a major improvement in the care environment (Garland 1991); they offer greatly increased scope for privacy, for the person to have more of their own possessions with them and to have a meaningful personal space to which it is worth being orientated. In the USA, units still tend to be large: often as many as 80–120 beds 'to optimise service-production costs and regulatory requirements' (Regnier & Pynoos 1992), although these may be arranged in clusters of say 8 or 12. However, as Carr & Marshall reflect, the trend in the UK and Australia is very definitely towards 'homely' care. What is achieved is always a compromise; there are many different conceptions of 'home'; even if there are only eight residents on a unit, one may be sure that there will be eight different sets of tastes and preferences; this again makes the issue of the person having their own room, some personal living space, so essential. In the UK, regulations for the registration of residential and nursing homes are such that further compromises are necessary, for example, to meet stringent fire and hygiene standards. In practice, it is clearly noticeable that changes have also occurred to existing facilities. Wards that once had huge dormitories, with high beds with cot-sides, lacking colour or personalisation; residential homes that provided simple, sparsely furnished shared rooms; nearly all are now much more homely and welcoming, with large rooms divided with room dividers, and fireplaces added to living rooms.

In France, a small homely unit for dementia care would be described as a 'cantou', a word meaning 'hearth', reflecting that home is around the fireside (Ritchie et al 1992). These units often have one large communal room, with the residents' bedrooms and bathrooms, etc. opening off the main room, dispensing with confusing corridors and reducing the load on spatial memory. The kitchen area might typically be in a corner of the communal room, with food preparation a central interest and activity. The notion of the kitchen as being the centre of a home is reflected in the design of a home in Leicester, where the home's kitchen is in a central position, with large windows so residents may watch the chef at work. Unfortunately, regulations do not allow residents there to participate in preparing the meal as they would in some homes in France.

Many innovations involve a change to the care-giving regime, as well as a change to the physical environment; arguably, it is the former that is more important, in that negative staff attitudes and practices would negate the effects of the best physical environment. The effects of the care regime will be reviewed below, but it is worth making the point that the design of the building can have a direct influence both on the regime and the residents more directly, if only by providing certain constraints on what may be attempted. Keen (1989), in a helpful review of architectural influences, argues that there has been little consideration given to the contribution the buildings themselves might make to the problems. In similar vein, Regnier & Pynoos (1992) state 'facilities that are managed well are often kept from pursuing their most effective work because negative aspects of the environment are antagonistic to therapeutic goals' (p. 782). They discuss 12 environmental and behavioural principles of design which they argue have an impact on the quality of life and function of older people with cognitive impairment:

- privacy, e.g. own room
- provide opportunities for social exchange and interaction
- control, choice and autonomy; promote opportunities for residents to make choices and control events that influence outcomes
- orientation and wayfinding; an environment that is easy to comprehend

- safety and security; ensure user will sustain no harm, injury or undue risk
- accessibility and functioning; can the person manipulate features of the environment?
- provide a stimulating environment that is safe but challenging
- sensory aspects; allow for changes in visual, auditory and olfactory senses
- familiarity; use historical reference and solutions influenced by tradition to give a sense of continuity and familiarity
- aesthetics and appearance; attractive, provocative and non-institutional designs
- personalisation; mark it as the property of a single, unique individual
- adaptability; flexible enough to fit changing personal characteristics.

These authors exemplify these principles in practice in the USA in relation to design features in residential facilities (and the person's own home). In the UK, Manser (1991) is among architects now taking an imaginative approach to designing environments for people with dementia. Norman (1987), from a study of a number of innovative units for older people with severe dementia, draws attention to a number of design features that appeared helpful:

- single storey buildings
- ample, safe space for walking indoors and outdoors
- individual private rooms
- easy orientation and identification of key facilities
- minimal distances between sitting, dining, bedroom and lavatory provision
- kitchenette facilities
- minimal boundaries between staff and resident 'territory'
- easy access to shops
- good transport facilities
- dignified non-institutional furnishing and decoration with opportunity to furnish/ decorate own room.

There is clearly considerable convergence between the various accounts, particularly in relation to privacy, through single rooms, safety and orientation aids. Indeed, a study requiring relatives of patients in hospital care to list in order of importance the 10 priorities for a satisfactory care environment produced a similar list (Holden 1991), although 'non-slip floors' was high on the list, perhaps reflecting relatives giving particular emphasis to safety.

However, despite considerable interest in design, and the significant changes that have been achieved, there is, as Parmelee & Lawton (1990) indicate, little empirical research specifically evaluating design features. This may be in part because of the difficulties inherent in examining such complex, interrelated issues. Therefore, it is not even established that reducing the size of the unit per se has beneficial effects; smaller units almost inevitably necessitate a higher staff–resident ratio, and this may be the crucial factor. Providing 'wandering paths' which safely return the person to their starting point, and using colour and architectural and other features to distinguish areas within the unit have also not been adequately evaluated. Netten (1989, 1993) has examined the relationship between architectural complexity of residential homes and the person with dementia's ability to find their way around. This study illustrated the complexity of these issues in that different factors were shown to operate in large, communal homes compared with those in homes where residents lived together in small groups; the latter tended to aid orientation, with the presence of meaningful decision points acting as helpful landmarks.

Most attention over the years in empirical studies has been given to arranging the environment in such a way as to encourage social interaction: arranging furniture to make communication easier, in small groups around coffee tables rather than around the walls of a large dayroom (see Woods & Britton 1985, Wattis & Church 1986). The emphasis in the past was on breaking up a large waiting-room type of space into smaller, more social areas; the new units described above are being designed so that the living areas are more immediately conducive to a social atmosphere. At mealtimes also, interaction is influenced by environmental factors. For example, Davies and Snaith (1980) found that when tables were set for groups of six (instead of patients sitting around the walls, with individual trays attached to their chairs) a more normal social situation was created. Table-cloths, water jugs and so on were provided, and, to make conversation easier, efforts were made to reduce the high level of background noise. There was an immediate increase in social interaction; patients began to help each other and converse more.

Little attention has been given as yet to adaptations to the person's own home, although Regnier & Pynoos (1992) have some suggestions. Care needs to be taken in seeking to render the home more 'suitable' for care in the community, for example by moving furniture to make the place less cluttered or by putting appliances out of action to reduce risks, that the essence of the familiarity and personal choice which is the advantage of care at home is not lost. It is quite conceivable that institutionalisation could occur in the home setting as elsewhere.

There is then, overall, rather little evidence that changing the physical environment per se brings about changes in function in the person with dementia; however, later sections will demonstrate that when these changes are embedded in changes in the way care is offered, the current interest in improving the design of physical environments for people with dementia is more than justified.

Prosthetic environments

For a variety of physical disabilities, aids or prostheses are available to help in the restoration of a competent performance, e.g. dentures, glasses and hearing aids. As long ago as 1964, Lindsley advanced the notion of creating a prosthetic environment for geriatric patients in which their disabilities are compensated for by special features of that environment.

It is not necessary to re-train a person, but there may be an element of learning involved in order for the person to be able to use these aids effectively. For instance, if a patient has difficulty in finding the toilet and becomes incontinent because of this, a coloured line leading to the toilet could be marked on the wall. (Floor markings should be avoided as they lead to poor walking and other difficulties.) The person would then have to be taught to use the line and so would need to learn that, for example, the blue line leads to the toilet.

It is important to appreciate that it is the environment that requires modification to meet the needs of the individual, not vice versa. If behaviours or physical disabilities prevent people from functioning effectively, then something needs to be changed or added to their environment. The kitchen, toilet, bath, bedroom and living room need to be examined in order to identify influential factors which either aid or retard physical, behavioural and cognitive abilities.

Occupational therapists and others have designed special implements for this population which will assist poor eating and dressing skills: non-slip mats for plates, thick handles for utensils to assist grip, Velcro fastening to replace buttons, etc. There have been hopes that microprocessor technology could lead to the use of more sophisticated memory aids. A minicassette recorder, for instance, could store information for later use to prompt recall (Lincoln 1989, p. 653); however, for many, a notebook or diary will perform the function of providing an external information store equally well. Generally, memory aids need to be as simple and as familiar as possible if they are to be used to remind the person to do something; they need to be as specific as possible, in order to avoid the situation where the alarm clock rings at a preset time, but the person has forgotten what they must do when it rings!

Some efforts have been made to increase the person's safety and security. For instance, on some wards a system has been installed which alerts staff when a patient wanders off the ward. This operates on the same principle as alarms used in shops and libraries to indicate when goods and books are being removed without being checked out. The system allows the ward door to be unlocked, so that patients not at risk of getting lost outside are free to come and go as they please. The system works well in practice with patients who wander through the ward door without any particular intention of 'escaping' from the ward. They are easily guided back again onto the ward (Stokes 1986a). However, patients who are very determined to leave may be much more difficult to persuade to return. This system then runs the danger of precipitating a number of unhelpful confrontations when patients of this type are on the ward. Concerns have also been raised regarding the ethics of 'tagging' the person with dementia, and this approach raises important issues regarding the rights of the person with dementia, which must include the right to be in a safe environment. Less contentious approaches to the same problem of patients leaving the safety of the ward or home have been evaluated. Hussian & Brown (1987) showed that marking a grid pattern on the floor in front of the exit door reduced the frequency of patients leaving the ward; it is suggested that the two-dimensional grid pattern is perceived as a visual barrier by the person with dementia. However, Chafetz (1990) showed that if the person could see beyond the exit door—through the door itself or adjoining windows—then the grid pattern did not appear to have any impact. Possibly, the person's vision is drawn to the external view rather than to the floor. Mayer & Darby (1991) used a full-length mirror in front of the exit door, with some success in reducing frequency of patients leaving, providing an alternative visual distraction.

Another focus has been enhancing mobility. More stable furniture on a ward can assist mobility. The vast empty space on many wards must seem like an eternity of space to a frail old person faced with the prospect of finding her way to the toilet. Observations have shown difficulty in negotiating 'highly polished' non-slip vinyl flooring. To old eyes, it appears dangerous and it is walked upon as though it was a sheet of ice; the assurances of the designers are not enough to promote confidence! Willmott (1986) has demonstrated empirically that such flooring reduces the length of stride and speed of walking of elderly patients, in comparison with a carpeted surface. It is unfortunate that,

despite a greater awareness of special needs, studies continue to show that these needs are often not met. Benjamin & Spector (1990) found that, in a sample of care environments studied, safety features and prosthetic aids were, on the whole, poorly represented. Facilities were particularly unsuitable for those in wheelchairs. It was pointed out that many aids could have been incorporated for little cost; their findings indicated a failure to recognise the needs of prospective residents in providing an environment which would not provide support for the person's remaining abilities. Mountain & Bowie (1992) report, in a hospital context, that 'a large number of patients only possessed a core of toiletries ... and did not have items such as ornaments, pictures or jewellery'. Patients are then denied the support to memory and awareness of familiar items. Of even more concern is the implicit denial of basic human rights, and it is efforts to move away from such institutional care practices that are the focus of the next section.

Changing the pattern of care

In order to bring about changes in function of elderly people with dementia, it is necessary not only to modify the physical environment but also to concentrate on improving the social and interpersonal atmosphere of the ward or home and the expectations of staff and patients/residents. This approach is, of course, dependent on staff attitudes. It can be difficult for staff to accept patients being given more control and choices and being allowed to be more independent. So often the old pattern of care re-emerges. Davies (1982) reports how, a year after the successful intervention discussed above (p. 18), 'only token symbols of the "changes" remained'. This happens even though the new regime may involve a less apparent burden for the staff (e.g. in not feeding patients unnecessarily). Staff attitudes can be extremely resistant to change, and sources of reinforcement may be complex and subtle. They may, for example, involve a desire to care for someone physically (Godlove et al 1980) which becomes difficult to satisfy with this sort of change of regimen. Practical aspects of staff attitudes will be discussed in Chapter 10, but suffice to say here that in many ways they are the key to implementing and maintaining this, and other approaches. Where attitudes are positive and appropriate, changes to the regimen are more likely to retain their initial effects. In the UK, with the fragmentation of care that is following the greater emphasis on care in the community, there is great potential for developing services based on more positive attitudes; however, there is also the danger of staff in isolated residential units or visiting the person at home being unaware of the person's psychological needs and reverting to the practices that brought institutional care into disrepute. Careful monitoring, supervision and training of all staff involved is required if these developments are to be really beneficial to people with dementia.

Several evaluative reports of changes to the pattern of care are available. Melin & Gotestam (1981) reported an evaluation of a change of regime emphasising choice and encouraging self-responsibility for patients with dementia in a Swedish hospital. The changes took place around three specific areas: first, allowing residents more autonomy in helping themselves to coffee and cakes, creating more choice and a more natural social situation; secondly, mealtimes were altered so that free choice and unlimited time were offered instead of patients being fed if they were too slow; finally, activity materials— games, books, jigsaws, etc—were provided as was the necessary encouragement to use them. The 21 elderly patients, most having dementia and a high level of behavioural disability, were divided into an experimental and a control group. The changes were introduced sequentially, allowing a multiple baseline design for the experimental group. Changes in social interaction, eating skills and level of activity were monitored by direct observation of time-sampled behaviour.

The results of the study are clear-cut and dramatic. Social interaction during afternoon coffee increased greatly in the experimental group and eating skills improved following the mealtime changes; their level of activity increased when compared with the control group when they were encouraged to use the materials. The results provide strong support for the use of such an approach, encouraging independence and choice, particularly where the existing milieu may have led to underfunctioning and patients not using all their skills and abilities to the full. Significantly, relating to the previous discussion of staff attitudes, Ingstad and Gotestam (1987) showed positive changes in staff attitudes following these changes to the ward environment.

A second Swedish study (Brane et al 1989) evaluated 'integrity-promoting care'. This involved staff in a nursing home being trained and supported in implementing individualised care, with patients encouraged to participate more in decisions and activities, and more time being allowed for these so that they could go at their own pace. Changes to the physical environment aimed at achieving a more home-like atmosphere with domestic-style furnishing, and personalised clothing and possessions were encouraged. Changes over the 3-month intervention period and at a follow-up 6 months later were compared with those of a control group in a second nursing home. Patients in the integrity-promoting care group were reported to have become less confused, anxious and distractable; there were also improvements in mood and motor performance. Many of the benefits remained at the follow-up evaluation.

From France, Ritchie et al (1992) reported an evaluation of the impact of the cantou units, described previously, on people with dementia, in comparison with long-term hospital care. Residents in the cantou units were more mobile and less dependent in daily activities, had better language skills and interacted more with other residents. However, there were indications that these differences arose from differences in the patients admitted to the two types of care; although there was considerable overlap in degree of dementia, it appeared that the benefits of the cantou became less evident as the condition progressed. Ritchie et al conclude that both types of care are required, and the issue becomes who is more appropriately cared for in each setting; they suggest the hospitals could benefit from incorporating some of the features of the cantou, such as the involvement of families.

Two groups in the UK have published evaluative findings regarding new forms of dementia care. Lindesay et al (1991) describe 'the domus philosophy' aimed at tackling staff attitudes and fears which lead to poor quality of life in institutional settings for people with dementia. Emphasis is given to seeking to maintain the independence and to preserve the abilities of the person with dementia, through allowing the person to have an active role in the life of the domus, where the intention is to apply domestic rather than hospital standards of safety and hygiene. The domus philosophy contains a number of features:

- the domus is the person's home for life
- the needs of the staff should be considered equally with those of the residents
- the domus aims to correct the avoidable consequences of dementia, and accommodate those that are unavoidable
- residents' individual psychological and emotional needs may take precedence over the physical aspects of care.

The first evaluation of these principles in practice compared a new (but not purpose-built) and relatively large (27 beds) unit using this philosophy with two typical psychogeriatric long-stay wards, on a cross-sectional basis. Although the populations of each unit would be expected to be broadly comparable, and indeed were in terms of cognitive impairment, age and length of time in long-term care, residents of the domus were rated as less impaired in self-care and in communication and orientation. Higher levels of activity and staff–resident interaction were observed in the domus setting. The acknowledgement of staff needs in the domus is perhaps reflected in their reporting higher levels of job satisfaction than staff in the hospital wards.

Dean et al (1993a) reported a prospective evaluation of two further domus units; only one of these catered for people with dementia, and so the results in relation to that unit alone will be presented here. Patients were assessed in a long-stay hospital ward prior to moving to the purpose-built domus (12 beds) and then were monitored at intervals during their first year of residence. Improvements were identified in cognitive function, self-care and communication skills; again, increased levels of activities and interactions were observed. Some dramatic changes were observed; one patient spoke for the first time in 5 years within a week of moving to the domus. The increases in staff–resident interaction have been demonstrated to have been of good quality (Dean et al 1993b), with a marked reduction in negative interactions by the end of the first year of operation of the domus in comparison with the hospital ward. The improvements in quality of life do have a cost: staff to resident ratios are higher than in the hospital wards, and the costs are accordingly higher (Beecham et al 1993). This is in contrast to the cantou units in France, which were established in part to lower the costs of care.

However, a caution that additional resources are not a simple guarantee of positive care is provided by the research group evaluating three experimental NHS nursing homes for people with dementia (Sixsmith et al 1993a). Like the domus units, the new homes aimed to provide a homely living environment and individualised care. Comparing these homes with two other homes and a hospital ward, using techniques to estimate the amount of staff time spent on various activities, it was found that the additional resources were used in routine care, rather than in what the authors describe as life-enhancing care, such as social interaction and group activities. In a further article, Sixsmith et al (1993b) show that in one of the three homes 'rementia' could be observed. After admission to the home, residents' functional level tended to improve for some time, before beginning to gradually decline, as would be the expectation in dementia. It is difficult to draw conclusions from these data, as it is not clear what were the factors leading to this pattern of change in one home and not in the other two. We would also want to emphasise that positive care has not been seen as additional to other 'routine' care by other researchers, but as an approach that transforms every type of interaction; it is not just reflected in numbers of activity sessions with people at this level of impairment, but equally in the way the person is helped to dress, bath and have a meal. Therefore, the way staff resources are deployed is vital, but it is the use to which each interaction is put that is of prime importance.

Group living

The group-living concept combines changes to the regime with some fundamental changes to the physical environment. It has attracted much interest in the UK and has been implemented in many residential homes for older people. Evaluation of its effects has been mainly anecdotal; Booth & Phillips (1987) review most of the relevant empirical research.

The crux of this approach is the size of the living unit. In contrast to the large living groups of many traditional old people's homes—often 40 to 50 people—seen as inhibiting personal interaction and preventing individualised care, group-living homes are divided into living units of 8 to 12 members. One might speculate that people with dementia in particular would be adversely affected by larger groups, in view of their greater difficulty in remembering who people are and in forming relationships. For a group to work, it requires a shared interest, activity or purpose, manifestly lacking in many homes. The rationale for having groups at all is the often reported loneliness and apathy experienced in many homes. If effective groups can be established then resident-to-resident interaction will increase. Together with this aim, choice and involvement of individuals in their own self-care were identified as objectives in raising quality of life for residents.

Typically a home with 40 residents is split into four or five groups. Each has its own lounge/diner, with tea-making facilities, TV, etc. Each group shares the range of self-care activities. They can get up in the morning at any time and help themselves to a light breakfast. At lunch and evening meal the group members set the table, serve themselves and afterwards wash up. They make their own drinks and have a choice of food, and are consulted regarding menus.

They are encouraged to participate in the choice of furniture and decoration for their rooms. It has proved possible to adapt older homes at very little cost to this system which certainly does not need to be confined to purpose-built homes. Residents with dementia are integrated into the groups and are helped by their fitter peers whilst carrying out what tasks they can. Rejection of the less able seems to occur less frequently in smaller groups.

Anecdotally, results were promising and exciting. Residents who were thought to be confused began to play leading roles in the life of some homes. The dormant abilities of some residents were revealed. They became more vocal and active, with activity centred on the domestic tasks rather than craft work etc. Staff had more time to spend with residents and knew them much more closely. Relatives, volunteers and neighbours were said to come into the homes more—being entertained to tea by the groups, who were now in a position to offer hospitality.

One empirical study has documented the effects of introducing group living in a home where a number of residents suffered from dementia. Rothwell et al (1983) reported a marked increase in purposeful activity, from observations made in the home before and after the implementation of group living. A proportion of the residents completed brief tests of verbal orientation and life satisfaction. Only the latter showed significant change, with residents reporting greater contentment under the new regimen. Booth & Phillips (1987) reported the results of a large-scale study comparing dependency levels over a 2-year period in 292 residents living in group homes with those of matched residents in traditional homes. Essentially, there seemed to be little difference in outcome between the two types of home, in terms of number of residents becoming more or less dependent over the 2-year period. If anything, group-living homes seemed to lead to more improvement and less deterioration on a rating of mental state, which focused on orientation and wandering. However, differences were very small.

This study has several drawbacks. The 2-year

comparison meant that only the 50% surviving were considered; the dependency-rating scales were probably not very sensitive to change, with the majority of residents showing no change; and the scales certainly did not cover some of the quality of life aspects important in any evaluation of group living. What does emerge is that group homes are more likely to have a positive approach to the residents' capabilities, but that a number of traditional homes were adopting similar policies without the group-living format. The physical changes in themselves did not always provide a good indication of what went on within the home!

In Sweden, group-living homes have developed slightly differently; typically they consist of a group of four flats in an ordinary housing block, in which eight people with dementia live, each having their own room and possessions, with 24-hour staff cover for the unit as a whole. Wimo et al (1991) indicate that such a project can be a cost-effective alternative to institutional care, with anecdotal reports of enhanced function. Such units are unable to manage severe physical disabilities, which may be a problem as a resident's condition deteriorates, with a number of residents eventually moving on to nursing home or hospital-type placements in view of decline in physical health and mobility (Malmberg & Zarit 1993). A more detailed evaluation of similar units by Annerstedt et al (1993) compared a group of people with dementia moved from institutional care with a control group who remained. Cognitive and mood changes favoured the group-living group over a 6-month period; although both groups declined over a full year, there were indications of this being less marked in the group-living residents.

The Swedish units illustrate how incomplete the attempts in the UK to provide a more domestic setting have been; older people with dementia can be looked after in a small cluster of ordinary living accommodation (adapted as necessary) with considerable success, particularly for those with a moderate degree of dementia. In the UK, group living has been a way of structuring an old people's home rather than a radical shift in care provision. However, it does achieve a smaller scale of provision, which sets the scene for, but does not guarantee, many of the more desirable features of positive care.

BEHAVIOURAL APPROACHES
Introduction

Behaviour modification has been extremely important in a number of areas of therapeutic endeavour: mental handicap, chronic schizophrenia, various problems of children, etc. It is based on an empirically derived body of knowledge and related to psychological models of how behaviour is learned and maintained, such as operant conditioning. In essence, behaviour is broken down into specific, clearly defined components—this makes programme targets easier to establish. The conditions under which the behaviour will occur are ascertained (the discriminative stimuli) and the consequences of the behaviour are examined. If the result is something the person wants or desires then the behaviour has been positively reinforced and is more likely to occur again. If following the behaviour something unpleasant is removed then this is described as negative reinforcement. Again the likelihood of the particular behaviour recurring is increased. By comparison, if something pleasant is removed, or something unpleasant added, then the behaviour is punished. For further details of the behavioural approach see Patterson (1982).

Since pioneering work by Lindsley (1964) and Cautela (1966, 1969), a number of authors have advocated using behaviour modification with the elderly, e.g. Hussian (1981, 1984), Wisocki (1984) and Carstensen (1988); there are now a number of examples of its application to older people with dementia. Stokes (1986a,b, 1987) and Stokes & Goudie (1990) provided a practical account of behavioural approaches to working with problems common in dementia care, such as wandering, screaming and aggression.

Although biological processes do occur in ageing and dementia, the elderly person's actual function is always a result of interaction with the environment. If any learning is possible for the dementing person, then the behavioural approach will facilitate the learning process. It will indicate the environmental conditions needed for new behaviour to be learned, or for existing behaviour to be maintained, which is just as important. The environmental changes here are very finely regulated and individualised. They relate to the setting and events that precede the behaviour in question, and to what happens subsequently: all features of the environment in its broadest sense —the physical and social context. Barrowclough & Fleming (1986a) have produced a simple manual which helps staff to examine these aspects so that retained skills and interests can be used to develop the positive aspects of the person's behaviour.

Although Woods & Britton (1985) have argued that many of the other approaches reviewed in this chapter can be usefully conceptualised in behavioural terms, there is still disappointingly little systematic research on the use of behaviour modification per se with patients clearly diagnosed as having dementia; many studies are case-studies with small numbers, and, particularly in earlier studies, diagnostic details were often rather vague. However, before reviewing relevant literature, it is important to outline the learning potential of the person with dementia in order to clarify how an approach based on principles of learning may be used in a disorder where difficulty in learning is a primary symptom.

Can elderly people with dementia learn?

The response of elderly people with a dementing disorder to environmental conditions suggests some learning ability may be retained. The characteristic of dementing conditions—a deficit in learning new material—is easily observed, for example, by providing a patient with a fictitious name and address and asking for a recall in 5 minutes. Such tests reveal the existence of a learning deficit and are not designed to provide evidence of any retained ability. What is of interest is to examine what conditions are most favourable for learning to take place.

Miller & Morris (1993) identify four areas where learning is relatively well preserved in patients with Alzheimer's disease.

Classical conditioning. Here the person learns to associate a simple stimulus–response relationship with a conditioned stimulus; an example would be a puff of air producing an eye-blink response; when the puff of air is combined with a buzzer, eventually the buzzer alone will suffice to produce the eye-blink. This most basic type of learning has been shown to be only slightly reduced in people with dementia.

Operant conditioning. Here the person is rewarded for making a particular response; at first there is a reward for every response, but subsequently a certain number of responses or a response at a certain interval after the last reward are required. The person learns to respond in order to maximise reinforcement. In a laboratory task of operant conditioning (Ankus & Quarrington 1972) involving 48 patients with dementia-related memory disorder, the response trained was pulling a lever—rather like on a fruit machine—to obtain a 'prize'. It appeared that the effects of the training depended on the individual's preference for the particular reward; when an appropriate reinforcer was used relatively normal learning took place of the relationship between lever pulling and reward operative at any particular time, particularly if only gradual increases in the ratio of pulls to reward were made. Burgess et al (1992) have followed up this work, training five patients with dementia to press a lever, the 'reward' being a visual pattern appearing on a TV screen in front of the person accompanied by a sequence of tones; subjects were asked to 'make the music come'. Four out of five patients showed clear evidence of learning to make the response, and there was evidence in most cases that responding varied according to the schedule of reward being operated. Morris (1987) used a 'matching to sample' paradigm, where the person is presented with a coloured shape, then has to choose it when later presented with it alongside another one. Patients with moderate to severe dementia were able to learn this discrimination, but it is suggested that learning consisted of making specific associations rather than learning an abstract rule.

Implicit memory. This is where performance of a task is enhanced without conscious or explicit recall of material. An example is learning on a motor skills task, where rate of learning has been shown to be preserved in people with dementia. Another example is 'priming', where exposure to an item facilitates later processing of that, or a related, item. Miller & Morris (1993) reviewed a number of studies indicating that priming effects occur in patients with Alzheimer's disease; often the effects are as large as those in normal subjects. One example involves showing the person a list of words, then giving the patient the initial letters of the words to be recalled (Morris et al 1983). Word completion occurs more readily after prior exposure to the word; the effect in patients with dementia is near normal. A further—very practical— example of the preservation of implicit memory arises from a study by Sandman (1993). Carers of dementia sufferers planned with them a significant event, standing out from the usual routine. This might be a picnic, trips out or a meal at a special restaurant. Patients were subsequently asked about details of the day, not directly related to the event, such as what they were wearing, who they met that day and so on. Patients showed normal recall for items from these special days, whilst being significantly impaired on items from ordinary days.

Verbal learning and retention. There are indications that when information is adequately registered, forgetting rates after the first 10 minutes or so may be virtually normal. Little et al (1986) have shown that even patients with a moderate degree of dementia may retain information over a 1- or 2-month period. After at most five repetitions of a pair of words, patients showed significant retention of the association even after this lengthy delay. This was demonstrated by better performance on repeated pairs than on new pairs of words. Backman (1992) suggests that learning is enhanced where greater support is given both at the time of learning and at the point of retrieval; therefore, the person with dementia may need more trials, learning fewer items at a time, with more guidance in coding the material as well as more retrieval cues. For example, Sandman (1993) showed that people with dementia improved their recall of a TV programme when they worked on creating their own test questions on it.

These findings have some immediate practical implications. One is to 'de-emphasise memorisation as a goal' (Sandman 1993). By making the experience as rich and meaningful as possible, memories associated with it will be enhanced. Helping the person to work on the material (but not asking them to remember it) and using retrieval cues gives the best hope of enhancing performance. Using, and building on, well-preserved skills will increase function and achieve more success. However, it should not be assumed that such techniques help the person achieve 'normal' memory. The person, in fact, may have little or no conscious memory of the event; what is being accessed are more automatic processes, achieving the goal by a different pathway.

People with dementia do have some learning potential on which behaviour modification may build, alongside its support for preserved skills and behaviour. Particular attention will have to be given to creating the best possible conditions for learning to take place and be maintained.

APPLIED STUDIES OF BEHAVIOUR MODIFICATION

Self-care

A series of studies (Baltes 1988) have demonstrated clearly that attempts by residents in nursing homes to be independent in self-care are usually ignored by staff, whilst dependent behaviour is systematically reinforced. There is tremendous scope for reversing these contingencies. Rinke et al (1978) used prompting and reinforcement to improve self-bathing in six nursing home residents, aged from 67 to 90 years, diagnosed as having 'chronic brain syndrome'. Each of five components of bathing (undressing, soaping, rinsing, drying and dressing) were in turn the focus for intervention. This multiple-baseline design allowed for the specific effects of the behavioural intervention strategies on the person's self-care to be monitored. As a further control, two of the subjects received no intervention. These control subjects showed little change throughout. The other four residents responded well, with each component of the overall task reaching near maximum levels when it was prompted and appropriate reinforcement given. The respective contributions of reinforcement and prompting were not established, but there were suggestions from the data that either might have been sufficient alone in some cases to bring about or maintain improvement. Prompting included physical prompts, e.g. handing the resident a towel, and verbal instructions. Among the rewards offered were praise, a choice of 'grooming aids' (powder, lotion, etc), visual feedback on a wall chart and a choice of things to eat. A certain number of appropriate responses were required to earn the tangible rewards.

In a family setting, Pinkston & Linsk (1984) reported teaching family members to use differential attention to reinforce the self-care of a 70-year-old lady with dementia. They praised her when she brushed her teeth, combed her hair, had a bath or remained dressed for several hours. They ignored inappropriate behaviour. In this case, prompts had proved ineffective and had been seen as nagging, resulting in a number of negative interactions between the patient and her family. The intervention led rapidly to a near maximum level of self-care function.

Josephsson et al (1993) reported an intervention with four patients with dementia, seeking to support everyday activities such as preparing and consuming a drink or snack. The programme was set up in such a way that it was more dependent on external memory aids and motor skills than on the person's own memory ability. Verbal prompts and cues and physical demonstrations of components of the activity (for the patient to repeat), together with signs on drawers and cupboards were among the forms of support offered. Three of the four patients showed improvements in performance, although for two of these the environmental guidance

continued to be required for these gains to be maintained. The fourth patient showed a high level of anxiety throughout, which may have interfered with learning.

Mobility

Burgio et al (1986) successfully applied a prompt and praise procedure to increase independence in walking in eight nursing home residents (four reported to have a dementia). For six of the residents, the improvement was evident as soon as the intervention began; the other two residents improved within a few days of baseline observations—before the intervention! Not only did most residents walk further, but most progressed to more independent means of mobility, e.g. needing less staff assistance, using fewer prosthetic aids, not using a wheelchair, etc. An important component of the intervention (and of the baseline observation procedure) appeared to be the opportunity it provided to the resident to walk. The authors suggest that immobility was related, at least in part, to 'environmental contingencies that either discouraged walking or failed to prompt and reinforce the behaviour'. Efforts were made to teach the nursing home staff to adopt the intervention procedure, and gains were generally maintained at a 4-month follow-up.

Social interaction and participation in activities

Lack of activity and social interaction are frequently features of institutions for elderly people (see Woods & Britton 1985, Ch. 9). Several studies have used behavioural methods in an attempt to increase the amount of social interaction. For example, Gray & Stevenson (1980) gave positive feedback for accurate statements to patients during weekly group sessions. Social interactions between patients increased significantly in three groups, each of around six members, all of whom appeared to have been disorientated.

An application of social skills training is described by Praderas & MacDonald (1986).

They taught four moderately cognitively impaired nursing home residents telephone-conversational skills, expressing common courtesies, asking questions, etc. Results were generally positive, with marked improvements in skill in two residents when assessed in a role-played telephone conversation. Unfortunately, none of these residents had any contacts in the community who they could telephone (two had been in institutions for many years), but the aim of helping residents to be skilful enough to maintain their community links is laudable.

Green et al (1986) reported a single case where a wife was able to learn to use contingent reinforcement (touch, praise, smiles) to increase her husband's spontaneous and appropriate verbal behaviour. He had had a stroke 3 months previously and seldom conversed unprompted. The intervention was maintained at a 6-month follow-up; its success was a great encouragement to the wife, who had been distressed by the apparent permanence of her husband's disabilities.

Three patients with dementia were taught to use a 'prosthetic memory aid', with the aim of improving the quality of their conversation with their primary care-giver and others well known to them (Bourgeois 1990). The aid essentially consisted of relevant photographs and drawings mounted in a plastic wallet. There were improvements in conversational quality, making more statements of fact and fewer ambiguous statements. Gains were maintained at a 6-week follow-up. Interestingly, whilst the changes were confirmed by independent judges, the care-givers themselves noticed little change, perhaps being too familiar with the conversational content to be impressed by it.

Burton (1980) reported an increase in the purposeful activity of patients with dementia during occupational therapy (OT) sessions. This was achieved through staff consistently prompting patients to use materials and reinforcing them when they did so. It was also noted that patients slept less during the OT sessions following the introduction of this approach! McCormack & Whitehead (1981) reported similar increases in engagement (and reduced sleeping) on a geriatric ward when individual or group activities were provided and encouraged. Bracey (1989) describes the application of an approach called 'room management' with patients with dementia. This involves a systematic approach to offering activities to the patients in a dayroom and offering support and encouragement to use them. Rather than two staff trying to run a large activity group for, say, 10 patients and probably failing to hold their attention, the staff rotate around the room; some patients may be involved in an individual activity, others in a small group. The rotation is arranged to minimise the interval between contacts with a staff member, giving enough help to keep the person involved in the activity. Results indicate quite dramatic increases in activity levels when this approach is adopted.

An intervention aiming to increase both participation in an activity and social interaction was attempted by Carstensen & Erickson (1986), who sound a cautionary note. They increased attendance and social interaction by serving refreshments at the activity event, but showed that most of the dramatic increase in interaction between residents was accounted for by 'ineffective vocalisations', i.e. nonsensical and unreciprocated speech. In future studies it is essential that both quantity and quality of interaction and activity are considered.

Continence

In our experience, incontinence is one of the most difficult and disturbing problems facing those caring for elderly people. It need hardly be said that the problem is deeply disturbing for the elderly patient. It is also a very common problem in dementia. The widespread use of absorbent pads has assisted in managing the problem for care-givers but does not resolve completely issues of dignity for the patient.

Results of a number of early studies were disappointing (see Hodge 1984), perhaps because of a tendency to use an overly simplistic behavioural analysis of a complex chain of behaviour, to neglect the role of physical factors and to be over-ambitious in their goals. Some positive findings have been reported. Hussian (1981) attempted a programme of regular toiletting with 12 'regressed institutionalised geriatric patients'. Prompts and reinforcement for toiletting and praise for being dry led to a dramatic reduction in incontinence in only a fortnight! Prompting alone was sufficient in maintaining the behavioural change. The rapid toilet-training method developed for use with people with a learning difficulty was used successfully with two elderly patients with dementia by Sanavio (1981). For over 2 years, both had been incontinent of urine and/or faeces day and night and never used the toilet independently. One patient began within 4 days to use the toilet without prompting, with a corresponding reduction in the number of episodes of incontinence. This improvement was maintained 8 weeks later, and Sanavio was able to demonstrate its relationship to the intervention method, using a reversal design. The second patient's faecal incontinence virtually disappeared, and again independent toiletting was reinstated.

This level of independence may not be attainable for all patients: for those with physical disability and mobility problems remaining dry may be the more realistic goal. Schnelle et al (1983) reported a programme used to teach 21 immobile patients with dementia to ask for help from staff when they needed to urinate. The programme included prompting, social reinforcement for asking to be taken to the toilet and for being dry, and social disapproval for being wet. The results indicated that incontinence decreased and appropriate toiletting requests increased compared with controls. The results were so rapid (from the first day) that the authors attribute the improvement to better staff–patient management, rather than to patients re-learning skills that had been lost. A necessity in this instance was for staff to actually respond to patients' requests for help. Further reports from this group (e.g. Schnelle et al 1989, 1993) and from Burgio et al (1988) indicate the effectiveness of this prompted voiding procedure with a large number of patients in a number of different nursing homes; patients are asked on a

regular basis if they would like to go to the toilet, and are assisted with toiletting if they answer positively. Two-hourly checks are identified as adequate for many residents; Burgio et al have succeeded in increasing the interval between prompts for a number of patients. The predominant issue has now become how to ensure staff do persist with this procedure of proven effectiveness after the research team complete their input; quality control procedures are being evaluated in this respect (Schnelle et al 1993).

Less positive results have emerged from two studies involving psychogeriatric patients with a severe degree of dementia, reported by Rona et al (1984, 1986), perhaps because independent toiletting, rather than remaining dry, was the objective. In the first study, following baseline assessments of the level of incontinence on three wards (involving 2-hourly checks), each ward was fitted with signs, distinctively painted toilet doors and floormarkings leading the way to the toilet. On one ward, baseline measures were continued for a further 3 weeks, in case the regular checks were helpful in themselves; one ward had no further intervention; and the third ward had a toilet-training programme based on each patient's individual peak times for voiding. Verbal and tangible reinforcement were provided for appropriate responses. The results in terms of the number of episodes of incontinence favoured the ward where training had taken place. Although the improvement there was only slight, it became significant when compared with the large increase in wetting episodes on the other two wards. The authors point out that the differences may have been, in part, the result of differences between the three wards, and so in their second study they compared a training group and a control group drawn from the same wards. Here the results were less positive. Improvements were only noted for patients who were incontinent less than once a day, with patients who had been more frequently wet not improving with the training procedure.

Clearly, a behavioural approach to incontinence in people with dementia has had only limited success. In view of the importance of incontinence we will discuss some factors that may contribute to these mixed results.

First, incontinence is the most difficult, practically, of the target problems so far reviewed. All the previous interventions could possibly be confined to an hour or two a day, and intensive work carried out in that period. By its very nature, incontinence has to be modified throughout the day and throughout the night, and so limited intervention is more difficult. This in turn means much greater commitment and cooperation from care-staff on the ward.

Secondly, correct toileting requires a number of skills: dressing, mobility, ability to find the toilet, ability to recognise it, to control urination until the toilet is reached, etc. This chain of behaviours can break down at any point and so an individual analysis of problems will be required in order to identify the problem in each case. Specific neuropsychological impairments, such as a dressing dyspraxia or an agnosia (see Ch. 6) may lead to incontinence, for example.

Thirdly, goals of treatment need consideration. An ideal goal might be complete continence and independent toileting. With patients suffering from a severe degree of cognitive impairment, a more attainable goal might be remaining dry with regular prompting. If the individual's micturition pattern guides the toileting programme, it could be more efficient and rewarding for all concerned.

There is a need in this area for both medical and psychological intervention to maximise the chances of success with such a complex problem. Smith & Smith (1986) provide a detailed discussion of these issues, together with other important aspects, e.g. should fluids be restricted in the evening? Is 'habit training' effective? They conclude that behaviour modification has much to offer in maintaining continence in people with dementia, but that there is room for improvement in the quality of behavioural methods being applied.

Behaviour problems

There have been few recent examples of programmes to reduce behaviour problems (or 'challenging behaviour'). Perhaps this reflects a welcome change of emphasis away from the problem per se towards a more constructive approach aimed at building up positive behaviour and function, rather than simply removing the negative aspects. There is also a trend towards a broad-based approach, incorporating behavioural principles alongside a range of other individualised interventions (e.g. Hinchliffe et al 1992, Mintzer et al 1993). Certainly there is a recognition of the diversity of problem behaviour; that aggression and wandering, for example, may result from a variety of different factors, which need to be assessed and defined for the individual (Ware et al 1990, Hope & Fairburn 1990, Stokes & Goudie 1990). Some examples of programmes in the literature will, however, be described.

One of the most difficult problem behaviours for staff (and other patients) to live with is a patient persistently shouting and screaming. Some success in reducing (but not necessarily eliminating) screaming and shouting has been reported in single cases by Baltes & Lascomb (1975) and Birchmore & Clague (1983). In the latter study, the patient was a 70-year-old lady with dementia, who was also blind. The plan was to reinforce her when quiet, but finding an effective reward proved difficult. Touch, in the form of rubbing the patient's back, proved most helpful in this case. Hussian (1981) reduced a patient's self-stimulatory stereotyped vocalisations, providing reinforcement for 10-second periods without noise. The impact of the intervention was increased by employing 'artificial discriminative cues', i.e. brightly coloured, large cardboard shapes, which were specifically paired with reinforcement in brief training sessions. These perhaps serve to highlight the difference between behaviour judged appropriate and inappropriate. Garland (1985), reporting findings from a series of 11 'noisemakers', pointed out the variety of factors to be considered in a behavioural analysis, and the range of treatment options available. Apparent causes included delirium, communication difficulties, self-stimulation, in the context of sensory or social deprivation, echoing noise made by others, and seeking attention from carers, some of whom responded to noisemaking but ignored the person when quiet. A further factor that should always be considered is pain: when the person is unable to communicate the experience of pain verbally, shouting or screaming may be a way of expressing discomfort. Garland notes that in the 11 cases examined, most seemed to be affected by several of these factors. Four patients died within 3 months of referral, reflecting perhaps physical health problems. Three of the patients showed no response to psychological interventions, whilst the remaining patients showed some response. In four of these cases there was a marked reduction, maintained at a 6-month follow-up. Garland reported that among the most useful therapeutic strategies identified were the use of distracting auditory stimulation (e.g. playing relevant music through headphones), carers differentially reinforcing appropriate behaviour and ignoring noise, and brief periods of removal to a quiet area when noise occurred. In each case, it was important to develop an individual package of interventions. Hallberg et al (1993) drew attention to the self-stimulatory aspects of 'vocally disruptive behaviour'; they also identified this occurring in association with strong negative emotions and recommend more attention be given to patients' emotional state. Stokes (1986b) provided a guide to examining the various possibilities resulting in a person screaming or shouting, coupled with practical suggestions on management.

A related problem arises from inappropriate verbalisations. For example, Pinkston & Linsk (1984) describe the case of a 73-year-old man with Alzheimer's disease, living at home with his wife. The patient expressed a number of 'worried statements' each day, e.g. repeatedly asking 'Do I have money in the bank?'. By training the wife to reinforce positive statements with praise and attention and ignore worried statements, worried statements were reduced markedly, the patient spoke more positively and the wife's subjective level of burden in caring for her husband at home was also reduced. Similar methods reduced the frequency of accusations in a further single case (Green et al 1986). Tarrier & Larner (1983) reported an intervention with a group of four immobile stroke patients, who repeatedly asked to be taken to the toilet

(although not needing to urinate). The patients seemed to have found an effective way of capturing staff attention, although the staff were becoming frustrated by the frequent false alarms. The intervention consisted again of differential attention to appropriate behaviour: staff spent time with the patients at other times than toiletting. The frequency of false alarms was reduced, and patients called for help less often. In this instance the staff did not perceive the objectively measured changes.

Finally, Hussian (1981) has reported the use of the 'artificial discriminative stimuli' mentioned above in relation to several other sorts of problems, with apparent success. Thus wandering was reduced in three patients with dementia. Here one form of cue was paired with reward and another with an unpleasant stimulus (a loud handclap). The two types of cue were then placed in appropriate places: the latter at danger points, those with positive associations in the patient's room. Another target in one case was the reduction of inappropriate sexual behaviour. The patient, who frequently masturbated in public, was taught to masturbate only in private places. A further two patients repeatedly manipulated any objects in reach in a stereotyped manner. They were reinforced for a similar but appropriate activity (clay modelling), again in the presence of an artificial cue. It remains unclear how these cues work; fading the cues by reducing the size seemed effective in maintaining improvement in some cases; some patients required booster sessions after a few months to re-train the association between cues and consequences. It is debatable whether they should be preferred to cues with overlearned associations (e.g. a red sign saying DANGER). Their size and colour may aid concentration and attention to the relevant aspects of the learning situation. As yet this work lacks widescale replication.

Individual planning

In the early 1970s, a series of publications emanating from a research team at the Philadelphia Geriatric Centre highlighted the subject of individualised treatment of excess disabilities of mentally impaired elderly people. Excess dis-abilities (EDs) are those functional incapacities that are greater than expected in view of the patient's level of impairment, in other words the discrepancy between the potential and actual level of function. Brody et al (1971, 1974) provided individualised therapy for EDs; although general health deteriorated, there were improvements in relationships and activities over a period of a year. Nine months after the end of the treatment year, the treated group deteriorated, indicating the need for some form of maintenance inter-vention.

This study is an early example of an indivi-dualised approach, with clearly specified, graded treatment goals and explicit treatment plans, which help to ensure a consistent approach across disciplines. This is an approach which will be described in more detail in Chapter 5. A couple of more recent studies are available to give some indication of its practical usefulness.

Miller (1985) reported a comparison of geriatric wards in the UK, some of which used indivi-dualised care-planning (based on nursing process models) whilst others used a system of task allocation, where nurses were responsible for particular tasks, e.g. toileting, bathing, feeding, etc, for a large number of patients.

Observations on the different types of ward suggested that on the task-allocation wards 'nursing practices were pushing patients into dependency', whereas 'when a nurse had to . . . write out a care plan for every patient, she was . . . more likely to take the patient's real needs and self-care skills into account'. Empirical support for these observations comes from assessment of the functional abilities of patients on the three wards of each type included in the study. Patients admitted to the six wards had similar dependency levels, but patients who had been in hospital a month or more were signi-ficantly more dependent on the task-allocation wards. On both types of ward, patients' scores on a test of verbal orientation fell into the impaired range, but patients scored higher on the individualised care wards. Miller also shows that dependency levels fell on one ward when a nursing process approach, emphasising indivi-dualised care, was introduced.

Obviously, research of this kind is fraught with difficulties. Did the wards differ in other ways? Were the patients or staffing or resources different? Miller recognises these problems; wards were matched carefully, and the absence of differences in short-stay patients adds credence to the results. What cannot be answered from this study is whether it is the whole indivi-dualised approach or rather certain attributes of it or the people implementing it that leads to these results. *Something* about this indivi-dualised approach, on wards in three different hospitals, seems to have led to lowered dependency levels.

Barrowclough & Fleming (1986a) have devel-oped a training manual for the implementation of an individual programme-planning approach with elderly people. It involves careful indi-vidual assessment, an understanding of the person's strengths as well as their needs and the setting of relevant and specific goals aimed at meeting selected needs. The use of this approach with staff in residential care homes has been evaluated (Barrowclough & Fleming 1986b), with the results demonstrating its feasibility in this context.

In our view, it is within the context of an individual-centred approach that psychological approaches to older people with dementia will have their greatest impact. This is borne out in work with people with dementia in the com-munity, where individualised assessment and care-planning is emerging as feasible and valuable in a number of community support schemes (e.g. Challis et al 1988).

REMINISCENCE

In recent years there has been a surge of interest in using reminiscence with older people. Coleman (1986) and Bornat (1994) provide comprehensive accounts of theoretical and therapeutic aspects. One important factor has been the influential work of Butler (1963), developing the concept of 'life review' as a task to be accomplished in the last phase of life.

The person is seen as actively attempting to make sense of her life, its value, its purpose, the accomplishments, the disappointments, the joys and the sorrows. Acceptance is the goal of a successful life review, despair the consequence of a life seen as useless and worthless. Encouraging the person to reminisce was seen as a valuable therapeutic activity which helped the person get to grips with and put into perspective a lifetime of experiences. Reminiscence began to be seen as a positive activity, rather than as a negative attribute of old people, forever saying 'When I was young ... !' At least two other factors have also been important. First, the increasing availability of aids to reminiscence. In life-review work, often old photographs and other memorabilia would be used to stimulate the person's recall of experiences from different phases of their life. In the UK, following the original *Recall* pack produced by Help the Aged in 1981, a wide variety of reminiscence materials have been produced which, by their wide availability, have encouraged the use of this approach, much to the enjoyment of staff and clients. These materials include pictures, artefacts, music and archive recordings, newspapers, and videotapes of newsreels (see Appendix 3 for major suppliers).

Secondly, many people working with older people with dementing conditions have discovered that talking about events in the person's past often helps communication and interaction, and that the more they understand the person's past life and experiences the more they can make sense of the person's current conversation and behaviour. As we shall see in Chapter 7, these findings form part of a practical approach to communicating with people with dementia.

These different factors have all led to 'reminiscence therapy' being widely used, but there is still considerable confusion as to the aims, target population and techniques of the 'therapy'. As Merriam (1980) points out, the life-review process, where memories are analysed and evaluated, is only one form of reminiscence work. Other types include *informative* reminiscence, 'telling a story' about past events and experiences and *simple* reminiscence, recalling the past. Reminiscence has been used extensively with patients who are depressed as well as those with dementia; it should be recognised that the aims and techniques may need to be different in

each case. Norris (1986) provides an excellent description of the practical application of a variety of reminiscence techniques. There is an accumulation of evidence for the effectiveness of various types of reminiscence work in reducing depressive symptoms in older people (Scogin & McElreath 1994).

Coleman (1986) reported findings from a 10-year study of the use of reminiscence by elderly people, which have important implications for its therapeutic use. He identified four groups for whom reminiscence had different implications. Group I enjoyed reminiscing and maintained high morale throughout. Group II reminisced compulsively, but as their past had been full of troubles, this increased their depression and anxiety. The third group did not reminisce at all, as they found the present and future more stimulating. Like Group I, this group enjoyed high morale. The final group found the past a depressing topic, not because of past difficulties but because of the contrast with a less fulfilling present. There is clearly a need to be aware of these individual differences, to learn as much about the individual as possible and to anticipate individual differences in response to reminiscence-based activities.

Haight & Burnside (1993) stressed the need to distinguish between 'reminiscence' and 'life review'. Whilst the two terms have often been used interchangeably, they suggest that life review be solely used to describe an intervention where the therapist is seeking to assist the person in achieving a sense of integrity. This involves the older person recalling and evaluating events and experiences throughout their life, usually in a one-to-one setting with the therapist, who acts as a therapeutic listener. Garland (1994) provides a useful account of life-review therapy. Reminiscence, by comparison, is seen as having a variety of goals, including increased communication and socialisation, and providing pleasure and entertainment. It may be individual or group based; structured or free-flowing; it may include more general memories than specific events or experiences; themes and prompts are frequently used; evaluation of memories is not specifically encouraged; and the focus is on a relaxed, positive atmosphere. Sad memories may emerge, but support is available from the group leader and other members or from the worker in individual work to contain any distress and pain associated with such memories.

Life-review therapy, as described here, is much more likely to involve working through difficult and painful memories and experiences; it should be undertaken—like any other personal therapy —with the person's consent, with a clear aim, by properly trained and supervised workers. Generally speaking, it is a more appropriate approach for older people without cognitive impairment. Reminiscence work is appropriate for people with dementia, but some caution is still required, taking into account Coleman's report of large individual differences in attitudes to reminiscence amongst older people and the need to avoid an intrusive approach that invades an individual's privacy. Particularly in a group setting, awareness of participants' life histories is important, to ensure appropriate support can be given if events that have traumatic connotations for certain individuals are being raised by other members.

Empirical research on reminiscence with people with dementia is scarce, despite many positive anecdotal reports. Thornton & Brotchie (1987) and Woods & McKiernan (1995) provide detailed reviews. Goldwasser et al (1987) compared reminiscence and support groups with a no-treatment control; sessions were held twice a week for 30 minutes for 5 weeks. The reminiscence group showed improvement in depression, although this was lost at a follow-up 6 weeks after the groups ended. None of the groups changed in behavioural or cognitive function. There was a suggestion that the less impaired patients showed most response.

Baines et al (1987) have evaluated reminiscence in relation to RO. Staff involved in a reminiscence group acquired much more individual knowledge of the residents in the group than they did of residents in a control group who received no additional treatment. Residents were rated as deriving a great deal of enjoyment from the groups by both staff taking part in the groups and staff who saw the residents only outside the groups. Attendance at the reminiscence groups was consistently high. The elderly people in the study were living in a residential home for the elderly and all had a moderate to severe degree of cognitive impairment. Some effects on cognitive and behavioural function following reminiscence sessions were apparent in a group of five residents who had previously responded well to a month of RO sessions. They showed a reduction in scores on a problem behaviour rating scale, as well as an increase in verbal orientation. A group who had a month of reminiscence sessions before going onto RO sessions showed far fewer positive changes in relation to the untreated controls.

Baines and co-workers' evaluation of a number of aspects of their treatment approaches is commendable. Enjoyment of sessions and greater staff knowledge of the residents may be just as important aims as improved cognition and behavioural function. They may indeed be more appropriate goals in working with people with dementing conditions.

Other studies have looked at what happens in the group session. Head et al (1990) contrasted reminiscence work with alternative group activities in two day-centres. In one, there was a clear increase in the contributions made by group members during reminiscence as opposed to other activities. This appeared to be related to the other day-centre having a much more stimulating range of alternative activities, rather than any failure on the part of the reminiscence work to elicit communication. In an initially unstimulating environment, the results of any intervention will appear much more dramatic. Woods & McKiernan (1995) reported the results of work by McKiernan, Yardley and Bender indicating increased engagement of patients with a moderate to severe degree of dementia during reminiscence groups in three different units, confirming 'that it provides a meaningful, appropriate and stimulating activity for people with even a very severe impairment'.

Gibson (1994) reported an evaluation of a number of 'general' reminiscence groups in a total of four residential homes and two day-centres. Some groups were specifically for people with dementia, whilst others had a mixed membership. In relation to people with dementia, in mixed groups they showed pleasure and enjoyment and rarely exhibited within the group any behavioural disturbance; outside the group some individuals were reported by staff to be less agitated and restless. Where only people with dementia were in the group, the interaction tended to be between leaders and members, rather than between members, as had more commonly been the case in the mixed groups. Small, structured groups seemed to be most effective for people with dementia.

Gibson (1994) also reported a series of five case studies, indicating the effects of individual reminiscence work with people with dementia. These cases were selected as the most 'troubled or troubling' residents of nursing homes. The approach involved the compilation of a detailed life history, from which a care-plan was evolved, including 'special' reminiscence-type work. The aim was to use 'life-history as a working tool to enrich the quality of social exchange in the present'. Trips and activities that related to the person's interests and experiences were planned, and the environment was personalised and individualised according to the person's own style. Residents are reported to have shown increased sociability, decreased aggression and less demanding behaviour following the implementation of this approach. Staff were also very positive about the work, recognising more of the 'personhood' of each individual. This life-history work is an important development, and should become a major influence in care-planning (see also Woods et al 1992; note that what they describe as 'life reviews' are better regarded as life histories). Life history differs from life review in that it does not require an evaluative aspect; it is not directly aimed at changing the view of himself/herself held by the person with dementia, but rather at helping care-staff to see the whole person, in the context of their lifespan. This perspective should assist in modifying the care-givers' interactions with the person with dementia, resulting, potentially, in a significant change in the person's quality of life.

A number of questions remain regarding reminiscence work. What styles of group leadership are most helpful in increasing residents' participation in discussion? Are particular prompts—music, pictures, objects—especially helpful for different people? Then there are a number of other techniques to be examined further. One-to-one work with more impaired people; life-history books for each person, telling the person's life story in words and pictures, illustrated with appropriate personalised photographs from family albums and local history collections (e.g. Jones & Clark 1984); reminiscence outings, visiting places of interest and relevance from the person's past; and reminiscence theatre, enacting events and experiences from the person's life.

Reminiscence opens up many horizons in work with older people with dementia. There is a pressing need, not for research which tells us whether or not it is a 'good thing', but rather for work that shows how best it can be carried out with different people, in different settings and for particular purposes.

VALIDATION THERAPY

This approach was developed in the USA by Naomi Feil, a social worker, partly as a result of dissatisfaction with approaches such as RO. Feil found that insisting upon the person being orientated to the present reality often led to the person withdrawing and even becoming hostile (Feil 1992). Jones (1985) summed up the approach as 'communicating with disoriented elderly persons by validating and supporting their feelings in whatever time or location is real to them, even though this may not correspond to our "here and now" reality'. Although Feil has been developing the approach since the 1960s, it was in the 1980s that the approach began to attract wider interest, initially in the USA and then further afield. Several publications describe aspects of the approach (Feil 1989, 1993). The 1993 book *The Validation Breakthrough* gives the most detailed description of the techniques involved.

There is a recognition of the individuality of the person with dementia and respect for their value as a person at the core of this approach, which accords well with other approaches based on a clear statement of values (see Ch. 5). There is also an emphasis on the importance of what has gone on previously in the person's life having a major influence on their current state; specifically, the person with dementia is seen as endeavouring to resolve 'unfinished business' before the end of their life. Four stages of this 'resolution' phase of life are identified: malorientation, time confusion, repetitive motion and vegetation. People with dementia are viewed as progressing through these stages, showing increased physical deterioration and withdrawal inward. The aim of validation is to restore dignity and prevent the deterioration into vegetation, through the provision of an empathic, non-judgmental listener, who accepts the person's view of reality. Painful feelings from the past that are expressed, acknowledged and validated in this way are thought to decrease in strength; whereas if ignored or not expressed they are said to heighten.

Feil (1993, p. 31) acknowledges that people do not remain neatly in one stage or another, and that considerable fluctuation occurs. However, by detailing different techniques for different stages she is offering some insights into what may be more or less helpful in particular types of situation. The specific techniques include many aspects of non-verbal communication—use of touch, eye-contact, tone of voice—as well as using music and reminiscence. The loss of recent memory, combined with sensory losses, is seen as leading to the retrieval of earlier memories and familiar faces, and 'the need to go back to mend torn relationships' (Feil 1993, p. 30). There is thought to be a reason behind all behaviour, and an important technique is to link the person's behaviour with the unmet human need underlying it. Three needs are seen as universal: the need to be loved and nurtured, the need to be active and usefully engaged and the need to be able to express deep, raw emotions to an empathic listener.

The core technique is to recognise the person's communication of feelings and emotions and to acknowledge and validate these, verbally and non-verbally. Whatever the person's current reality, whatever the facts of the matter, their feelings have their own validity. To respond to emotions only on a cognitive level is to ignore a whole dimension of communication—indeed probably the most significant aspect of communication. For example, many people with dementia talk often of their parents, as if they were still alive. To respond at a cognitive level, to set the record straight, may well miss a key issue for the person with dementia. Miesen (1992, 1993) has shown the importance of attachment for many people with dementia, reflecting a need for security and safety in a perplexing and, at times, frightening environment; this need for attachment returns to the parents, the original attachment figures, in the person with dementia who develops a 'parent fixation'. This should then be seen as an expression of need, not simply as a sign of confusion.

The techniques are often applied in a group setting but can be used effectively on a one-to-one basis. Even a few minutes several times a week is thought to be a worthwhile input; much could be done during routine care-giving, although validation is seen as demanding work in its own right. More severely impaired patients, in particular, will require an individual approach. In group settings, there is an emphasis on comfort and of the time together being 'special'. Music is used as a uniting activity, and every effort is made to minimise communication difficulties. Group members are encouraged to take on responsibilities within the group: song-leader, welcomer, giving out refreshments and so on. The wisdom of group members is drawn upon, placing them in the position of having something to give from their extensive experience of life; for example, 'what advice would you give a young person who doesn't want to stay on at school?' Issues for discussion are chosen to reflect real concerns and issues; controversy is not avoided.

Although there are a number of anecdotal reports attesting to the effectiveness of validation therapy (see Feil 1992, 1993), there are very few published studies documenting its effects. An exception is an evaluation of a validation group reported by Morton & Bleathman (1991). The group was run over a 20-week period in a residential home. Five residents with dementia participated; for 10 weeks beforehand, their behaviour, mood and interaction levels in the dayroom of the home were monitored. These measurements continued during the period of the validation group, and for 10 weeks afterwards when reminiscence techniques were used in the group. The group sessions were held for 1 hour, once a week. Three residents completed the study; the results were examined individually and suggested that for two residents verbal interactions increased during the validation-therapy period, with a decline during the reminiscence period; while the remaining resident showed the opposite pattern, with an increase apparent during the reminiscence phase. It should be emphasised that these interaction measures were taken outside the group setting in the home's dayroom; perhaps the most remarkable finding of the study is the contrast between how little these residents interacted—during any phase—and the depth of interaction apparent during the group sessions (see Bleathman & Morton 1992, for a fascinating selection of transcripts from the sessions). Whether this is the result of validation techniques per se, or of the carefully structured small group context, cannot be determined, but would be worth further exploration.

Validation has attracted some criticism. There has been some confusion as to whether or not it was intended to be used with people with dementia (Stokes & Goudie 1990). This has arisen in part from the idiosyncratic and changing terminology adopted by Feil. Feil (1993) makes it clear that people with dementia are the focus. Younger people (i.e. under 70) with Alzheimer's disease are identified as generally continuing to deteriorate despite the use of validation, unlike older people with dementia (Feil 1993, p. 24). However, the techniques are still recommended as having some transitory effect.

Kitwood (1992a) pointed out that its emphasis on past life, on unresolved conflicts and difficulties, means that current sources of devaluation

and impoverishment may be overlooked. Indeed each behaviour may have a reason, but it may not be necessary to go back 50 years to find it; many people with dementia daily experience all manner of unhelpful, unsupportive interactions which may have as great an impact.

This emphasis on the role of 'unfinished business' tends also to lead to an implicit assumption that if one can learn to cope with life's problems in an adaptive way, dementia can be avoided; or conversely that people with dementia have, in a sense, brought it upon themselves, by the way they have lived their life. There is no evidence to support this notion, and it must serve to accentuate further the 'them and us' divide between cared-for and care-givers, if dementia is attributed to the person's own actions.

RESOLUTION THERAPY

Resolution therapy is described by Stokes & Goudie (1990). Like validation, the aim is to tune in to the emotional communication of the person with dementia, adopting empathic listening skills. There is less emphasis on unresolved issues from the past and more on the need for careful listening to identify feelings relating to making sense of the current situation, or expressing a current need. What the person says may, on the surface, not make 'sense'; but using counselling skills—warmth, acceptance, reflective listening, etc—the concealed meaning may become apparent, reflecting the underlying feelings. The focus is on what the feeling is, not on why the person feels it; demanding explanations is seldom helpful in any context. Having identified the feelings, the next stage is to acknowledge them, verbally and non-verbally, and to modify the environment and the pattern of care to respond to unmet needs.

As well as counselling approaches such as this, there have also been developments in the application of dynamic psychotherapy (Hausman 1992, Sinason 1992) and cognitive behaviour therapy (Thompson et al 1990) to older people with dementia. These developments reflect the earlier recognition and diagnosis of dementing conditions, resulting in a growing number of individuals with a clear awareness of what is happening to them. As yet detailed studies of these approaches with these patients are not available; the application of a range of therapeutic-listening techniques to people with dementia is long overdue.

3

Reality orientation

RO—THE ARCHETYPAL POSITIVE APPROACH

We have decided to devote a chapter to reality orientation (RO), as we believe it merits detailed consideration. This is not because we see it as the way forward for dementia care, but rather that the extensive development and evaluation it has undergone over a long period has generated much to inform and to enhance positive approaches in general. The difficulty of evaluating the effectiveness of positive approaches and defining appropriate targets for change is particularly well illustrated by the literature on RO.

Origins

Reality orientation can be traced back to 1958 when an 'aide-centred activity programme for elderly patients' was set up at a Veterans' Administration Hospital in Topeka, Kansas, USA, where Dr James Folsom was then working. Almost certainly RO existed before then, but at this time a structure and a name began to be applied. The programme went with Dr Folsom to the VA Hospital at Tuscaloosa, Alabama via Mount Pleasant, Iowa and was further developed and refined. By the mid-1960s, published descriptions began to appear (e.g. Taulbee & Folsom 1966) and the methods were beginning to crystallise. In 1969, the American Psychiatric Association published a short booklet, outlining the methods of RO, together with the comments of a psychologist and a physician, entitled *Reality Orientation: a Technique to Rehabilitate Elderly and Brain-damaged*

Patients with a Moderate to Severe Degree of Disorientation (edited by Louise Stephens). An RO training programme was established at Tuscaloosa and nurses and others working with the elderly from all over the USA and from other countries participated in short training courses there. In 1978, the training team there published a practical guide to RO (Drummond et al 1978). By 1975, the methods were in use in the UK, with the first published controlled study carried out at Warley Hospital in Brentwood, Essex (Brook et al 1975). Subsequently it has been used worldwide and continues to be used in a variety of forms.

It has also been applied to other populations, e.g. younger people with head injuries (Corrigan et al 1985), people with learning difficulties (Hong 1989) and patients with chronic psychiatric problems (e.g. Wallis et al 1983). Several practical manuals are available, detailing techniques used in different implementations of RO (e.g. Cornbleth & Cornbleth 1977, Hanley 1982, 1988, Rimmer 1982) and countless descriptive articles have appeared over the years.

Varieties of RO

Three major components of RO are usually identified. The first is 24 hour RO (sometimes called 'informal RO' or the 'basic approach'). This is a continual process whereby staff present current information to the person in every interaction, reminding the patient of time, place and person, providing a commentary on events and responding to the person's questions with accurate information. Confused and rambling speech is not reinforced. The environment is structured with signs and cues to help the person remain aware of the surroundings. RO classes, or intensive sessions, are a supplement to 24 hour RO but in some centres these have been used in isolation. These sessions are also variously called 'intensive RO', 'formal RO', and 'RO groups'. Sessions are held daily for half an hour to an hour with three to six patients depending on the level of impairment.

Group leaders do not require particular professional expertise, and qualities such as enthusiasm and a positive, flexible and creative approach are more important. Specific training in the procedures is needed, however. Sessions may be divided into different levels according to the degree of deterioration. Often basic, standard and advanced levels are described for those at differing levels of function. In basic group sessions ('classes') the emphasis is on presentation and repetition of current information and orientation material related to simple information on day, weather, names and months. The standard group uses sensory stimulation and past/present discussion to develop interpersonal relationships and learning. In the advanced group, there is less emphasis needed on basic orientation so activities are wider ranging; the groups, in fact, became virtually indistinguishable from other forms of group work. In some hospitals in the USA, 'graduation' ceremonies were arranged when patients had benefited as much as possible from RO or were being promoted to an advanced group. A diploma is presented to a group member by a senior staff member. In the UK, the emphasis has been more on a social setting than a classroom, with, for example, the use of simulated pubs. Possibly the creation of a social environment helps the patient to feel less pressured, more comfortable and less likely to withdraw than in a potentially threatening classroom situation. However, this factor may well be closely related to cultural aspects. In the USA, graduation has greater social implications and connotations of increased self-esteem, which are not operable in the UK or in other countries that have their own situations associated with social pleasure, esteem and relaxation.

The final traditional component of RO is the use of one of a number of prescribed attitudes (attitude therapy) to be used by all care-staff with a particular patient. These include kind firmness, active friendliness, passive friendliness, matter of fact and no demand; the attitude is chosen according to the patient's personality and needs. Their use is thought to facilitate staff consistency in approach to each patient. However, their actual use has been little documented and with some patients different attitudes may be required by different situations, thus complicating their use considerably.

Application of RO and relationship to other approaches

It should be noted that RO was specifically designed and developed for people who are disorientated and have severe problems in memory and learning (despite a few of the earliest case reports including people with chronic psychiatric problems). It is appropriate for use with people suffering from the range of dementing conditions, although it is not limited to them. It is a flexible approach. Different levels of groups are described and it is appropriate for different degrees of impairment.

RO is based on interaction between staff and patient, both in 24 hour RO and in RO sessions, and provides, of course, many opportunities for prompting and social reinforcement of desired behaviour (often correct verbal orientation), as in a behavioural approach. It also involves environmental changes through the use of memory aids, signs, etc. Above all, it is a communication approach that enables care-staff to make contact with people with dementia and gives the staff member some principles to apply to a situation that is often fraught with difficulties and where crossed wires are more common than true communication.

RO involves attitudes of both staff and institutions; it involves positive attitudes which indicate that talking and explaining things to a person with dementia is worthwhile even if it seems to be forgotten immediately. It also involves a respect for the elderly person. Communication implies listening as well as talking, and listening applies to what is unspoken as well as to what is verbalised. Without this respect, no communication takes place and RO becomes a pointless exercise.

RO can operate in some ways as a prosthetic environment. In the group or outside, the person is enabled to succeed. Clues and prompts are given; he or she is shown where to find the answer to the question. The person is asked questions that he or she is still able to answer. The effects of any memory problems are minimised rather than emphasised, as it is so easy to do. Perhaps by succeeding in this way, the person will in fact function better as he or she gains confidence; certainly it will be a refreshing, enjoyable change from the repeated failures which characterise the process of dementia.

Reminiscence is often used in the course of RO. A major difference is that it is easier to envisage RO being applied in a continuous fashion, outside specific sessions (although Gibson (1994) has shown how reminiscence work can form the basis for a comprehensive care-plan). When past events are used in RO they are typically brought up-to-date so that the person is able to integrate past and present. There is a similarity with activity and stimulation approaches; in RO sessions it is activity and stimulation that are often as apparent as the continuous orientation to current surroundings. Although validation may, at first sight, seem to be at odds with the basic RO approach, Woods (1992) shows that the central validation technique has been incorporated in sensitive applications of RO for some time. There is, then, much common ground between approaches, with perhaps differences in emphasis and language but many similarities in practice.

THE EFFECTIVENESS OF RO

Establishing the effectiveness of health and social care approaches has become of increasing importance in a climate where accountability and cost-effectiveness are of prime concern. Evidence is required to justify the way in which resources are deployed, to ensure that time is not devoted to procedures that have no impact or that make little or no difference. It is also important not to raise false expectations and for programmes to be developed on a rational, rather than an impressionistic, basis. The question we have been asked many times over the years regarding RO and other positive approaches is 'do they work?' 'We shall see that this is not a simple question to answer. The evaluation of the efficacy of any treatment method is fraught with difficulties. Debates continue about the effectiveness of many well-established therapeutic methods with other client groups. In some ways, the task is more difficult with elderly populations; patients fluctuate a great deal more and have more risk of becoming physically ill and even dying, perhaps quite independently of the treatment procedures being used. Other difficulties will become clear as the literature is reviewed, but these general considerations do emphasise that a definitive, unqualified answer is almost impossible. We can, however, be clear about some of the key issues in evaluating positive approaches.

It could be argued that there is no question to answer; for example, Hanley (1984) suggests that RO and other positive approaches are to be valued on humanitarian grounds in that they give emphasis to interactions based on respect, concern and recognition of individual identities. In this light an approach may be a 'good thing' whether or not it changes the patients. What may be important is that staff and others concerned treat patients in a genuinely caring fashion. However, the question of impact remains; the emphasis is shifted from impact on the elderly person to changes in the behaviour and attitudes of the care-giver.

Does RO work?

The final point above indicates the need for amplification of this apparently straightforward enquiry. Additionally, it should be asked on whom it works, and also what is meant by 'work' in this context. What criteria should be applied? Taulbee & Folsom (1966), pioneers of RO, noticed that with some of their patients 'their look of hopelessness changed to hope-fulness' when they began RO. If changes are occurring then it is necessary to define along what dimensions these changes are taking place, whether it be facial expression, memory for current events, self-care skills or whatever. As far as staff are concerned, the changes might be in their attitudes to their patients, or changes in the way interactions are made with patients. In the future, Kitwood's definition of indicators of psychological well-being in people with dementia (see Box 5.2, p. 82) may form a basis for evaluative studies. The choice of appropriate areas in which to examine the effects of the approach is all-important; indeed the indicators of psychological well-being are much more likely to pick up a change from 'hopelessness' to 'hopefulness' than all the memory tests and behaviour rating scales that have dominated studies to date.

A further complication with people with dementia in particular arises over our concepts of change. Suppose measures of some attribute of the patient are made and then 1 month after they have begun RO that attribute is reassessed. If it is exactly the same as before, this could be thought of as indicating no change; but suppose that if that person had not had RO he would have deteriorated—as over a period of time patients with a dementia are often considered to do—then absence of change may still indicate a positive effect of treatment. Thus, even a deterioration could still be consistent with a positive effect of treatment, as long as the deterioration is less than it would have been without treatment!

So changes are being sought—in patients or staff—that are more positive than they would have been without RO. 'Positive' can be difficult to define more precisely; it is straightforward enough if memory is being assessed: improved memory is a positive change. However, 'amount of complaining' is another matter; some might see it as a good thing if the person becomes more complaining and asserts himself more; others might see it as an unnecessary nuisance. Value judgements may then come into play; generally changes in the direction of more independence on the part of the patient and more recognition of the elderly person as an adult individual by the staff are viewed as positive, but there will, of course, be grey areas, open to debate and interpretation.

Does RO change those employing it?

The effects on care-staff of using RO have been relatively little explored. Effects on relatives using it have not been examined in any systematic way. Taulbee & Folsom (1966) described how RO could involve nursing assistants, who spend much more time in contact with the patients than any of the other professionals, becoming members of the rehabilitation team. Through RO they become more than simply agents of physical care, they become, in effect, therapists; clearly in some instances this could lead to greater job satisfaction and morale.

Bailey et al (1986) attempted to assess such a change in staff involved in implementing 24 hour RO on a ward in a geriatric hospital. Using an established questionnaire of attitudes to elderly people, no change was evident over a 5-month period. However, there are a number of difficulties in assessing attitude change in this way. Neither before nor after the study were the scores of the staff in the range which would imply a negative attitude to the elderly. The questions may well not relate to the particular group of elderly people with whom the staff are working. It would be quite possible for someone to have positive attitudes towards 'the elderly' and negative attitudes towards the actual patients on the ward, with all their disabilities, demands and needs. Finally, as the authors point out, such questionnaires may readily be answered in the positive, socially desirable direction and may show little relationship to actual practice (see also Adelson et al 1982, Saxby & Jeffrey 1983). It is noteworthy that Ingstad & Gotestam (1987), who showed positive changes in staff attitudes following changes to the ward environment (see Ch. 2), used a much more specific attitude measure.

In an interesting and detailed study, Baines et al (1987) used an information questionnaire and semi-structured interviews to explore staff reactions to leading RO and reminiscence sessions. They showed that both types of group led to staff having much more personal knowledge of the residents involved—an important step towards individualised care. After 4 weeks of group sessions, staff were able to answer correctly an average of 25 items about each resident, compared with five items initially. After a further 4 weeks of group meetings, staff scores had increased to an average of 29 items per resident. The effect was specific to know-ledge about residents within the groups. There was no change in scores relating to information about patients who had not been involved. The interview data suggest that staff reappraised

their view of the ability of residents with dementia to respond to a small group. They found the sessions more beneficial than they had anticipated in improving their communication with and their knowledge of the residents. Job satisfaction was also reported to be increased.

Staff morale, sense of achievement and job satisfaction have been reported to be improved in several studies (e.g. Merchant & Saxby 1981) and would merit more systematic attention in future research. Some of the studies of new-style dementia units (see Ch. 2) have included these areas; for example, Dean et al (1993b) suggested that domus staff had higher levels of morale than their counterparts in hospital units.

Although it is, of course, highly desirable to see changes in these aspects, part of their value has to be in increasing the elderly person's quality of life, by improving the quality of staff–patient interaction. In fact there is remarkably little evidence to show that staff carrying out RO actually behave differently from their previous practice. It has usually been assumed that because staff have been trained in the methods they will implement them in practice. Clearly if long-term beneficial effects in care-giver attitude and morale are to be attributed to involvement in RO, there must be some indication that RO is actually being implemented. Change in a person's behaviour is often a precursor to attitude change.

An increase in the proportion of time during which the care-worker acts in a manner consistent with RO may well be seen as a desirable aim, if the RO approach to the person is seen as incorporating humanitarian values. Particularly with 24 hour RO, it can be difficult to ensure RO is being carried out appropriately. If the frequency of staff–patient interactions is very low, the amount of 24 hour RO that is possible must also be low. Woods & Britton (1985, Ch. 9) show that many institutions are indeed characterised by low levels of staff–patient interaction. Even in the group setting, staff may deviate from the intended approach. The Quality of Interactions Schedule, used by Dean et al (1993b) in their evaluation of a new domus unit, would be one method of evaluating a change in the quality of interactions between care-givers and the person with dementia.

In an unpublished study, one of us (R.T.W.) has examined the quality of RO carried out in RO sessions before and after specific training in RO techniques as employed in a controlled study (Woods 1979). Training consisted of a talk illustrated with slides, discussion, a handout summarising the major points, some demonstration and role play of RO techniques. RO group sessions were recorded on audiotape and then analysed to assess changes in RO behaviour. Using operational definitions, each staff statement on the tapes was categorised as an RO statement (i. e. aiding RO), as a negative RO statement (hindering RO, giving incorrect information), or as neutral (neither orientating or disorientating the person). Table 3.1 shows the findings. There was a significant increase in the proportion of RO statements made after training. The proportion of negative RO statements showed little change; training seemed to help these staff be more efficient RO leaders, with fewer remarks being 'wasted' (from an RO viewpoint) following training. Some of the post-training recordings were made some 1 to 2 months after training, so this effect is probably not merely transitory, although its duration is of course uncertain. It proved impossible to carry out a similar exercise outside the RO group room and to evaluate the effects of training on the amount of 24 hour RO carried out. A high proportion of the staff–resident interaction occurred in relation to bathing, dressing, toiletting, etc, and not in the 'public' areas of the residential home where interactions might be observed relatively unobtrusively.

However, Hanley (1984) has been able to attempt such an investigation and reports considerable difficulty in implementing 24 hour RO in a hospital setting. He devised a system to assess both the quantity and quality of 24 hour RO being carried out, before and after the implementation of 24 hour RO. He found no change in the number of interactions staff had with patients (approximately nine interactions per patient in an 8-hour period) and, even more disappointingly, no change in the quality of the interactions, measured by the mean number of

Table 3.1 Mean proportions of staff statements consistent with RO, inconsistent with RO and neutral in RO sessions carried out by five staff members before and after training

	Before training (%)	After training (%)
RO statements	77.4	89.4*
Neutral statements	21.1	9.4*
Negative RO statements	1.5	1.2

*Before–after difference significant at 5% level (correlated t-test, 1 tailed).

the following six features of 24 hour RO present per interaction:

- engages patient verbally
- names patient
- names self
- refers to time or place
- explains procedure
- refers to orientation aid.

Most discouraging of all was that when staff rated their own interactions with patients, they indicated that they thought they were carrying out many of these procedures. The direct observation of interactions indicated clearly that they were not. For example, all 15 nursing staff involved said that most of the time they called the patient by name, whereas, in fact, this only occurred in 48% of the interactions. All staff said that most of the time they explained procedures to the patients, but this only occurred in 14% of the interactions; 13 of the 15 nurses stated that they named themselves and the same number said they referred to aids at least once in a while. Neither of these interactions occurred in any interactions observed. Hanley's work raised serious doubts as to the extent to which 24 hour RO is actually implemented.

In Australia, Reeve & Ivison (1985) and Williams et al (1987) have evaluated a slightly modified form of 24 hour RO, where the emphasis is on staff responding appropriately to patients' requests for information, rather than initiating discussion of orientation in every interaction. In both studies they used direct observation of staff–patient interactions to assess the extent to which the procedure was carried out (Reeve 1986, personal communication). Their results showed adherence to the modified 24 hour RO procedure following training; both the quantity and quality of interactions were satisfactory. Over 90% of staff responses to patients' requests met the requirements of their modified 24 hour RO (Williams et al 1987).

As has been demonstrated in other settings (e.g. Milne 1985), it is not sufficient to train staff in a particular procedure and then simply to expect that staff behaviour will change in relation to their patients. Nor is it sufficient to ask staff whether they are putting the procedure into practice. Ways of ensuring that the training has had an effect and of developing more effective training are of great importance. Studies intending to show the outcome of any positive approach must demonstrate the extent to which staff apply the approach in practice.

Positive approaches are not implemented in a vacuum. In different institutions they will already be applied to differing degrees; there will be different types of staff, diverse attitudes and a multiplicity of institutional goals. Evaluating these aspects is a complex matter. The extent to which the institution values staff–patient interaction and patient independence, is patient- rather than staff-centred, and is rehabilitative rather than custodial, will all have an impact. Environmental assessment procedures are available which aim to quantify these aspects (see Ch. 6).

Does RO change the person with dementia?

Controlled trials of RO

The early literature on RO consisted mainly of anecdotal reports or studies without a control group; as mentioned above, the likelihood of decline in people with a dementia makes a control group essential in order to assess whether or not the treatment is having any effect. The first controlled trial of RO was carried out by Brook et al (1975) at Warley Hospital, England. Eighteen patients were assigned either to daily RO sessions

or to control groups. The control patients went to a specially equipped RO room for half an hour a day but simply sat in a circle and, unlike the RO group, received no encouragement from the therapists to use the RO materials; their questions were answered as briefly as possible. Ratings of the patients' self-care, orientation, socialisation, etc, were made fortnightly by nursing staff who were not aware to which group particular patients belonged and so could not be inadvertently biased in favour of RO. Results were presented for three levels of initial functioning, high, medium and low, so that any differential effects of RO at different levels of patient functioning might be seen. The results are shown in Figure 3.1 : all groups seemed to improve in the first 2 weeks. After this, the control groups deteriorated while the RO groups either maintained progress or continued to improve. The most deteriorated patients showed the least improvement in RO.

This first controlled study clearly favours RO with this group of elderly psychiatric patients, all but one of whom had a diagnosis of dementia. This finding was at the time an exciting antidote to the prevailing therapeutic hopelessness that surrounded dementia care. That an intervention for only 3 hours a week could be associated with such changes in function on the ward appeared a major breakthrough. The results of a number of other controlled trials were published by 1980; since that time the rate of reports has declined markedly. We have identified in total 21 controlled studies that included subjects with an apparent diagnosis of dementia. These are summarised in Table 3.2. It is important to notice the many differences between the studies.

1. Only seven studies included 24 hour RO; only two demonstrated that these procedures were actually being implemented.
2. All studies included small group sessions, except Williams et al (1987). Two of the most recent studies have described their groups as 'cognitive stimulation' (Breuil et al 1994) and 'the 3R mental stimulation programme' (Koh et al 1994), rather than as RO groups. However, the programme descriptions are consistent with RO-type activities.

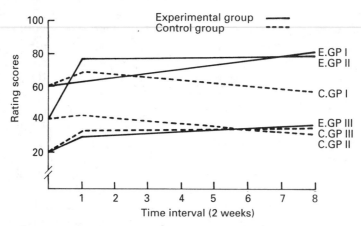

Figure 3.1 Ratings of intellectual and social functioning of patients in RO (experimental) and control groups by nursing staff unaware of group membership over the 16-week experimental period. Reproduced, with permission, from Brook et al 1975, British Journal of Psychiatry 127: 42–45.

3. The studies have been mainly carried out in hospital (geriatric and psychiatric), nursing home or residential home settings; some of the more recent studies have used out-patient and day-patient populations. Subjects' diagnoses have been variously described, reflecting changes in diagnostic practice over the years, but dementing conditions have predominated. Wallis et al (1983) had the most mixed sample, including patients with other psychiatric conditions.

4. A variety of control groups have been used; most commonly no-treatment. About a third of studies have attempted to control for the effects of the additional attention received in RO groups by offering an alternative group activity, in a few cases in addition to the no-treatment control. Some of the alternative groups have been equivalent to a placebo—a pure control for attention, with no specific therapeutic intent; a few have been potentially effective in their own right, e.g. reminiscence groups (Baines et al 1987). Some studies have randomly allocated subjects to the different groups; others have had the treated group in one ward/home and the control group in another. In the latter case, there is the risk that other differences between the units will distort/obscure the effects of the intervention. However, operating different programmes for different patients on the same ward can be problematic; it is difficult for staff to practise 24

hour RO with one person and not with another! Offering different groups for subjects from the same ward is more feasible, however.

5. A variety of measures have been used. These fall into two main groups: first, cognitive tests, typically an orientation/information test, in some cases backed up by further neuropsychological tests; and second, behaviour rating scales, covering a variety of areas of function. A very few studies include a measure of life satisfaction, and the two Australian studies that focus more on 24 hour RO have a measure of the ability of the person to find their way around the ward. A particular issue with the behaviour ratings has been their completion by staff on the wards concerned, who may be influenced by the intervention, or by different expectations in different wards. Ideally, raters should not be aware of whether the person is in the intervention or the control group, and the same raters should rate both groups. This is difficult to achieve in practice, and again is easier for group comparisons, rather than 24 hour RO.

6. The length of projects has also varied greatly, from 3 weeks to a year, with the frequency of sessions similarly varied from once a week to twice daily. Two-thirds of studies had RO sessions at least five times per week.

7. There are differences in study design. Most are a simple comparison of intervention and

Table 3.2 Controlled studies of RO

Authors	Location	Setting	Mean age (years)	Mean length of stay (years)	24 hour RO	No. of RO sessions per week	No. and sex of subjects	Control groups	Duration	Assessment methods
Brook et al 1975	Warley, Essex UK	Psychiatric hospital Dementia (1 head injury)	73.3	1.9	No	Daily	18 10F 8M 9 RO 9 Control	Group taken daily to RO room; no active therapy	16 weeks	Behaviour rating scale
Harris & Ivory 1976	Florida USA	State hospital CBS, OBS, others	66.6	24.6	Yes	Daily	29 RO 28 Control all F	NT	5 months	Florida State Hospital behaviour rating scale (i) Ward behaviour (ii) Verbal orientation (iii) Aides' impressions
Citrin & Dixon 1977	Nebraska USA	Nursing home Moderately disorientated	84	–	Yes	Daily	12 RO 13 Control	NT	2 months	RO information sheet Geriatric rating scale (GRS)
MacDonald & Settin 1978	New York USA	Nursing home	64.4	–	No	3	10 RO 10 SW 10 NT 21F 9M	SW NT	5 weeks	Life satisfaction index NOSIE (nurses' rating) Behavioural mapping index
Voelkel 1978	Ohio USA	Nursing home Moderately/ severely mentally impaired	80+	2.67	No	3	10 RO 10 RS 19F 1M	RS	6 weeks	Mental status questionnaire PSMS physical self-maintenance scale
Holden & Sinebruchow 1978	Leeds UK	Geriatric hospital CVA, dementia others	77	1.43	Yes	5–6	46 13M 33F 30 RO 16 NT	NT	3 months	Stockton geriatric rating scale Clifton assessment schedule

Table 3.2 Continued

Authors	Location	Setting	Mean age (years)	Mean length of stay (years)	24 hour RO	No. of RO sessions per week	No. and sex of subjects	Control groups	Duration	Assessment methods
Woods 1979	Newcastle-upon-Tyne UK	EMI homes Dementia	76.6	Less than 3	No	5	14 12F 2M 5 RO 4NT 5 SA	SA NT	5 months	Wechsler memory scale Concentration test Information and orientation test Gibson spiral maze Crichton geriatric rating scale
Holden & Sinebruchow 1979 unpublished	Leeds UK	Geriatric hospital CVA, dementia others	80.3	0.9	Yes	5–6	16 6M 10F	NT	3 months	Crichton geriatric rating scale Holden communication scale
Hogstel 1979	Texas USA	Nursing homes Confused, senile or disorientated	82.2	–	No	5	20 RO 20NT	NT	3 weeks	18 item orientation questionnaire
Johnson et al 1981	Dundee UK	Psychiatric hospital Dementia	80.1	–	No	5–10	75 RO 23 NT	NT	1 month	26 item orientation questionnaire
Zepelin et al 1981	Detroit USA	Nursing homes Dementia, CVA	82.4	–	Yes	5	36 32F 4M 22 RO 14 NT	NT	1 year	24 item orientation test 7 activities of daily living scales 3 appropriateness of behaviour scales
Hanley et al 1981	Edinburgh UK	Psycho-geriatric-hospital Old people's home Dementia	79 81	–	No	4	57 53F 4M 28 RO 29 NT	NT	3 months	Geriatric rating scale Koskela test (includes verbal orientation) Orientation test

Table 3.2   Continued

Authors	Location	Setting	Mean age (years)	Mean length of stay (years)	24 hour RO	No. of RO sessions per week	No. and sex of subjects	Control groups	Duration	Assessment methods
Merchant & Saxby 1981	Plymouth UK	Geriatric hospital 'Mildly to moderately confused'	83	3	No	Daily	10 4M 6F	NT	8 weeks	Clifton assessment procedure Crichton geriatric rating scale Holden communication scale Slater and Lipman confusion scales
Goldstein et al 1982	Pittsburgh USA	VA Medical Centre Dementia, neurological disorders	59.1	1.46	No	5	14M	NT	3 weeks	18 item orientation test Activity level rating
Wallis et al 1983	Yorkshire UK	Psychiatric hospital Dementia (20), schizophrenia (14), affective (4)	69.8	Organics: 3.7 Functionals; 19.7	No	5	38 25M 13F 18 RO 20 OT	OT	3 months	Crichton geriatric rating scale Orientation test
Reeve & Ivison 1985	Sydney Australia	Psycho-geriatric ward Dementia	Over 65	–	Yes	3	19	ST	3 months	Crichton geriatric rating scale Holden communication scale CAPE orientation test Mini-mental status test Ward orientation scale
Baines et al 1987	Plymouth UK	Old people's home Moderate/ severe cognitive impairment	81.5	3.3	No	5	15 14F 1M	REM NT	4 months	CAPE cognitive tests CAPE behaviour rating scale Holden communication scale Problem behaviour rating scale Life satisfaction index

Table 3.2 Continued

Authors	Location	Setting	Mean age (years)	Mean length of stay (years)	24 hour RO	No. of RO sessions per week	No. and sex of subjects	Control groups	Duration	Assessment methods
Williams et al 1987	Sydney Australia	Psycho-geriatric ward Dementia	70.4	–	Yes	0	20	NT	3 months	As for Reeve & Ivison 1985
Zanetti et al 1993	Brescia Italy	Day hospital Alzheimer's disease/multi-infarct dementia	74.4	–	No	5	13	NT	4 weeks	Mini-mental state test Activities of daily living Neuro-psychology test battery
Koh et al 1994	Singapore	Day care centre Primary degener-ative dementia	71.9	–	No	1	30 22F 8M	NT	8 weeks	Mental status question-naire
Breuil et al 1994	Paris France	Out-patient Dementia	76.1	–	No	2	61 37F 24M	NT	5 weeks	Mini-mental state test Neuro-psychology test battery Behaviour adaptation scale

OT, occupational therapy; NT, no treatment control; OBS, organic brain syndrome; CBS, chronic brain syndrome; REM, reminiscence; CVA, cerebrovascular accident; SW, sheltered workshop; RS, resocialisation; EMI, Elderly mentally infirm; SA, social attention.

control groups over a specific period; a few use a crossover design, where the intervention group becomes the control group and vice versa, at a specific point (e.g. Holden & Sinebruchow 1979, unpublished). Others have a more complex design; for example, Reeve & Ivison (1985) split their group receiving RO sessions into two after 4 weeks with one sub-group continuing to attend (less frequently) and the other attending the control discussion group; this was to assess the benefits of continuing RO sessions at reduced frequency in maintaining initial gains.

Despite the considerable differences between studies, it is now possible to draw some fairly firm conclusions from the results which show a surprising degree of convergence.

Cognitive changes

There is overwhelming evidence that RO sessions are associated with improved scores on measures of verbal orientation. This is a remarkably robust finding. Virtually all the studies that have compared RO with no-treatment and that have used an orientation test have found significant changes in verbal orientation favouring the RO group. An exception is the study by Hogstel (1979), which had one of the briefest intervention periods (3 weeks). Given the emphasis on orientation in many RO sessions, such a result may not be seen as so surprising, although it does reflect the learning potential of people with dementia. Only one study (Williams et al 1987) associates cognitive change with 24 hour RO.

Does more general cognitive change occur? Here there are more mixed reports: Goldstein et al (1982) suggest that only those orientation items that are actually taught are learned, suggesting a very restricted form of learning; Hanley et al (1981) only found cognitive improvements on orientation tests. Others (e.g. Reeve & Ivison 1985) suggest that observed improvements on tests such as the Mini-mental State Examination reflect broader cognitive change. However, these tests include such a mix of items (including orientation) that, without a breakdown of items showing improvement, it is not possible to be certain that other cognitive abilities have, in fact, changed. More recent reports (Breuil et al 1994, Zanetti et al 1993) confirm the suggestion from Woods' (1979) study that changes in aspects of new learning ability may follow this form of cognitive stimulation. Significant differences were found on a concentration test and on the Wechsler Memory Scale (Fig. 3.2), as well as on an information/orientation test. Detailed analysis of the Memory Scale results showed that improvements in new learning ability formed a major component of the change observed.

Does general behavioural change occur?

If changes in verbal orientation have been the rule in RO studies, changes in aspects of behaviour, social function, activities of daily living and so on have been the exception. Study after study has failed to replicate the original positive findings of Brook et al (1975) in this area. Indeed, at least one study found changes in behaviour favouring the control group over a 12-month treatment period in social response, continence, dressing skills and mobility (Zepelin et al 1981). This is an important issue. Changes in verbal orientation are interesting and potentially have some usefulness, but there is no doubt that it is improvements in a wider range of activities and function that workers and relatives would prefer to see; one might speculate that these general changes would also do more to increase the person's dignity and self-respect.

A number of factors merit consideration. First, evaluating these areas satisfactorily has proved difficult at times. In the study by Zepelin's group, two out of five behavioural measures had to be abandoned because of poor inter-rater agreement. Breuil et al (1994) used a behaviour rating scale which proved to be at too low a level for their subjects, leaving little scope for improvement. Some measures may be too insensitive to show small changes. Zepelin et al also point out that comparing ratings made by different raters in the homes at different times can lead to difficulties; this is particularly so where the control group comes from a different ward or

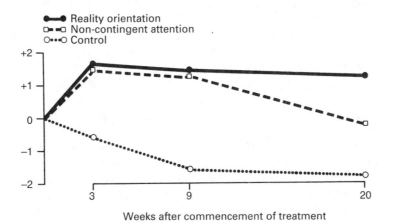

Figure 3.2 Mean change in total score on Wechsler Memory Scale over time in Woods' (1979) study. RO significantly more improved at 9 and 20 weeks than in control groups combined, which do not differ throughout.

home. Where this is the case, as it was in the project of the Zepelin group, the differences between the two care environments must also be considered. Harris & Ivory (1976) described different staff expectations on the two units in their study having an important influence on the ratings made.

Differences between care environments may also contribute directly to the discrepant results reported. The degree to which the institution has in the past 'encouraged' dependent behaviour may be significant. Therefore, for example, if the particular group has been underfunctioning in self-care then a comprehensive RO programme may tip the balance, whereas if the institution is already encouraging independence there may be less scope for improvement. Alternatively, if there continues to be no encouragement of independence outside RO sessions, then potential changes in general behaviour may be nipped in the bud. The extent to which staff carry over into 24 hour RO reinforcement of appropriate functioning is probably a major factor, and will be related to differences in attitudes and practices between institutions. Some wards or homes may be more receptive than others to RO. For some it may fit well into the ongoing development of the ward; in other places other interventions may have more chance of bringing about positive changes (Haugen 1985). There may well be a complex interaction between the level of development of the institution and the type of intervention that will be most appropriate. Once again, this could be a particular problem where the comparison group is drawn from another home or ward. The control ward may be evolving as a result of other influences, independent of the introduction of RO elsewhere.

Another factor to consider is that the emphasis on group average scores may obscure changes in the individual's behaviour; Woods (1979), for example, pointed out that the variation in behaviour rating scores increased greatly over the course of his study, indicating that individuals were changing in different ways. Negative findings regarding change in ward activities were reported by Goldstein et al (1982); however, they note that individual responses to the treatment were quite varied and show that for at least one patient an increase in purposeful activity did occur. In a later section, the limited amount of research looking at individuals in depth rather than at groups of patients will be reviewed.

It has been suggested that the degree to which the RO session is a formal classroom teaching session rather than a social setting where learning is encouraged and where it is possible to capitalise on previously learned social responses may be important. For example, Merchant & Saxby (1981) report improvements in orientation, awareness of others, communication, conversational ability and in socially acceptable behaviour following 8 weeks of RO sessions, compared with control subjects drawn from the same ward. The emphasis was on a social atmosphere, and Merchant & Saxby emphasise the enjoyment their patients gained from the RO sessions. If change in social behaviour and communication is an aim, clearly creating a conducive social climate is essential.

Woods (1979) and Woods & Britton (1977) argued that direct training of a particular skill would be needed if more general changes are to occur. Hanley et al (1981) applied this approach to ward orientation, i.e. the patient finding his way from one place to another on the ward. Patients received either no-treatment, RO classroom or RO classroom plus some sessions of ward orientation training. This last procedure involved the staff member taking the patient individually round the ward, asking him to locate different areas and giving clues and directions when the person was unable to do so. This last group did much better than the RO classes alone or no-treatment on a behavioural test of ward orientation. The groups did not differ on amount of verbal orientation assessed in the usual way (Fig. 3. 3).

This type of training, it might be argued, should be part of 24 hour RO, and Reeve & Ivison (1985) were able to demonstrate similar improvements in ward orientation following the introduction of signposting on a psychogeriatric ward, together with a form of 24 hour RO. This involved staff responding to residents' initiatives according to RO principles, but not seeking to increase the number of interactions. Improvements were also

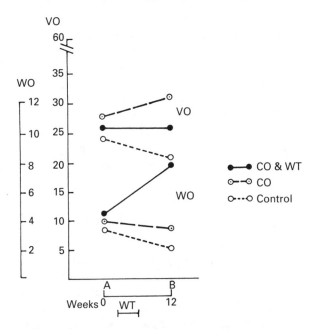

Figure 3.3   Change in mean verbal orientation (VO) and ward orientation (WO) after RO sessions (CO) and ward training (WT). Reproduced, with permission, from Hanley et al 1981, British Journal of Psychiatry 138: 10–14.

noted on the Holden Communication Scale and the Crichton Behaviour Rating Scale as well as in verbal orientation after 4 weeks of RO sessions. This improvement remained statistically significant for those patients who continued to attend RO sessions for a further 8 weeks. Control patients, again from the same ward, attended discussion groups for an equivalent amount of time. They showed some improvements from the changes to the ward environment and from the modified 24 hour RO, despite not attending RO sessions. In a subsequent study, Williams et al (1987) demonstrated, by using a control group from a separate ward, that the introduction of signposting and modified 24 hour RO was sufficient to lead to changes in ward orientation, and general behaviour (on the Holden Communication Scale and Crichton Behaviour Rating Scale), as well as cognitive improvements, without any RO sessions at all.

Improvements in ward orientation may then be feasible if the RO programme specifically includes procedures and modifications to the environment that are likely to be directly helpful. It is of interest that three of the most striking studies reporting behavioural change were those able to demonstrate implementation of the approach outside RO sessions: Hanley et al (1981) in direct training sessions; Reeve & Ivison (1985) and Williams et al (1987) in modified 24 hour RO. It is quite probable that more general behavioural changes occur when RO stimulates staff and patients to likewise focus on other aspects of self-care and social activity.

We have to conclude that changes in general behaviour are much more elusive then improvements in verbal orientation, but have now been demonstrated sufficiently often for them to be acknowledged as a possible consequence of implementation of RO. There are a number of indications of factors that need to be addressed in order to increase the likelihood of progress in this important area.

RO in comparison with other approaches

Two early studies compared RO sessions with a sheltered workshop approach (MacDonald & Settin 1978) and re-socialisation groups (Voelkel 1978). The results of both studies tended to favour the alternative approaches; the sheltered workshop was associated with higher life satisfaction scores and greater social interest, re-socialisation groups with more improvement on an orientation test. It has been suggested that these studies were not a fair test of RO; for example, Scarbrough et al (1978) asserted that MacDonald & Settin's interpretation of RO was erroneous. Voelkel's description of her re-socialisation group resembles closely activities other workers have used in RO. MacDonald & Settin's sheltered workshop group would certainly be beyond the capabilities of many patients included in other RO programmes. They comment that their RO residents mentioned to staff that 'the sessions seem boring and useless'. Similarly Voelkel states that most of her RO participants read the RO board without any difficulties and several were irritated at having to read the information, the approach, therefore, appearing child-like. It seems clear that in both studies the RO technique may not have been pitched at the appropriate level for the residents concerned and the alternative therapies may have been much more rewarding and satisfying for the residents. There is an indication here that approaches must be adjusted appropriately for the residents involved, and that the effects of a range of approaches need to be evaluated, in terms of for whom they are most appropriate.

Baines et al (1987) conducted a comparison of RO and reminiscence groups in a large residential home for the elderly. One group of residents attending RO sessions showed a significant improvement on the Clifton Behaviour Rating Scale compared with untreated controls and residents attending reminiscence sessions. However, when there was a crossover of treatment and the group originally receiving reminiscence sessions took part in RO sessions, they did not show corresponding behavioural improvements. In fact the group that received RO first continued to improve on verbal orientation during the phase of the study when the residents were attending reminiscence sessions. Therefore, in this study, the positive changes seemed to relate more to a particular group of residents rather than to the specific form of treatment, although the authors attribute their findings to the sequence of the treatments with RO followed by reminiscence being superior to reminiscence preceding RO.

We have to conclude that, at the present time, the status of RO in relation to other approaches in terms of outcomes for people with dementia is not clear; different approaches may have particular benefits for individuals at different times.

Other research findings

1. The relative contributions of 24 hour RO and RO classroom sessions

As mentioned above, the form of 24 hour RO and environmental modification used by Reeve & Ivison (1985) was sufficient to bring about changes in ward orientation in patients not attending RO sessions, together with some cognitive and behavioural change. However,

patients who did attend RO sessions throughout the experimental period showed a wider range of cognitive and behavioural improvements. This study is particularly important in that staff were observed to be actually carrying out the 24 hour RO as intended. A further study from this research group (Williams et al 1987) confirms that this form of 24 hour RO is superior to no-treatment on both cognitive and behavioural measures, even without RO sessions.

2. The use of memory aids in the environment

One aspect of 24 hour RO is the provision of visual aids in the environment giving items of information. Hanley (1981) has additionally shown that, with respect to ward orientation, large signposts identifying different ward locations were not sufficient to improve patients' orientation. Behavioural change was only evident when the signposts were used as part of the ward-orientation training procedures outlined above. Similarly, Bergert & Jacobson (1976), in a Swedish study, concluded that environmental cues were useful in re-orientating the person to time and place but that the person had to be taught to use the cues provided; they suggested that when the cues were not present, orientation decreased again. Reeve & Ivison (1985) and Williams et al (1987) incorporated colour-coding of doors according to function, verbal and non-verbal signs, signposting and large RO boards in their 24 hour RO procedure, but they did not evaluate their effectiveness in isolation from the staff interactions with residents. There is a need for 24 hour RO to include the active use of these memory aids, with staff drawing the attention of patients to them, as they may well not make use of them on their own initiative.

3. Intensity of RO sessions

As can be seen from Table 3.2, the frequency of RO sessions used in various studies has ranged from once per week to seven times per week. The ideal frequency must depend to some extent on the subject population used, with, presumably, the frequency of sessions being related to the degree of disorientation. Positive changes have emerged from studies using only three sessions a week (Reeve & Ivison 1985, although this was backed up by 24 hour RO). A puzzling finding emerged from Wallis and co-workers' study (1983) where sessions were offered 5 days a week. Patients attending RO most frequently during the initial 2 weeks improved least on both cognitive and behavioural measures. The authors suggest that early in treatment daily half-hour sessions were over-demanding for some patients. Much may depend on the previous level of stimulation and activity: patients in this study were those who were unable or unwilling to attend the occupational or industrial therapies already available.

In virtually every study, sessions have been given once only on any particular day. Johnson et al (1981) raised the possibility of whether additional RO sessions each day would be of benefit, particularly where 24 hour RO could not be implemented. They found the same range of improvements on verbal orientation with one or two RO sessions per day, with no apparent benefit from doubling the number of RO sessions each day.

4. Group v. individual sessions

At times a person cannot be included in group RO, perhaps because of severe deafness or restlessness. In these situations, individual RO sessions are often recommended. Johnson et al (1981) compared the efficacy of group RO sessions with 10-minute individual RO sessions. They were equally effective in improving verbal orientation, but individual sessions did not appear to be more effective. Where a person cannot be included in a group for some reason, these extremely brief individual sessions have then been shown to be of use.

5. Maintenance of effects of RO

How long-lasting are the effects of RO? Does it have to be continuously applied in perpetuity or is a brief intensive period of RO sufficient to produce lasting change? Holden & Sinebruchow

(unpublished) followed up their patients 6 months after RO sessions finished. They reported significant behavioural deterioration on both the Crichton Geriatric Rating Scale and the Holden Communication Scale. Although cognitive improvements were maintained 1 month following the end of treatment in the study by the Wallis group (1983), the general impression appears to suggest an absence of maintenance, certainly in the longer term and in some instances within a month (e.g. one group in Baines et al (1987) showed a clear cognitive loss to baseline level following 1 month without RO sessions). It has been suggested that less frequent RO sessions may be helpful in maintaining change. Reeve & Ivison included one group who had in successive months three, two and one RO sessions per week. They remained significantly better than their matched controls, but did not differ from patients who had only the initial month with 12 RO sessions in total. Again the supportive 24 hour RO environment may be important here, in perhaps aiding maintenance. Given that most gains from RO sessions appear to occur fairly early in the course of treatment, the use of reduced frequency RO sessions for maintenance purposes deserves further exploration.

6. Components of reality orientation

When RO has been applied in practice, it has comprised a number of elements, which vary from study to study, most obviously in relation to 24 hour RO and RO sessions but in other aspects also. There is very little research evaluating the relative effectiveness of the various components. Individual RO (Johnson et al 1981) removed many of the social factors operative in RO sessions; its efficacy shows these are not necessary for cognitive improvement to occur. Riegler (1980) compared the effects of RO sessions with and without music on a small number of nursing home residents and found a clear superiority for the music group in terms of improvement on a basic orientation and information test. The use of music included 'singing and playing rhythm instruments to accompany songs and jingles dealing with names, members, day, date and year'. Other activities included listening to and discussing music concerning particular times and places. It may be that the music helped group members participate more, relax more and enjoy the sessions more, making the sessions less serious, classroom-like and formal.

Hart & Fleming (1985) report a modified procedure for RO sessions, using shaping and reinforcement to encourage verbal orientation and using role play to increase conversational skills. This procedure was compared with traditional RO sessions, based around repetition of information from an RO board. The results indicated an improvement on verbal orientation by patients receiving the modified RO. Both groups had been attending traditional RO sessions for the previous 18 months. Disappointingly, no difference was observed in social interaction on the ward between the groups, using a time sampling technique.

Finally, there is the suggestion from the work of Baines et al (1987) that reminiscence sessions should be preceded by RO sessions. The RO sessions did, in fact, include some reminiscence activity, but comparisons with the present day were always made, and historical accuracy emphasised. The generality of this finding remains to be established.

7. Patients benefiting most from RO

As Table 3.2 shows, RO has been applied in a wide range of settings: nursing homes, residential homes, geriatric hospitals, psychiatric hospitals, etc. Although it might at first sight seem obvious that less severely impaired people with dementia will make a better response, the evidence on this point is mixed. Brook and co-workers (1975) did show that the lowest functioning group benefited least. Contrary results are provided by Johnson et al (1981), who found changes in verbal orientation of comparable size at each of three levels of functioning in a long-stay psychogeriatric population. Hanley et al (1981) similarly report that degree of dementia did not appear to be a significant determinant of change, and Wallis et al (1983) found that initial scores did not correlate with degree of improvement. The discrepant

results may reflect differences in how severity is defined; Brook et al were using a behavioural rating, whereas the other studies were using a cognitive measure. Although it is often not made explicit, it is a reasonable assumption that most studies, in fact, exclude those with the severest impairment, where there is little response to the environment or verbal communication and where group work of this kind is not really viable.

8. Use of RO in community settings

Day-hospitals and day-centres have an important role in the assessment, treatment and support of elderly people with dementia, allowing them to remain in their own homes longer and providing much-needed relief for relatives and friends. There has been little study as yet of RO in such settings, and no studies at all of teaching these techniques to family care-givers. The report that comes closest to relatives using RO techniques is from Bourgeois (1990) (see Ch. 2). Three care-givers were taught to use a 'prosthetic memory aid' with the person with dementia, resulting in improvements in conversational quality. The aid consisted of photographs and drawings of people and events and might not have been out of place in an RO session.

In a day-care setting, Greene et al (1983) have reported the results of RO groups in a Glasgow day-hospital. This followed some moderately successful individual interventions (reviewed in the next section). Groups of four to six patients met twice a day on the 2 days per week that they attended. Patients had a mild to moderate degree of dementia. All were living with a relative who could monitor any changes in their behaviour in their own home or had a relative who lived close by. The relatives completed rating scales on the patient's mood and behaviour at home and also on their own degree of stress and their own mood. The 13 patients involved were also cognitively and behaviourally assessed at the hospital. Assessments were carried out at the beginning and end of a 3-week baseline period, then after 6 weeks of RO sessions and, finally, after a further 6 weeks where RO sessions were not held.

Results (see Fig. 3.4) showed a dramatic, significant improvement in verbal orientation following RO. The gain was lost at the 6-week follow-up assessment. Changes in relatives' ratings of the patient's behaviour and in their degree of stress were not significant, but relatives' mood did improve significantly with RO and deteriorated again at follow-up. This was despite the relatives being unaware of the procedure being followed in the project. These findings then hold some encouragement for the use of RO in day-settings in that not only was cognitive change found, but also a beneficial effect on the supporting relative.

The individual case

So far in this chapter we have been examining group changes, group differences and group effects. Even when changes have proved to be significant, the size of the improvement has often been small over the group as a whole. Group studies have their place, but if the extent to which the approach works and its attendant limitations are to be really understood, individual cases need to be examined, preferably where objective measures have been taken over a period of time. In the behavioural literature particularly, single-case designs are used a great deal and can be extremely powerful in comparing and contrasting different aspects and phases of a treatment approach.

The first published case studies of this type were carried out by Greene et al (1979). Three cases are reported, all females showing severe to moderate impairment in all areas of cognition and having a diagnosis of dementia. RO sessions were highly structured; they consisted of a standard list of questions of general and personal orientation given in conversational manner over a 30-minute period. Each patient was seen individually twice on each attendance at the day-hospital. In baseline phases, correct answers were not supplied when there was no response or an incorrect response. In RO phases, correct answers were given where necessary. In both phases, the patient was told when correct

answers had been given. Patient 1 was seen four times a week for 7 weeks: weeks 1, 4 and 5 baseline conditions; weeks 2, 3, 6 and 7 RO phases; then followed up once a week under baseline conditions for a further 5 weeks. Improvements in orientation score were apparent in the RO periods. These were lost in the return to baseline phase and gradually returned to initial levels 5 weeks after the end of the RO sessions. General changes in the patient's behaviour during RO phases were suggested by anecdotal reports; for example, her husband temporarily stopped demanding her admission.

The second case study attempted to systematise the more general effects by including ratings made by the unit occupational therapist of the patient's performance and social functioning in occupational therapy (OT) sessions. The patient was 52 years old and had pre-senile dementia. She was seen on 3 days per week, and a similar design was followed to that used with patient 1, except that, in the final phase of once-a-week sessions, RO was included. The results showed a clear improvement in orientation in RO phases. This was maintained in the return to baseline phase, and orientation remained at a high level during once-a-week RO sessions. The OT ratings were made without knowledge of the experimental phase and showed that ratings of performance of activities paralleled the changes in orientation. The patient's social rating increased steadily in all phases. The authors speculate that this may be related to general stimulation effects whereas the changes in performance scores seem more likely to be related to changes in orientation.

The third patient was an older (72 years), more severely demented lady, seen 3 days a week. Results for this patient were similar with respect to orientation, with a decline in performance, however, at the return to baseline phase. Changes in OT ratings were not quite as marked, but did show some improvement. Generalisation to items not taught in the RO sessions was tested to ensure that the improvements noted were not simply from rote learning. These items, which included differently worded questions, photographs of people included in the orientation test

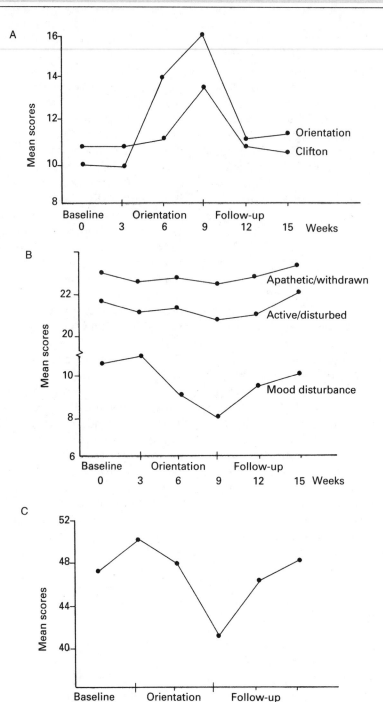

Figure 3.4   A. Patients' mean scores on verbal orientation tests.
B. Mean scores on sub-scales of the patients' Behaviour and Mood
Disturbance Scale (rated by relative). **C.** Mean scores of relatives on
self-rating of mood (note that RO sessions only took place during the
'orientation' phase). Reproduced from Greene et al (1983), with the
permission of the authors and *Age and Ageing.*

and new items, showed the same pattern of improvement in RO phases.

Greene et al (1979) introduced the concept of a gradient of generalisation; the more a behaviour depends on orientation the more change will be apparent in it following RO. This is a hypothesis well worth pursuing. Woods (1983) explored further the issue of generalisation from items of orientation that are specifically taught in RO sessions to items that are not.

The patient was a 68-year-old woman who had been an in-patient in a psychiatric hospital for 3 months with a diagnosis, supported by neurological investigation, of Korsakoff's psychosis. Twice-daily structured RO sessions (with specified information only being taught) were conducted by nursing staff. If the patient did not know an answer, a clue was given, followed by the correct answer if the patient could not make use of the prompt. The experimental design made use of a multiple baseline (Table 3. 3) in which all information items were assessed regularly. The RO sessions covered only a proportion of these items at any time. Assessment sessions took place at the beginning, middle and end of each phase, each of which was 9–12 days long, except phase IV which lasted 1 month. The results are shown in Figure 3.5.

Generally items showed most improvement during the phase of treatment when they were specifically taught. Two exceptions should be noted. The patient's performance on list I items did improve markedly in phase I but continued to improve during phase II, before falling off during phase III, after 3 weeks of other items being taught. The records that nurses kept of RO sessions suggested that the assessment at the end of phase I gave an underestimate of her

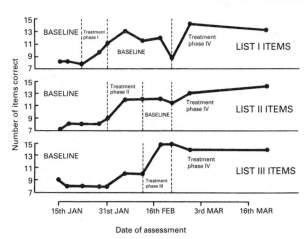

Figure 3.5   Learning of verbal orientation and basic information in a single-case experimental study. See text for details of multiple baseline design and the phase of intervention.

near-perfect knowledge of list I items at that time; the 'improvement' in phase II was, in fact, probably maintenance of improvement already made. The other exception is the slight improvement in list III items in phase II; these gains were made on items in list III that had similar content to certain items in list II. An overall 60 item personalised memory and information test showed gradual improvement over the experimental period (Fig. 3.6). The final phase, in which all lists reached near-maximum levels, involved staff teaching her to use her diary and to re-orientate herself using this aid; the improvements were maintained well in this phase.

Exactly this specificity of learning has also been demonstrated by Patterson (1982) with four clients receiving 'personal information' training, a procedure similar to that described here, and in a group study by Goldstein et al (1982). The evidence is accumulating that, to be learned, the information has to be taught!

Hanley & Lusty (1984) have taken further the use of a diary to aid orientation. In a single-case study, they taught an 84-year-old patient with dementia to use a diary and watch to answer orientation questions, reaching perfect performance on a 30 item personalised test after 2 weeks of training (Fig. 3.7). During this training, the

Table 3.3   Multiple baseline design of case study

Experimental phase	Treatment conditions
Baseline	No RO sessions
Phase I	List I taught
Phase II	List II taught
Phase III	List III taught
Phase IV	All unlearned items taught using a diary as memory aid

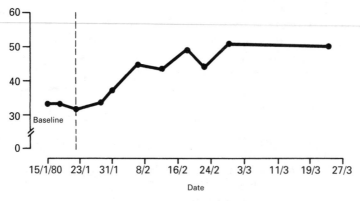

Figure 3.6 Scores an a 60 item information and orientation test achieved by subject in the single-case experimental study shown in Figure 3.4.

patient kept a third of her 'appointments' (e.g. having her hair done, collecting the daily paper, etc), whereas previously she had only kept one out of 36. The improvements were soon lost once training was discontinued, but the training period was very brief (2 weeks) and took only a few minutes each day, and so could have been continued indefinitely if necessary. This study did not require the patient to remember any items of information; she was able to refer to her diary and her watch to find out the answers, a skill this patient was clearly able to demonstrate, but only with specific, focused training and encouragement.

Hanley (1986) reports a further case study where once again a memory aid (a notebook) was used. Here, an 83-year-old woman with dementia was taught to use the notebook in conjunction with the RO board in order to improve her orientation, her knowledge of personal information and her awareness of her husband's death. The patient had become confused at times about whether or not he was alive, and she had asked staff during a lucid phase to remind her that he was dead. In correcting her on this sensitive item, staff took care to give her time to talk about her feelings and to give her the attention and care she needed in doing this.

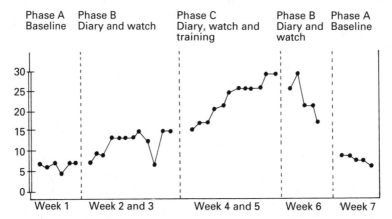

Figure 3.7 Patient's scores on a personalised orientation test during (A) baseline phases, (B) when provided with a diary and a watch and (C) when trained to use the diary and watch. Reproduced, with permission, from Hanley & Lusty 1984, Behaviour Research and Therapy 22: 709–712.

Regular visits to the cemetery were arranged as a tangible reminder. The results were clear-cut; when this approach was taken she was aware of the facts about her husband's death on 11 out of 15 days; beforehand she had no awareness of his death on any of five occasions. Similarly, her orientation and personal information scores improved.

Again, the patient was not required to remember information; she only had to use the RO board and the notebook in order to find all the answers required. However, before specific training in doing this was given, she showed little improvement. In fact, whilst she did rely on the RO board for answers to orientation questions, she soon re-learned the items of personal information and rarely had to consult her notebook.

A number of single-case studies have been reported in relation to ward-orientation training. Hanley (1981) reports eight cases. The results overall indicate a good response to active ward-orientation training, where the patient is requested to show the staff member to the next location on a set route. If correct, the patient was verbally reinforced; if not, appropriate prompts and cues were given to enable the patient to find the correct location. There tended to be little carry-over to locations not specifically taught, and following the cessation of training the im-

provements were gradually lost. Putting signposts up on the ward had little additional effect, until further training, incorporating the use of the signposts, was given. For some patients, the improvements seemed to be much better maintained once they had been trained to use the signposts that had been placed on the ward. Gilleard et al (1981) report similar findings with a further six patients. Although they are more optimistic regarding the effects of signposting alone, they confirmed the superiority of combining signposting with specific training. Their test was particularly difficult as it was carried out after the signs had been removed, so this was not just the effect of learning to use the signs.

Finally, Lam & Woods (1986) report a single case where an 80-year-old female patient with dementia, with marked difficulties in finding her way around the ward, was trained to find a number of important locations—her room, the toilet, the lounge, etc. Instead of learning a set route around the ward, as in previous studies, the sequence of locations was chosen at random on each day. The training involved giving predetermined cues if a location could not be found, the cues making use of landmarks and signs on the ward. Figure 3.8 shows the clear improvement in the patient's ability to find the target locations, which was rapidly lost when

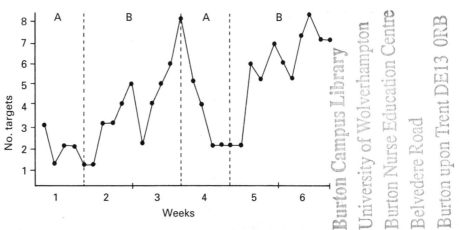

Figure 3.8 Number of target locations found on ward by patient during (A) baseline and (B) training phases. Reproduced, with permission, from Lam & Woods 1986, International Journal of Geriatric Psychiatry 1: 145–147.

the training was temporarily stopped and regained when the training recommenced.

These studies emphasise that re-learning can take place, and that the changes seen are directly related to the training given in verbal or ward orientation. They do not necessarily provide a model for how to carry out RO, but they do illustrate the potential of these techniques when they are harnessed to the needs of an individual case. A good example of this is provided by Hanley (1986) who shows how an 86-year-old lady with severe dementia was helped to become continent once again by a ward-orientation programme geared to helping her find her way to the toilet.

CONCLUSION

The evidence that RO is associated with improvements in verbal and ward orientation is considerable. The question of changes in other areas of functioning remains contentious; changes in behaviour have been reported much less frequently. However, with modified, responsive 24 hour RO there are more encouraging indications. Many questions remain: do the changes found actually make a difference to the quality of life or well-being of the person with dementia? Changes may be statistically signi-

ficant, but does, say, a two-point change on an orientation test really affect the person's life? How can changes be maintained? Can we develop ways of providing continued support and encouragement for people with dementia to be able to find the information, and the places, that are of importance to them?

Institutional differences are almost certainly of importance in our consideration of, at times, conflicting results; Woods & Britton (1985) discuss the power of institutions to overwhelm psychological approaches. In order for staff to behave and interact in ways consistent with RO, the whole ethos of the institution may have to change, and in this light RO may be seen as one vehicle for a dramatic change from purely custodial care to a care approach that firmly places the emphasis on the needs and potential of the individual. This is a theme to which we will return in Chapter 5.

Above all, the RO research literature shows that positive approaches can make a difference; the diagnosis of dementia does not mean that change is impossible. These findings should be used as a springboard to develop approaches that are even more effective in meeting the real needs of people with dementia and those who care for them.

4

How do positive approaches have an effect?

In the previous two chapters we have described a number of changes in people with dementia associated with the implementation of positive approaches. How could any beneficial effects arise in people suffering from dementing conditions? What possible mechanisms could lead to change, when we understand there to be generalised damage to the brain in these disorders? Several possibilities that have been suggested will be outlined, together with some of the supporting evidence. It should be borne in mind that in such a varied group of conditions, different processes may be responsible for improvement in different individuals, and, of course, several mechanisms may be operating simultaneously.

REACTIVATION OF NEURAL PATHWAYS

In her introduction to Folsom's work on RO, Stephens (1969) made a statement that could be equally applied to any positive approach: 'The process can reawaken unused neural pathways and stimulate the patients to develop new ways of functioning to compensate for organic brain damage that has resulted either from injury or progressive senility, or from deterioration through misuse'.

The issues arising from this statement are:

1. Can parts of the brain suffer from disuse? Muscles need to be exercised in order to remain efficient; do neural pathways require regular use for the same reasons?

2. If certain pathways in the brain are blocked, damaged or even dead can other connections be made in order to maintain function by using other routes or a by-pass system?

3. Can brain cells regenerate?

These are very profound and complex problems which have intrigued scientists for at least the past 150 years. The most controversial issue—which relates particularly to 1 and 2 above—is the extent to which particular functions are under the control of specific localised parts of the brain. The work of Paul Broca and Carl Wernicke in relating particular speech deficits to specific areas of the dominant hemisphere would seem to support a localisation viewpoint. However, as Hughlings Jackson has indicated, localisation of a deficit is different from localisation of a function. In the light of recent evidence, whilst there is probably considerable localisation of certain major functions, total localisation appears illogical, and theories now recognise that many psychological processes depend on several brain areas and their interconnections being intact.

To what extent is recovery from brain damage possible? Zangwill in his introduction to the classic work by Luria, *Restoration of Function after Brain Injury* (1963), states: 'in man, unfortunately, recovery from the effects of brain injury is apt to be a good deal less complete [than in animals] and residual defects are distressingly common'. However, despite quite extensive damage, persons sustaining head injury and other brain damage can obtain restoration of function, to some degree and sometimes to an incredible degree. Paralysis can disappear and motor and sensory function can all return to near normal. Even disorders of speech, understanding, recognition, or practical skills can improve dramatically.

In recent years, there has been a considerable amount of work concentrating on restorative techniques, mostly in relation to brain damage caused by a specific trauma rather than that caused by progressive deterioration. Therapy has been mainly geared to helping the person compensate for what was seen as permanent loss, instead of attempting to find a means of regaining an ability that has been damaged. There are a number of techniques employed which differ in approach, and the exact mechanisms of restoration of function remain somewhat unclear. The major theories are discussed in more detail by a number of writers, including Rothi & Horner (1983), Miller (1984), Craine (1987) and Fussey & Muir Giles (1988).

Briefly the four main theories are:

1. In superficial or temporary injury, where dysfunction arises temporarily from brain areas being 'bruised' and swollen from the trauma; recovery occurs naturally as the swelling and bruising subside (diachisis).

2. Substitution, where recovery occurs by the function being taken up by related, undamaged brain areas, perhaps achieving the same goal by different means.

3. Radical reorganisation, where a completely different, unrelated brain area takes up the function, setting up a new functional system; Luria (1963) believed that specific training programmes could be used to bring about this process.

4. Regeneration, where there is growth and development of brain structures and tissues to replace some of that which has been lost.

Neuropsychological re-training programmes have been established on the basis of there being plasticity in brain function. Craine (1987) offers a series of principles to be used as a guide to re-training. These include:

1. The cerebral cortex is a dynamic process of neurological organisation that can be completely halted or slowed down by injury or environmental deprivation, or it can be greatly increased or heightened by carefully planned environmental stimulation.

2. The organisation of learning within the cerebral cortex results from repeated activity on the part of the individual and becomes organised into functional systems of behaviour. In other words, practice, practice, practice until the subject matter is automatically employed.

3. The activities of training must recapitulate the developmental stages involved in the indi-

vidual's original acquisition of the learning or the skill that is being trained.

4. In order to successfully regain an ability, each stage must be thoroughly learned before proceeding; if errors are carried forward problems could arise.

5. Consistent and direct feedback to the patients about their performance is crucial to retraining.

In any re-training, it is vital to recognise the individual and his or her previous history and personality; no two people are the same. The loss of ability or function may seem identical, but the many variables lead to different needs and strengths to be taken into account in developing a strategy for re-training.

To return to the questions posed as a result of Stephens' statements about neural pathways, some answers are possible. Cells *can* regenerate, certainly in youth but probably also in older brains, through the growth of certain aspects of brain cells (Wilcock 1984, Sofroniew 1993). There are suggestions in the literature that function can be maintained by using other routes or strategies, or by using by-pass systems. The possibility of parts of the brain suffering from disuse and 'wasting' as disused muscles do is difficult to confirm; certainly, repeated practice is thought by many to be one way of re-establishing function.

The theories that have been outlined may not be mutually exclusive. They point the way for intensive research evaluating the effects and mechanisms of rehabilitative techniques. Behavioural strategies are being increasingly used in neuropsychological rehabilitation (Caplin 1987, Meir et al 1986).

In the context of dementia-related disorders, it is conceivable that some of these mechanisms could occur. Diachisis might occur in multi-infarct dementia, for instance. There are beginning to emerge links between environmental stimulation and biochemical changes in the brain in dementia. In the study of 'integrity-promoting care' (Brane et al 1989), described in Chapter 2, measures of the levels of various chemicals in the subjects' cerebrospinal fluid were made

before and after the environmental changes were introduced. Somatostatin, which has been implicated in relation to cognitive loss in Alzheimer's disease (Perry & Perry 1993), was shown to be present in increased concentration following the intervention, reflecting, according to the authors, 'an increased activity of neuromodulatory factors in the brains of the patients that are cared for in an integrity-promoting way'. Kitwood & Bredin (1992) pointed out that there is evidence from such studies and from work with ageing rats that an enriched environment may have a definite impact on brain structures and neurological development. Reorganisation and substitution are likely, however, to require more time and retained capacity than might be available once a deteriorating process is under way. Whatever the form of brain injury, Stephens' suggestions must remain speculative—although in the light of current theory not completely far-fetched.

INCREASED ATTENTION AND STIMULATION

Any form of research carried out in an attempt to change behavioural patterns should be questioned as to the effects of added attention. This has been called the Hawthorne effect, after the first researcher to be concerned about such a variable. This is akin to the placebo effect, which has to be carefully controlled for in drug trials. All investigators need to be aware of the inevitability of some degree of change arising simply because the system is the focus for much more attention than usual. Attempts to allow for this variable include the use of control subjects who, while not receiving the actual therapy, receive all the other extra attentions which arise because of the experimental situation. Untreated control groups have been used in several studies; while they match exposure to the measures being used, they do not allow for the non-specific effects associated with any intervention. For example, early RO studies did not control for the effects of attention, the stimulus provided for staff involved in special activity, or the extra engagement with the experimental as compared with the control group in any given study. In studies of RO, reported by Woods (1979) and Reeve & Ivison (1985), 'social attention' comparison groups were used. These group sessions aimed at encouraging conversation in group meetings held for the same amount of time and meeting as frequently as the RO sessions. In Woods' study, RO methods were not used in these groups and rambling or confused talk was not corrected. Both these studies found RO to be superior in terms of cognitive change, suggesting that the *form* of attention is of importance. Generalised attention may not be as beneficial as attention that specifically encourages and re-inforces orientated behaviour. These findings are not an artefact of staff realising that 'social attention' was a form of placebo. In Woods' study, the same care-staff led both groups and in fact preferred the 'social attention', believing it to be more effective. These results cannot then be related to the fulfilment of expectations. Non-specific effects do not seem to be sufficient to account for all the changes produced by RO. Staff attention is almost certainly an important and effective therapeutic tool, but it needs to be directly focused on appropriate behaviour, rather than supplied in an indiscriminate manner.

Although in research studies, 'placebo' effects are seen as a complication, in practice there is no reason why they cannot be used to maximise the gains produced by any intervention programme. Creating a 'special' atmosphere, boosting staff morale, enriching the environment, and ensuring people with dementia are offered more opportunities to engage with staff and in interesting activities are all worthwhile. However, the form of staff–patient interaction remains vital; here quality matters absolutely.

GENERAL COGNITIVE EFFECTS

If an intervention produced a general increase in the person's cognitive functioning—in alertness, concentration, and new learning ability, etc, as well as in verbal orientation—then performance in a number of other areas could be facilitated. These general effects could also result from practice at and reinforcement of being attentive and concentrating on cognitive tasks as are usually carried out in, for instance, RO sessions. If stimulation is varied and the sessions are carried out in such a way as to be enjoyable and rewarding to the participants, then motivation, attention and concentration can be maximised.

As reviewed in Chapter 3, there is, in the RO literature, some evidence for general cognitive changes occurring, although most studies have only assessed verbal orientation. For example, Reeve & Ivison (1985) report improvements on the Mini-mental Status Test (Folstein et al 1975), related to RO sessions. Breuil et al (1994) designed their intervention to be specifically a form of cognitive stimulation and did identify cognitive changes on the Mini-mental State and a test of verbal learning. In Chapter 2, we noted that cognitive benefits were identified in some studies of reminiscence and of changes to the pattern of care, although there are inconsistencies between studies.

At present, the efficacy of positive approaches in contributing to general improvement in the level of alertness and concentration of elderly people with dementia is open to question. If this could be established there would be the fascinating task of relating it to possible changes at a neural level, or to motivational aspects.

RE-LEARNING

As discussed in Chapter 2, elderly patients with severe memory disorders are capable of some new learning. Various programmes can provide good conditions for this limited learning to take place. For example, appropriate behaviour is elicited and reinforced in RO which may be viewed as a behaviour modification programme for orientation.

Single-case studies, described in Chapter 3, demonstrate clear-cut learning of verbal orientation under appropriate conditions. Studies of ward-orientation training also demonstrate clear specific learning of information taught to the patient. Comparisons of RO sessions with 'social attention' sessions have emphasised that attention has to be given to desired behaviour for improvements to be obtained.

All this strongly suggests that re-training and re-learning must be considered a possibility in the operation of any structured intervention with older people, just as with younger patients who have sustained damage to the brain. However, in all cases, there is a limit on learning set by the degree of actual damage to that ability; where a progressive form of dementia exists the problem can be intensified. This is probably the main factor in the relatively small gains that have been reported. Clearly, where capacity is limited, it is important that it is used as efficiently as possible, perhaps by learning to use memory aids (Woods 1983, Hanley & Lusty 1984, Hanley 1986). The patients involved in these single-case studies were all able to learn to use a notebook or diary to assist in the recall of personal information or of appointments. Similarly, with regard to ward orientation, the value of signposting as a memory aid, in conjunction with training, has been demonstrated by Hanley (1981). Bourgeois (1990) has successfully taught the use of a memory aid to enhance the conversational skills of people with dementia.

Hanley (1984) particularly emphasised the importance of cued recall, giving the person a prompt to assist in retrieving the piece of information required. In Chapter 2, we mentioned the evidence showing that people with dementia are less impaired when cued recall is used. However, Downes (1987), drawing on the extensive research on cued recall in amnesia, argues that the higher levels of performance in cued recall do not reflect *knowing* the day, place or whatever in any real sense. The person may well be literally *unknowingly* giving the correct response to the cue. Being correctly orientated for the day of the week usually involves re-collecting the activities of the current day and the previous day (Brotchie et al 1985), for example. The person with dementia does not go through such a process when cued to say 'Today is Wednesday' by being given the first two letters of the answer. The person achieves the right answer, but the process is completely different from the normal one. In relation to verbal orientation, it may be that rather than talking about re-learning we should see interventions as a means of compensating for dementia-related impairments. The 'correct' responses are arrived at from external cues, provided by the physical and social environment, rather than from the self-generated cues that we all normally employ. For tasks that can be less dependent on verbal reflections, as in finding the way around a ward, 're-learning' may be a more appropriate description. In effect, the person with dementia is becoming increasingly dependent on implicit memory for functions that might previously have involved more explicit processes.

Downes points out that a crucial test of the value of any 'improvements' is whether they can be observed outside the standard test situation. Does the person find his or her way around the ward better when on his/her own, following ward-orientation training? Does he or she use improved verbal orientation outside the structured setting? There is, unfortunately, little evidence for this sort of impact on the person's everyday functioning. However, in the case studies reported by Hanley (1986), there are interesting indications of some clinically significant changes. If we see change as less about the person learning and more about the environment compensating for deficits and cueing appropriate behaviour, the question of the generalisation of learning from the test situation becomes more of an issue as to what extent the environment can be adapted to replicate the conditions found helpful in the more structured situation.

OVERCOMING DEPRESSIVE WITHDRAWAL

Seligman (1975) argues that repeated trauma can lead some people to adopt a position of 'learned helplessness'. The person then fails to carry out tasks of which he or she is capable. There is withdrawal from active participation and a belief that control over the environment is lost: that nothing can be done to make any difference to the situation. Self-esteem becomes lower as everything seems more and more hopeless and useless.

These considerations are relevant for at least two major groups of patients. First, those with a dementia or other organic damage will be faced with many failures at tasks that were previously extremely easy and straightforward; for some of these patients, this failure will be distressing and perhaps traumatic. One way of dealing with this is to do less and less and thus avoid failure by not attempting any sort of task. As a result, they will function at a much lower level than their true degree of impairment necessitates.

The second group of patients are those who have also become depressed and withdrawn, but with only minimal, if any, cognitive impairment. They may have had a number of experiences of rejection, and suffered losses, isolation or other trauma. They may even have been diagnosed as having dementia, as diagnostic errors do occur (see Ch. 1). Studies indicate that such people may be placed in an institution for physical or social reasons.

Positive approaches which aim to help the person to experience success once again may begin to combat the helplessness and assist the person to function at a level more in keeping with his or her full potential. Increased self-esteem could be a powerful mediator of generalised improvement.

If an elderly person has withdrawn because of shame, depression, feelings of inadequacy and lowered self-respect and is then placed in an unpatronising situation where the demands are set so that it is guaranteed that some response will receive praise, self-esteem will improve. When someone is faced with the realisation that memory is failing and that abilities and status are also suffering, self-doubt and depression seem almost inevitable. Failure is the factor which becomes the focus of attention, not only by the self but also by others. If instead of concentration on the many failures—inability to wash and dress, inability to move about freely—these are minimised and there is praise for simple things, confidence can return. To praise a person for the positive things that he or she can do is an effective method of approach. To read what day or month it is from a calendar is a simple task, to be able to tell a story about a past experience is always possible to some extent, to be able to recognise a smell, to know the name of a flower or a fruit; these are simple aims on which to build. It is easy to say 'that's right' with some enthusiasm. To an elderly person becoming used to being always wrong, this is an achievement which will encourage further attempts towards self-expression and help.

What is being said here is that some people with dementia may be 'under-functioning', having greater disability than their neurological impairment necessitates. This is reflected in Kitwood's (1990) discussion of the way in which negative interactions and attitudes from those around the person with dementia serve to increase the person's apparent disability. Kitwood's work is discussed in more detail in Chapter 5; it is worth noting here that it is this mechanism which Kitwood & Bredin (1992) are elaborating in their theory of dementia care: 'a dementing condition tends to be compounded by depression or anxiety, a sense of apathy or disencouragement'. Feil (1992) is similarly describing validation as a means of preventing the person with dementia withdrawing inward, reducing anxiety and strengthening well-being.

Evidence that positive approaches have an impact on depression and withdrawal in people with dementia is beginning to accumulate. In the study of integrity-promoting care by Brane et al (1989), reduced anxiety and distractability were noted; improvements in mood related to a move to a group-living unit were noted by Annerstedt et al (1993); Goldwasser et al (1987) reported improvements in depression following reminiscence groups; Lord & Garner (1993) reported improved mood in patients attending a daily music session; there are numerous examples of increased activity and interaction.

It is of interest that two studies that have compared RO with other approaches (MacDonald & Settin 1978, Baines et al 1987) both suggested that RO was associated with lower scores on the LSI (Life Satisfaction Index). In the first study, the comparison therapy—a sheltered workshop—was clearly much more relevant and enjoyable for the people involved. In the latter, the trend was for attendance at RO sessions to be associated with lower LSI scores, although there was not a significant difference between the groups. These authors suggest that an apparent lowering of mood may relate to a more realistic self-appraisal; both positive and negative feelings were expressed openly in the RO sessions as they progressed. Both RO and reminiscence sessions were reported to be enjoyed by the residents involved.

There are difficulties in assessing mood in people with severe cognitive impairments. The reliability of self-report measures, like the LSI with more impaired patients, is open to considerable doubt. Another approach would be for someone who knows the patient well to rate the patient's mood using a suitable scale. This method was adapted by Greene et al (1983) in their study of people with dementia attending a day-hospital. A relative living with the patient completed a number of ratings regarding the person's mood and behaviour. During the period of the trial when RO sessions were taking place, an improvement in the patient's mood at home was noted. Other evidence is more anecdotal. Certainly, a large number of patients with a diagnosis of early dementia may, in fact, have depression or may have depression plus early dementia. Our impression is that such patients often do well on RO. Mrs B sat in her chair for some months, declaring that she was incapable of doing anything. She felt that she was useless, a nuisance and frequently wept with despair. She believed that she would not do anything right in RO, but, on the contrary, once there she found that she could do things she thought impossible. She required a great deal of re-assurance and encouragement, but smiles began to appear as success after success occurred. Her self-care improved, and she was well enough to be discharged within a few weeks.

Clearly these processes need systematic exploration. Is the withdrawal being described here appropriately described as 'depressive'; how important is anxiety and fear? Can Kitwood & Bredin's (1992) indicators of well-being (see Ch. 5) be used to systematically monitor the impact of positive approaches on people with dementia?

CONCLUSION

This chapter has of necessity been somewhat speculative. This reflects the current state of research on positive approaches to care; theories and practice seem to develop in an unconnected way, and there is more concern with establishing whether or not a programme works, with very little attention given to *how* it might elicit change. Many approaches seem to have developed as a practical coming together of methods and ideas, rather than having, from the start, a firm, reliable conceptual base. On the available evidence, the behavioural re-training/environmental compensation model and the combating of depressive withdrawal seem to be the most useful models for the operation of effective approaches. Indeed, the former may largely account for the small changes usually found in group studies, and the latter for the more dramatic changes which also occur. As Kitwood & Bredin (1992) comment: 'some individuals who had been seriously deteriorated in all their functioning, including some who had been written off as hopelessly demented, show considerable reversal or 'rementia' when their conditions of life, and especially their social relationships, are changed'.

PART 2

Positive approaches in practice

5

An integrated approach

How I long for a little ordinary enthusiasm. Just enthusiasm—that's all.

John Osborne

Chapter 1 ended with the hope that readers would take from this book an integrated, individualised, value-based means of working with and communicating with elderly people with dementia. With a very few exceptions, most of the research that has formed the basis of the intervening chapters has focused on specific techniques, rather than on developing an overall approach. Can any of these techniques form the basis for the integrated approach that is required?

RO, as perhaps the most studied of the approaches, has been the subject of numerous critiques over the years. In general these suggest that RO alone does not fit the bill (e.g. Burton 1982, Schwenk 1981, Powell-Proctor & Miller 1982, Woods 1992). Its emphasis on verbal learning by repetition (at least in the classroom setting) has been particularly identified as a limitation of the approach (Miller 1987, Bowlby 1991), with cognitively impaired elderly people being thought to respond better to a more systematic, multi-modal approach, including non-verbal material. Bowlby pointed out that RO was an important starting point, which in current use has developed to a point where it requires another name, having all but abandoned the classroom format and now having a positive influence in areas outside verbal orientation. 'RO is more and more commonly becoming understood as the provision of a reassuring foundation in reality for those who are unable to provide it for themselves' (Bowlby 1991). As the variations of approach develop, so evaluation becomes more complex, but it is, of course, vital that there is this development and evolution. We need to learn from experience and from the evaluative studies and incorporate new insights into practice. It is right to move on from the RO approach, which never could meet all the complexities of work with people with dementia, but not to leave behind all that has been learned in the process (Woods 1992). Similarly, critiques of other positive approaches, such as reminiscence (Thornton & Brotchie 1987, Woods & McKiernan 1995) and validation (Babins 1988) indicate that, while they may well have an invaluable role to play, they are not universally applicable to the whole range of people with dementia. Alone, they too are unable to satisfy the diversity of individual needs, responses and preferences shown by people with dementia.

What then should an integrated approach incorporate? Which findings from the various studies are essential to any approach? Here we describe those that, in our view, are most significant.

FEATURES OF AN INTEGRATED APPROACH

Attitudes

The first feature we would emphasise, and to which we give over-riding importance, is that the approach should be based on an explicit set of values regarding the elderly person with dementia. Any approach can be potentially harmful if applied with inappropriate attitudes that devalue or patronise the elderly person.

Gubrium & Ksander (1975) have illustrated this point clearly in relation to RO. They observed RO in two nursing homes and their findings led them to doubt the 'reality' of RO. One particular interchange they reported is indicative of what they observed. The aide leading an RO group had indicated on the RO board that it was 'raining'. He asked the patient what the weather was; she looked outside, saw that the sun was shining (the rain having abated) and said it was sunny. The aide disagreed with her until she

read 'correctly' from the board that it was raining, whereupon she was praised warmly. Buckholdt & Gubrium (1983) and Dietch et al (1989) similarly point out the danger of RO being applied in a mechanical, depersonalised fashion (see Ch. 10).

Other approaches too can be misapplied. For example, in the behavioural approach to incontinence reported by Schnelle et al (1983), social disapproval for wetting was given, e.g. 'I don't understand why you wet yourself and didn't ask for help. I come round every hour'. It is not difficult to imagine how such a statement could be turned into a vindictive reprimand with a particular tone of voice and inflection.

The dangers are clear. An explicit value system can go some way towards ensuring that bad practices do not slip through and that uncertainty is reduced. Staff have a clear yardstick against which to compare their interactions with those with whom they work. Attitudes are discussed in practical terms in Chapter 7. In Box 5.1, we list five principles set out in the important King's Fund publication (1986) on working with elderly people with dementia, which provide a sound basis for work in this field.

Box 5.1 Key principles (from King's Fund 1986)

- People with dementia have the same human value as anyone else irrespective of their degree of disability or dependence.
- People with dementia have the same varied human needs as anyone else.
- People with dementia have the same rights as other citizens.
- Every person with dementia is an individual.
- People with dementia have the right to forms of support which do not exploit family and friends.

Kitwood (1990) has elaborated on the types of negative attitude that may be identified in dementia care and that, he argues, lead to the person with dementia functioning less well than the limits set by their level of neurological impairment. These negative attitudes are described as forming a 'malignant social psychology' around the person with dementia, in that they may accelerate the progression of the dementia and certainly reduce the person's well-being.

Kitwood gives 10 examples of the types of attitude and behaviour that go towards forming a malignant social psychology, where the person is devalued and depersonalised:

- treachery: where deception is used to obtain compliance
- disempowerment: de-skilling the person by taking over—decisions, daily activities—that the person could still, perhaps with help, manage himself
- infantilisation: treating the person as a small child
- intimidation: the person is confronted by powerful others, who gain compliance using their power, emotional, psychological or physical
- labelling: the diagnostic label becomes the most important feature of the person, setting low expectations, 'explaining' everything the person does
- stigmatisation: the label becomes a cause of rejection, the person an outcast, an 'alien' being
- outpacing: the person is rushed, pressured to respond quickly
- invalidation: the person's feelings, emotions and experiences are ignored
- banishment: the person is rejected by others, sent away, physically or psychologically
- objectification: the person is no longer seen as human and is dealt with as though an object.

Anyone who has worked with older people with dementia for any amount of time, in the community as well as in residential settings, will be able to add further examples from their own observation. Why do the best intentioned of us continue to fall into these unhelpful practices? It seems that common sense and good intentions are not enough; understanding, empathy and imagination are required to gain the insight needed to see the world from the perspective of the person with dementia. It is not easy to reduce the pace of care-giving when there are so many other competing pressures. Perhaps there are features of dementia that particularly lead us to fail to recognise the person with dementia as being the same *person* as previously and deserving of the same respect. Possibly, our own fears of developing dementia lead some of us to main-

tain a distance, avoiding putting ourselves in their shoes, avoiding the closeness that would come from fully recognising the personhood of the dementia sufferer.

The adjective Kitwood uses for these attitudes, 'malignant', is very powerful. There has been increasing awareness of the strain experienced by care-givers, but the stresses faced by the person with dementia have tended to be overlooked, perhaps with the convenient assumption that the person is not aware of what is happening to them. Kitwood (1993) argues that 'the diagnosis of a primary degenerative dementia should not be regarded as a "sentence to death which leaves the body behind" ... now personhood can only be guaranteed, replenished and sustained through what others provide'. The analogy of, say, Alzheimer's disease as a 'living death' (cf. Woods 1989) reflects the depths of the care-giver's sense of loss, rather than a psychological model of the disorder. In an interaction with a person with dementia, two persons are involved. The person with dementia is not an alien; we respond to the person with dementia; he responds to us; we are not superior beings, at times we fail to grasp what is being communicated and that is as much our responsibility as it is that of the person with dementia. When we fail to notice the gestures, actions and phrases being employed as a means of attempting contact with others, the person is likely to feel (even more) lost, rejected and useless, as we would if we were consistently ignored. 'If their gestures repeatedly fall to nothing their predicament is a terrible one. They have only dwindling "inner" resources on which to draw, and their confidence to make an appeal to others is draining away' (Kitwood 1993).

The important point is that by noticing and responding to the attempts to make contact by the person with dementia facilitating communication, personhood can be sustained. By being aware of and seeking to avoid 'malignant' attitudes and practices, we have a way into working with the person that can influence well-being, response level, quality of life and function, so that they come closer to the constraints imposed by the person's neurological impairment.

Individualisation

As well as its justification as a basic principle, there are ample pragmatic grounds for developing individualised approaches. These include the great variability in people with dementia, the variability in response to treatment approaches, differences in appropriate target areas for intervention and differences in interests, preferences and attitudes. Kitwood (1993) provides an equation that shows the range of factors that contribute to individual differences:

$$SD = P + B + H + NI + SP$$

where SD = senile dementia; P = personality; B = biography; H = physical health; N = neurological impairment; SP = social psychology. For those who prefer words to equations: how the person's 'dementia' presents now will be influenced by their previous personality traits, their background, experiences, trauma and successes, their physical health and the environmental influences upon them, in addition to the level and type of neurological impairment which is present. Clearly with such a range of influences, the scope for individual variation is immense.

Any approach must take account of individual differences, be flexible enough to ascertain and respond to individual needs and build on the preserved abilities and interests of the person with dementia. Therefore, two patients with the same 'problem' might be best approached in quite different ways. Generalised treatment approaches to, say, incontinence or wandering will have less effect than approaches which recognise 'the same problem may occur in the same person at different times for different reasons' (Hodge 1984). A good illustration of this is provided by Snyder et al (1978), who identified at least three different patterns of behaviour that could all be described as 'wandering'; single individuals showed different patterns at different times. Detailed individualised assessment is needed to reach a sufficient depth of understanding of the person with dementia in order to really tackle their special needs.

We cannot expect the person with dementia to adjust to an environment or a programme that even comes close to meeting their individual needs; expecting adaptation and adjustment is putting an additional burden on the person whose resources are already stretched by the demands of moment-to-moment living. The onus is on those who work with the person to 'fine tune' their approach so that it is as close as possible to being just right for that individual.

Learning is possible

We reviewed evidence in Chapter 2 concerning the learning ability of people with dementia. The RO literature in particular provides confirmatory support for the view that some learning is possible. Re-learning to a small extent has been demonstrated with both verbal orientation and ward orientation. Obviously, new learning is not one of the major strengths of the person with dementia, but it is by no means impossible. There is little in the way of generalisation from one area to another, so it is important to focus directly on training the skill in question. Hanley (1984) suggests a number of ways in which the chances of learning occurring could be increased (see also Carroll & Gray 1981). These include:

• increasing the person's motivation by using relevant, interesting materials
• providing a number of opportunities for practice
• providing a number of retrieval cues in the environment, reducing the emphasis on free recall, using the person's limited learning ability to make use of further prosthetic aids which will reduce dysfunction further.

Moffat (1989) makes some additional suggestions, including a technique where only a small amount of material is learned at any one time, going on to fresh items only when this has been retained. The time between presenting the material and asking for its recall is cautiously increased, reverting to a shorter time if the person cannot retrieve it. Given that learning will never be easy for people with dementia, it is important that all the available findings from cognitive psychology on enhancing the efficiency of learning are considered when evaluating what may be achieved.

Selection of targets

Most positive approaches have been criticised for not being supported by compelling evidence for their efficacy. If changes are demonstrated, they are either too small to make a difference or not 'real' changes, i.e. they are not clinically relevant. For example, the emphasis of RO on verbal orientation has often been suggested as reducing its clinical relevance. Does the person with dementia really need to know what day it is? Is there any benefit in knowing the name of the prime minister? These considerations must lead towards the development of approaches where targets for intervention are selected for the individual patient such that a small realistically attainable change would actually make a difference to that individual patient's quality of life. For one patient, this might involve learning to find the toilet on the ward; for another, improving dressing skills. For others, increasing social contact may be an important target. For some patients in the community who receive different services on different days, learning to keep in touch with days and dates may be a priority. The often-noted lack of generalisation of learning means that targets have to be very carefully selected to be precisely and specifically relevant and appropriate.

When to stop

The poor maintenance of changes produced by all the various therapeutic approaches means that an approach must be developed where intervention is not simply for a fixed period of time. It must be on-going, and targets need to be regularly reviewed as the person's condition changes. An approach that assumes stability in the person's function is doomed to fail. The approach must, therefore, have a built-in monitoring and review procedure to allow the maximum flexibility. It must be seen as an overall long-term approach, not as a short-term intervention.

Effects on staff and carers

Schwenk (1981) asserts 'it is not clear whether RO is therapeutic for the staff or the elderly'.

The impact of any approach on those caring for the person day by day must be considered. If it is positive, staff or carers may usefully be aided in their difficult and demanding task, a worthwhile aim in itself. Improved morale and less strain and burden are likely to lead to more positive interactions between carers and patients, and so will be of benefit for all concerned. This area has attracted too little research attention so far, as we discussed in Chapter 3. The improvement in carers' mood reported by Greene et al (1983), coincident with their relative with dementia attending RO sessions at a day-hospital, is one of the most interesting positive indications. The increase in staff knowledge of individual patients reported by Baines et al (1987) is also important. An integrated approach must take into account the needs, strengths, perceptions, commitment and abilities of carers if practicable, realistic care-plans are to be developed. It is not sufficient simply to produce positive change in the patient's behaviour. As Tarrier & Larner (1983) discovered, staff may not perceive objectively measured change. Sometimes, interventions have to be developed in situations where carers' and patients' needs are discordant. Resolution of these differences is not always possible; approaches which fail to recognise them are likely to run into difficulties.

What can you expect?

What should be expected from psychological approaches to dementia? There is clearly no miraculous 'cure-all', no return to complete normality. It has been suggested that the term 'therapy' is inappropriate, in view of its curative connotations: 'management' has been preferred by many workers (e.g. Miller 1977). Yet Schwenk (1981) argued, for example, that approaches other than RO should be explored 'in view of the lack of strong evidence that RO is *universally* beneficial to the elderly' (emphasis added). Indeed great expectations! Could any approach in any sphere claim universal benefit? If workers in this field blind themselves to what they know about dementia and build up their hopes, expecting to see massive improvements in their patients when they begin to use a particular approach they will almost inevitably be disappointed. The approach is then likely to be consigned to the pile of approaches that have been tried and found wanting. What will be the next approach to follow the same path? People with dementia *are* likely to show overall deterioration; people with dementia do differ greatly from each other; people with dementia have many *different* strengths, retained abilities and resources, needs and disabilities. Changes are generally likely to be small, probably in specific areas.

Even when there is not an improvement in function, there can be important and valuable achievements in involving the person in a positive experience: a feeling of success, a moment of contact with another human being, a smile of appreciation … Kitwood & Bredin (1992) argued that the major aim of dementia care should be to maintain the personhood of the dementia sufferer, and that it is possible to recognise indications of (relative) well-being in people with dementia when this is being achieved (Box 5.2). These indicators are thought to be expressions of four 'global sentient states': a sense of personal worth, a deep self-esteem; a sense of agency, to have some control over their personal life, to achieve something; a sense of social confidence, of being at ease with others; and, finally, a sense of hope, feeling secure, trusting that all will be well. The expression of such states, however fleeting, is a worthy aim of dementia care.

Box 5.2 Indicators of relative well-being in dementia (Kitwood & Bredin 1992)

- The assertion of desire or will
- The ability to experience and express a range of emotions (both 'positive' and 'negative')
- Initiation of social contact
- Affectional warmth
- Social sensitivity
- Self-respect
- Acceptance of other dementia sufferers
- Humour
- Creativity and self-expression
- Showing evident pleasure
- Helpfulness
- Relaxation.

If targets for change and development are individually set, the rate of expected achieve-

ment of these targets can also be individualised. By setting it at a level where small successes are being achieved, staff do not become disappointed and the patient is not over-pressured. It is not universally effective approaches that are needed, but an approach geared to individual needs. Here potentially useful changes—in function and well-being—can become a reality.

AN INTEGRATIVE APPROACH

These considerations lead us to recommend an approach that has been described as 'individual programme planning' (Woods & Britton 1985), 'goal planning' (Barrowclough & Fleming 1986a), and which is closely related to most applications of the 'nursing process' (e.g. Stockwell 1985). This approach flows easily from the principles and values previously outlined, and which we believe are vitally important for any worthwhile approach. At the heart of this approach is the individual plan. This should cover all aspects of the person's life. A multidisciplinary team is a good setting to develop such plans, to ensure that medical, social, physical, emotional and psychological aspects are not artificially separated.

It is useful if certain staff members develop close contact with a designated patient or group of patients. Such contact provides the opportunity really to get to know and build relationships with a more manageable number of elderly people. As there is less staff change, staff are recognised by patients more readily. It is easier to spot the areas where something may be achieved in individuals that are known well by the staff member. It is easy to be discouraged when thinking about a ward of 30 dementing people, but once they begin to be seen as individuals, new horizons become apparent. There may be practical difficulties in allocating nurses to particular patients, but in many settings these have been overcome. A key-worker system is often established, giving one member of staff responsibility for ensuring individual plans are drawn up, carried out and reviewed regularly for a small number of patients. In some places two staff, on opposite shifts, may share this responsibility.

An integrated approach is just as important in community settings as it is in hospitals or residential homes. The individual approach to care-planning is equally vital for those people with dementia living in their own homes or with their families. All agencies need to work together—health and social services, voluntary and independent sector—in order to ensure that the person's needs are fully and holistically assessed, and that there is a key worker to co-ordinate the package of care. Having care provided by a consistent group of care-workers, as small in number as possible, is essential to this approach. In the UK, social services have the lead responsibility for community-care assessments, but the assessor must ensure that other agencies and workers are fully involved in contributing to the assessment and care-plan.

Developing an individual plan begins with careful and thorough assessment of the person's strengths and needs. This should include assessment of any medical conditions and sensory deficits. One of the first goals of the plan should be to correct and alleviate these as much as is possible. The assessment should include efforts to elicit the views of the elderly people themselves and of their relatives or other carers. As far as possible, the person with dementia and his or her family should be involved in this planning process. Finding out the wishes of the elderly person may not be easy, especially when communication is poor. Guidance from the person's past life and experiences should be helpful, together with information from relatives, friends of long standing and so on. Getting to know the dementing person in the context of his or her whole life is vital. Reminiscence-based activities may be a great help; preparing a life-chart of the important events, people and experiences in the person's life is a good starting-point (Woods et al 1992).

The assessment stage will include attempts to *understand* as well as to define the person's behaviour. The reasons for difficulties must be examined, including consideration of specific neuropsychological deficits. Generalised descriptions of behaviour such as 'attention-seeking', 'confused', 'incontinent' and so on must be replaced by detailed descriptions of the person's behaviour, the exact circumstances, its frequency and its intensity. The assessment process is described fully in Chapter 6, where particular emphasis is given to straightforward methods for identifying specific neuropsychological deficits. The discovery of such deficits should not lead to therapeutic despair, but should concentrate energies on finding ways of overcoming the effects of the problems and ways of compensating for the disability.

Once the initial assessment phase is complete, the plan is drawn up. The strengths and needs that have been identified are used to form the plan. The person's strengths and resources are used to help meet particular needs selected for intervention. These are not selected simply for the convenience of staff, but in relation to the quality of life of the person. It may be that where a particular problem behaviour has been identified, the targets will include the encouragement of activities that are incompatible with or which will reduce the frequency of the 'problem'. For instance, the target for a person who is frequently incontinent might be for the person to learn where the toilet is on the ward.

Goals for the person are broken down into smaller manageable steps. Which people will take what action under what circumstances is clearly specified. The criterion for successful achievement of the goal is made explicit and is set to be realistic, attainable and observable, so that confusion over what has been achieved is kept to a minimum. An indication of the actual frequency of the behaviour and the desired change may prove useful, e.g. 'improve dressing' would be an imprecise target; it would be hard to say when it had been achieved. 'Increase frequency with which patient puts on his shirt with only verbal assistance, from present level of once a week' might be better.

Accurate recording of the patient's behaviour is very useful indeed; for example, if the target is to increase the patient's rate of self-initiated visits to the toilet then each visit should be noted on a record sheet. Recording is invaluable in providing staff with both a reminder of the target and reinforcement for their efforts. In order to monitor change, it is, of course, essential to have an initial measure for comparison purposes. This could be done by daily recordings of the particular behaviour, until a fairly consistent picture of the person's function is attained. As different people tend to interpret observations in an individual manner, it is advisable that staff should discuss any discrepant findings so that a high degree of consistency is obtained. Some patients may benefit from having their own chart, showing their progress in graphic form.

Having established a plan for the individual patient consisting of targets and procedures for achieving them, the task is not complete. The plan *cannot* be an inflexible and unchanging statute for all time; it has to change to meet the changing events that occur once it is put into action. Responses may be unexpected or even undesirable; some targets may be quickly achieved, others may take longer or show no progress at all. The next stage is to review progress and to establish fresh targets where necessary. If previous targets have been realised, then more difficult ones can be set; if progress is slight, then the level of difficulty must be lowered, using, perhaps, intermediate goals. Realistic, attainable goals are important in all work with elderly people. The ideal aim is complete independence, but to be realistic more independence of functioning in a particular area would be a desirable improvement. Small changes can be of real practical value, but are too often overlooked. Their occurrence indicates a positive move forward. If encouraged, they can increase self-esteem, confidence and effort on the part of the patient and have a real effect on staff morale while also releasing more time for rehabilitative work.

Examples of individual plans

Obviously these examples are much abbreviated—with a range of goals sketched out. They are presented here to illustrate the points outlined above.

Mrs A

This 78-year-old lady was a resident in a residential home specialising in the care of

Table 5.1 Plan for Mrs A

General	Specific (these are aims not orders)
Increase domestic activity	To make her bed at least two days out of three To tidy and dust her own room at least one day in three To help with laying the table once a day To help drying up after meals once a day
Increase cooking activity	To make a pot of tea daily To make a snack (e.g. sandwiches) one day in three To cook a meal one day in seven
Increase social activity	To attend an Over-60s Club once a week outside the home
Improve and support memory	To participate in daily 'memory group' Pictures of important people/events to be used in the 'memory group' To use memory aids about the home To keep a diary as a memory aid To prepare, with help from her family, a life history book for use in individual reminiscence sessions with Mrs A

people with dementia. Her diagnosis was indeed dementia, probably Alzheimer's disease. She reported that she felt a bit of a failure as she could not remember things and often felt useless. She liked to be kept busy and to socialise with other residents. She had a family, and previously had been a fit, active person with a warm personality. As regards her abilities, her self-care was largely independent, her mobility and dexterity good. She socialised well, making relationships with particular residents, but had difficulty in learning their names and in recognising relatives when they visited. She knew her way around the home but tended to get lost outside. She only rarely took part in domestic activities such as preparing food, etc.

Mrs A caused no specific problems in the home. Although her memory was poor and she tended to ramble on in conversation, her behaviour only fluctuated when she suddenly became unhappy and weepy.

Mrs A's strengths included: good mobility, good dexterity, independent self-care, ability to find her way around the home, her interest in being active and sociable and her excellent social skills.

Mrs A's needs included: needing to feel useful by being busy in a way she would see as helpful; needing more opportunities to socialise, perhaps in settings outside the home; needing to learn to use memory aids and supports to overcome memory failures. A tentative plan would aim to use some of Mrs A's many strengths to meet her needs. Her good skills and mobility and her interest could be harnessed to increasing domestic and cooking activity; her warmth and social skills would make it feasible for her plan to include socialising outside the home; the same strengths would be an asset in group sessions of a suitable level, geared towards helping her use memory aids. Table 5.1 shows a plan devised to fit these needs. Record keeping would indicate the degree of success in reaching the targets and what level of prompting was required—with the aim of eventually reducing prompting.

Mrs B

Mrs B was another resident in a specialist home with the diagnosis of dementia. It was difficult to obtain a clear picture from her of exactly what she wanted. It seemed that her major goal was to be with her daughter: she had previously lived with this daughter and had been very dependent on her for physical care. The daughter's marriage had been jeopardised so she was unable to continue to care for her mother at home. Previously Mrs B had been socially very active and very much involved as an organiser in various charitable bodies.

The care-staff completed a detailed behaviour rating scale which showed that toiletting and eating were normal, that she communicated well and that orientation about the home was good. Poor mobility curtailed domestic activities. She lacked confidence in walking and would desperately hang on to people and things, sometimes so fiercely that people would fall over with her. She refused to dress herself and was resistant to

looking after her personal cleanliness.

The major problems the staff reported were her constant demands for somebody to come to her, her continuous shouting and her resistance when being helped. Her daughter spent a great deal of time at the home and whilst there her mother persuaded her to do everything for her. The daughter was so concerned about her mother that, as she told the staff, her marriage was still under strain, despite the fact that Mrs B had been removed from the scene.

The staff felt extremely angry with Mrs B; she played one off against the other and made them look uncaring in front of visitors. It was as though she was trying to exercise over them the same enormous power she had over her daughter.

Fluctuations were noted in Mrs B's behaviour; for some staff she would dress herself, sometimes. When not being overtly observed, it was felt she walked slightly better. When her daughter was present she lost all semblance of independence in her behaviour.

Mrs B's behaviour had been labelled as 'attention seeking' and—as is so often the case with such difficult patients—staff who were genuinely caring and warm to their residents were extremely angry with her. It would have been only too easy in what had become a tense home situation to establish a punitive plan; the suffering that other residents were undergoing in being deprived of *their* rights of attention could have made this seem justified.

Mrs B clearly had a number of strengths and resources, although the 'problems' being experienced by the staff threatened to obscure them! Her strengths included: an evident interest in social activity and in being an organiser; good ability to communicate, orientation, eating and toiletting; the concern of her daughter; some ability to dress and walk, in certain situations.

Mrs B needed to become more confident in walking, and to regularly dress more independently; she needed to have more opportunities to socialise (and so to receive 'attention') appropriately; finally Mrs B needed to develop more mutually satisfying relationships with her daughter and the staff at the home.

The plan developed aimed to use Mrs B's

Table 5.2 Plan for Mrs B

General	Specific
Increase mobility to unaided walking in home	Brief walking practice to be given, but staff support to be gradually withdrawn
Increase social interaction	Staff to employ 'chatty' conversation when she is sitting quietly, perhaps concerning past activities; Mrs B to be invited to take on organisation of small tea party with three other residents
Improve dressing to self-care level	Staff to encourage her to do a little more for herself each morning, providing lots of time, only a few prompts which are withdrawn as soon as possible, but praising every effort made
Increase physical independence from daughter	Daughter to be counselled to withdraw physical care and provide attention in alternative ways
Staff to feel less angry with her	Care for Mrs B to be shared among staff; staff to be free to hand over to someone else if they feel under stress with her; staff to discuss her difficulties and her qualities and seek to understand her point of view

strengths to help meet some of her needs (Table 5.2). It aims at building up positive behaviour, whilst not ignoring the negative feelings of the staff which it was important to have in the open to be discussed and acknowledged.

Notice that no specific attempt is made to stop Mrs B shouting. One might consider ignoring her shouts, but the problem with this is that even if the staff manage this consistently other residents or visitors will respond from time to time and thus spur the shouting on even more. The plan aims to meet Mrs B's needs for her daughter's attention and that of the staff by increasing her positive behaviours and providing some attention for these. Mutual staff support is important too; not all patients are easy to love and yet care-staff can feel guilty if there is an inward feeling of distaste, anger or active dislike for a particular person. Open discussion of these feelings helps to see that other people can experience the same emotions and negative feelings. Together it may be possible to see

beyond the problem to more likeable attributes; here a previously highly competent lady, faced with the frightening reality of failing abilities, found a way of maintaining great power by taking on a demanding, dependent and manipulative role.

Mr C

Our third example is a man with a moderate degree of dementia, also resident in a specialist home. He had previously been interested in music, lived alone and had been an avid reader. Socially affable, he would willingly join in group activities, although he had yet to form any real relationship with any particular residents. Mobility and eating skills were generally good, but he was quite disorientated, becoming completely lost in the home. Occasionally he was incontinent, at night in particular. He joined in some domestic activities but required some verbal prompting for dressing and washing.

The one problem which concerned the staff was his temper and they reported that he 'was prone to temper outbursts and some aggression'. This was usually verbal, but at least once a day a blow was struck. Staff carefully recorded the events leading up to these incidents; they seemed to be of two types. The first was in relation to personal care, at a point when a member of staff had *told* him to do something, upon which he would become angry and impatient. The second was where a member of staff had corrected him, and a confrontation had resulted. For example, if he announced he was going to work or looking for his wife and was reminded he no longer worked or that his wife had died, he would argue, become angry and lash out. Afterwards he would be a little apologetic and then act as if the incident had never happened. There was no real evidence of fluctuations in his behaviour.

Mr C's strengths included his interest in music and in reading, his sociability, his good mobility and eating skills, his ability to be continent most of the time during the day and his ability to wash and dress with only verbal prompts.

A clear need for Mr C was to be able to find

Table 5.3   Plan for Mr C

General	Specific
Develop recreational interests	Explore Mr C's previous interests, obtain some of the music or books that he likes; draw him into daily recreational activities
Develop home orientation: aim to achieve independent ability to find his way	Guided tour of home, pointing out his room, toilet, dining-room, lounge, etc, indicating signs on doors, using colour as a clue, special pictures and particular characteristics as memory aids; repeat this at least twice daily, gradually asking him to do the guiding, prompting with clues only when he is uncertain
Develop independence in dressing and washing	Give praise to each phase of these performed correctly; ensure there is an order in laying out the clothes; gradually fade the prompts as the sequence is learned; eventually use mime as a clue until hopefully no prompt is needed
Develop relationships with other residents	Introduce him to other residents, slowly and appropriately, those sitting near him in the lounge, at the table; ask him to repeat the names when introduced
Basic approach to Mr C	Ask and do not tell him what to do; praise him for cooperation; avoid confrontation; validate his feelings, e.g. wanting to work, missing his wife, but do not correct him; respond factually to his questions

his way around the home, and to improve his dressing and washing skills, so even fewer prompts would be needed. More opportunities for pursuit of his interests and for developing relationships were also needed. Finally, Mr C needed staff to ask him to do things—not to give him orders—and to respond to him in a non-confrontational manner, acknowledging his feelings rather than correcting facts. A preliminary plan for Mr C might then include the features in Table 5.3. Again there is no specific resolve to deal with the problem behaviour; instead attempts are made to avoid situations in which it might occur. This is achieved by the staff consistently adopting an approach that Mr C is able to accept.

Mr D

Mr D is 68 years old; he had a mild stroke that left him with some weakness in his left hand and leg. He had recovered from this weakness very well, but there were other signs which caused his wife and family some concern. The cerebrovascular accident had affected the right tempero-parietal areas so that, although his speech was unaffected, he did have difficulty in finding his way about, showed evidence of dressing apraxia and had problems with maps and spatial organisation. Sometimes he had a little difficulty with finding his way around the house. He used to have a fairly responsible job with the Gas Board, used to drive one of the vans and was required to travel around the region. He had been a member of several clubs and sports associations and was regarded as an outgoing person. He had insight into the changes and was becoming increasingly depressed. His wife still worked and so he was alone in the house during the day except when he went to a day-centre twice a week. He had some difficulty remembering important information, or what he was meant to be doing, especially when he was on his own.

Mr D had many assets and strengths, despite his disability. His speech was good; he had always been a sociable person with interests in various sports and clubs. He had a concerned wife and family who could help in his plan, as could staff at the day-centre he attended twice a week. His own insight may be used for him to take an active role in finding ways around his disabilities.

The list of needs was shorter: he needed to learn to find his way around, to dress more independently, to use memory aids and to be engaged in activities and interests that would lift his mood. The plan illustrated in Table 5.4 might tackle these needs. Guidance on the plan should be given here to all the family (grandchildren included). The overall aim is to use preserved abilities in order to increase function in the more impaired areas.

Table 5.4 Plan for Mr D

General	Specific
Help recent memory	Notice board in kitchen—day, month and weather every morning, important information to be remembered; also notebook always in top pocket; memory games: name of newsreader on TV last night, one main headline from news, then increase in number of things to remember as successful; items from paper, TV, visitors, etc; games related to interests, cards, bought games, etc.
Help dressing	Clothes placed in order; tags denoting front, back, left or right; practice with buttons, encouragement, written instructions if necessary; modelling, verbal instructions, as little actual help as possible in order to build routine
Help him to find his way about	Use of three-dimensional games (useful type is 3D noughts and crosses); drawing maps of increasing difficulty, starting with home, then street, then shopping street Using words as cues, i.e. names of rooms, street names, house names, any signposts, shops' names and commodities; at home use colour and words to denote toilet, bedroom, etc. Play games, e.g. Scrabble to increase confidence; slowly move on to shapes, house colours, postboxes, buildings, etc; routine of putting things away in set place, washing up, clothes, etc.
Assist depression	All successes to be noted and encouraged; bouts of 'low' behaviour to be ignored, but alternatives to be offered—'let's go to the club' Interest to be encouraged, friendships used, routine way to the club, involvement in activities outside and at home

Mrs E

Mrs E was 65 years old and had been running the village shop with her husband for as long as anyone can remember. She was a well-known and respected member of the local community, active in local politics, a regular church-goer and involved in a number of charitable organisations.

Changes took place over a few months that alarmed her husband and family; she made impetuous decisions, showed considerable lack of judgment and was unable to plan ahead as she would have done previously; she seemed no longer capable of handling business matters. In the shop she got distracted when serving a customer, or sometimes she ignored them or was even quite rude; she guessed the cost of items rather than adding them up properly. In addition, strange rituals and fads appeared; she would go into the shop and walk around counting all the tins; or, at a meal, would sometimes stuff food into her mouth without stopping, and at others refuse to eat items she used to enjoy.

She changed physically too; her face became almost expressionless, and she appeared unfriendly; she echoed things that people said and was often apathetic. Apart from these changes, she functioned normally, and her understanding was unimpaired; in fact, many aspects of her intellectual capabilities seemed unchanged. Neurological investigations suggested the presence of a frontal lobe dementia; the family became very upset after being given this diagnosis, and began to regard Mrs E as a hopeless case.

Mrs E's strengths included many retained abilities, including memory, her concerned family, her numerous local contacts and interests and her general physical health. Her needs were quite complex: she needed help and support to ensure that her, at times, impetuous and ill-judged behaviour did not result in alienating friends, in her being humiliated or in threats to her safety; she needed the support of a family who would not write her off, but who were able to understand what was happening and recognise her retained abilities; she needed help to maintain previous interests and activities at a level which would not be over-demanding for her (Table 5.5). Essentially the plan aims to encourage her to use all her untouched abilities

Table 5.5 Plan for Mrs E

General	Specific
Explain to family the nature of Mrs E's condition, emphasising how much is retained	Hold family sessions; provide relevant information; consider with family how best to involve Mrs E in these discussions
Maintain abilities	Assess what shop tasks she is able to do; give more prompting and monitor more closely; encourage and prompt to continue with previous activities such as cooking, reading, listening to radio, etc, with more help where needed, particularly with sequencing the task correctly
Maintain social contacts	Encourage friends to continue to visit; prepare them regarding Mrs E's changed reactions and advise these are not deliberate; continue to take part in church and social activities, where possible, with support
Prevent harm arising from errors of judgment	Ignore as far as possible those rituals that do not do any harm; intervene and distract where harm might result; for food, give smaller portions

and help her to maintain self-esteem and confidence by noting her successes and preventing damaging failures.

Mrs F

This 78-year-old widow had been in a continuing care ward in hospital for several years and had a severe dementia. She required a great deal of physical nursing care and had always been a popular patient, smiling and appreciative, although unable to speak at all clearly. She had a daughter who visited several times a week and several grandchildren. Mrs F worked in a laundry for many years, and until recently often appeared to be trying to fold sheets and clothes.

Over the previous 2 months, staff had great difficulty at mealtimes with Mrs F; they said she had become aggressive and resistive; she would forcibly push aside the food when they tried to feed her and would begin to scream; similarly when the staff dressed or undressed her, she

began to struggle with staff, and often started to scream, upsetting other patients and the staff.

The change was quite unexpected; staff were beginning to assume it was caused by her dementia progressing further, an inevitable step on the inexorable decline. Observation of her behaviour at mealtimes showed she would open her mouth, push away helping hands and then scream; it was suggested that she may have developed a dyspraxia, so that she was not able to coordinate the movements of her arms to achieve the desired results; she might, in fact, have been trying to help, but only succeeding in doing the opposite; the screaming then might have arisen from the frustration of such a situation.

Mrs F's strengths could be identified as having a warm, helpful personality; a concerned family; a response to affection and to music. Her needs included receiving physical care (feeding and dressing) in a way that she did not find so frustrating; and a need for well-being, security, contact and control. Table 5.6 illustrates a plan that would try to answer these needs.

Table 5.6 Plan for Mrs F

General	Specific
Physical care to be less frustrating	Feeding: staff to discuss effects of dyspraxia, so they are aware Mrs F is not being resistive; staff to have a trial of *not* giving verbal instructions whilst feeding, but instead to rely more on her automatic response Dressing: talk about things other than the task; distract her; compliment her on her clothes
Enhance well-being	Staff to talk with Mrs F as often as possible, despite her lack of verbal response; her non-verbal response, a smile, holding a hand, will indicate her appreciation of contact; staff to make a point of putting on some of her favourite music and including her in a music group; look together at photographs of her daughter and grandchildren; give her small items of clothing, tea towels, etc. to fold

Summary of plans

In each of these six cases, fairly lengthy plans have been suggested: in the real-life situation, these would be likely to evolve over a period of time, with particular parts of the plan being reviewed, changed, extended, or abandoned according to circumstances. In our view, the decision-making progress outlined above should be followed through, even if the ultimate decision is to attempt no change at all to the person's functioning or their environment. In this way, patients are seen as individuals and not just as part of a large group.

CONCLUSION

In this chapter we have sought to outline an approach that seeks to produce effects in specific areas of functioning. The plans outlined above show how various approaches can mesh well together. We suspect that the behavioural principles of prompting and rewarding appropriate behaviour also play a part in the successes of other types of general treatment programme outlined in Chapter 2. This approach makes explicit what is often implicit in other programmes; this must help to bring about desired changes in a more efficient manner.

The setting of specific objectives tends to simplify the process of evaluating results and the ever-growing volume of knowledge of human learning, from experimental psychology, will in years to come generate techniques to be developed to facilitate learning further.

A danger of the 'individual plan' approach is that it may focus attention on changing the individual patient's behaviour and ignore the wider context in which that behaviour occurs. The behaviour is always an interaction between the person and the environment and we cannot ignore this interaction.

The environment is, of course, made up of many parts: the physical surroundings, other patients, the staff and their behaviour. Often in our individual plans we are changing aspects of the environment, e.g. by changing our response to the patient in different situations.

Whenever we come across a person with a deficit of those skills needed for independent living, we need to make a decision to try to, at one extreme, re-train these skills or, at the other end of the spectrum, change the environment so that these skills are rendered unnecessary. Therefore, for a person with dementia living at home who cannot care for herself/himself any more, do we re-train cooking skills or provide meals on wheels so that the skills will not be required? The behavioural approach in the community would seek to identify those skills that are and are not retained; only supports that are necessary should then be provided. A general package of services should not be given; it may not meet specific needs and may, in fact, deny opportunity for expression of some skills that are retained. For the elderly person living alone at home, it is this environmental modification that will be of prime importance as there is no one present to repeatedly reinforce appropriate behaviour. What is needed is a prosthetic environment, an environment that fills in the gaps in the person's skills and abilities. The use of memory aids is part of this, as are home-carers and meals on wheels. In the not too distant future the deteriorating person's environment could be monitored by a control system so the flat is kept at an even temperature, cookers are turned off automatically if left on or if saucepans boil dry and help is alerted if the person has a fall. Those controls the person can operate would be made as simple as possible. In this way risks to those living alone could be diminished, which would allow both personal choice and relief for the worries of relatives.

This approach is consistent with the application of the pilot Community Care Schemes (Challis & Davies 1985, 1986), discussed in Chapter 10, to people with dementia. A package of care is established which seeks to reduce the risks of both gradual self-neglect and the risk of accidents, establishing a regular pattern of prompting to maintain the person's function.

In a residential setting, the environment should be enriched with features that tend to prompt appropriate, valued behaviour by the person with dementia, that give full scope for the personhood of the dementia sufferer to be elicited. Thus, the environment should be arranged physically to facilitate social interaction, and appropriate materials should be readily available for valued activities. Where particular themes occur again and again in individual plans, e.g. orientation, domestic skills, social activity, a case can be made for establishing groups to work on these areas. Groups should always arise from needs identified from individual care-plans, rather than trying to fit patients into existing groups which may not meet their particular needs. Within any group, there is still a need for individualisation, according to the person's capabilities, interests and personality.

This integrative approach is founded on three central components: an agreed, explicit value system; a careful, thorough holistic assessment of the person; and an individualised care-plan, with clear, realistic, regularly reviewed goals. From this base, there is scope for work with individuals, for work with groups and for environmental change. In the remainder of the book, we will describe the practicalities of assessing and working with people with dementia in this way.

6

Assessment: some possibilities

We care what happens to people only in proportion as we know what people are.

James Henry

THE NEED FOR ASSESSMENT

In this chapter, we are concerned with the type of assessment that would be helpful in the individual planning process discussed in Chapter 5. Assessment for its own sake, or which produces scores or labels that do not add to an understanding of the patient as a person, are of dubious value and relevance. Test batteries applied without sensitivity and thought regarding the aims and purpose of the assessment and without consideration for the level of stress produced run the risk of 'battering' the older person (Holden 1984a).

Why assess?

There are a number of cogent reasons for making an assessment of an older person. These include:

- finding retained abilities
- isolating particular disabilities
- selection for particular purposes, e.g. group work, research, treatment, placement
- monitoring change
- diagnosis and prognosis.

It should be appreciated that assessment methods that are excellent for one purpose, e.g. in contributing to the information required in making a diagnosis, may be of little use for others, e.g.

monitoring change. Here, we will not be supplying a full account of test procedures for elderly people or discussing their relative merits or demerits, nor will we examine the issues involved in diagnosis, prognosis or placement (see Woods & Britton 1985, Beech & Harding 1990). The focus here is on holistic assessment leading to individualised care and support for the older person.

Without intruding on a person's right to privacy, it is important to have a wide knowledge about the individual with whom we are working. To know that there is a particular problem is not enough. In order to set realistic goals for improvement, to correct deficits—medical or sensory—and to gather relevant information about lifestyle, interests and abilities, it is necessary to involve a variety of disciplines. Nurses, doctors, occupational therapists, physiotherapists, speech therapists, social workers, clinical psychologists, care-workers, friends and relatives all have something to contribute to the store of information which will provide guidelines for intervention best suited to that individual. All the different disciplines that are available in a particular setting or team can feed into this wide ranging assessment. A first goal of any plan should be always to alleviate and correct any medical condition or sensory deficit as far as is possible. A competent medical evaluation is a vital aspect of a holistic evaluation.

The team needs to collect information, ideas, views and opinions in order to address the following questions:

1. What does the elderly person want?
2. What assets, abilities, skills, resources and interests does that person have?
3. What problems does the person experience? What needs does he or she have? What difficulties for others does his/her behaviour cause?
4. Are there any behavioural inconsistencies?
5. What are the person's previous daily routines and social history?

1. What does the elderly person want?

What are his or her objectives? What are seen as problems? What does he or she want from us? It is hard to believe that the necessity of posing such questions can come as a surprise. Those 'in charge' sometimes take it for granted that they know best and so ignore the wishes and needs of the person whose life is being organised. Even if poor memory, poor decision-making capacity or other problems exist, the right to be heard must be retained. Respect does not imply complete subservience to the needs and demands of the person. There are wishes which are totally unrealistic, practically impossible or even encroaching on the priorities of others. However, the views of the individual must be considered when any decision is being discussed. This question is placed first deliberately.

To make a decision about what an elderly person wants based on 'when I'm 85, I will want to . . .' is to impose our own, possibly faulty, conceptions and fantasies on the individual. It is essential to discuss the situation with the individual concerned and to take into account biography, abilities and personality in order to fully appreciate the situation. To accept at face value expressions of helplessness and weakness can lead to further misunderstanding about real needs and feelings. These first impressions may be signs of depression and withdrawal that can prove misleading and which may well recede as the person becomes more active and more in control of life once again.

2. What are the person's strengths?

Detailed observations of behaviour are of importance. There are various methods available to assist in achieving this, for instance rating scales (see Woods & Britton 1985). These can provide information on a variety of functions. It is vital to ascertain what a person can still do, what skills are retained: self-care, social, other acquired skills, capacity to perform domestic tasks and so on. The emphasis is on assets not deficits. It may be that tasks are carried out slowly, or some prompting is needed; what is important is to recognise that the person does have some skills and abilities and the eventual plan will seek to capitalise on these.

It is equally important to know what the

person's interests have been, what was enjoyed and some idea of background and life history. An outline format for this is provided by Woods et al (1992). This provides valuable information in building up a picture of what the person would be like without the present disabilities, in individualising recreational and constructive activities, in providing guidance as to topics for conversation and in selecting suitable rewarding items and events.

The question of the very deteriorated patient is often raised. What skills, abilities, and interests can possibly be retained? Here a more basic level must be considered; perhaps the person cannot use utensils for eating, but succeeds well with fingers; perhaps verbal communication is poor, but a smile is offered in response; despite apparent total withdrawal a sudden noise elicits a turn of the head; music and rhythm lead, perhaps, to joining in a dance or a song. Under these conditions, very careful observations are necessary. There is a need to stand back and allow the patient to attempt something for himself or herself before automatically doing it for him or her. This permits the expression of whatever remaining skill there may be. Above all else a patient must be seen as a living being who must not be 'written off' no matter how deteriorated appearances suggest him or her to be.

3. What are the person's needs? What are the areas of difficulty?

Again, the placing of this question is deliberate. Too often it comes first—understandably enough—as it is the problem behaviours that make life difficult for those in the caring role. It is placed low down the list of questions to avoid the possibility of perceiving individuals only in terms of problems. Frequently, patients are described as personifying a particular behaviour. As a result they become known as 'the screamer', 'the wanderer', 'the hoarder', etc. In any plan, the emphasis must be on the person's assets if the problem behaviours are to be improved at all. Negative aspects of behaviour cannot be seen in isolation from neutral or positive features. If the aim is to reduce the frequency of

a problem behaviour, e.g. wandering, the aim should be to increase the frequency of other—preferably incompatible—positive behaviours. In this example, the amount of sitting, reading a magazine or joining in a group singing session could be usefully increased.

In specifying the possible problems of each patient, several issues need to be examined:

1. The problem should be stated clearly.
2. The frequency of its occurrence.
3. The situation in which it occurs.
4. Any clues about events preceding its occurrence, or which could act as a catalyst.
5. What follows as a result of the behaviour. In other words what are the reactions of staff and others in the situation, what benefit or gain does the person obtain and what are the losses?

It is necessary to say much more than 'Mr Jones is aggressive'. A more correct account might be 'Mr Jones hits other patients once a week. This occurs when someone sits in his chair in the living area. The staff try to restore peace by removing the other patients from the lounge so that Mr Jones can have his seat back'.

Specific descriptions of behaviour are required; this is essential for an individual plan to be developed. Abbreviated notes, such as 'confused', 'attention seeking', 'demented', etc, are insufficient and may have quite different meanings for different staff members and disciplines. The word 'confused' can be used by one member of staff to describe continual wandering about the ward, whereas to another it would imply an inability to name the day and time of year. Particularly misleading is 'attention seeking' which can even be used as a derogatory term for unpopular patients. It rarely proves informative; after all, human beings are all seeking some form of attention! Problems can arise over the way in which attention is sought and the amount demanded. Once again the nature of the problem, in each case, should be explicitly specified.

Mrs R and Mrs S were both described as 'attention seeking'. Mrs R was an obese diabetic who found it impossible to stick to the prescribed diet and so had a constant thirst. She would call for water whenever a nurse passed within earshot—even though she might have a glass already in her hand. Her call was loud and insistent. Enumeration of this behaviour indicated that she shouted 'nurse, nurse' approximately 30 times in an hour. The appearance of a nurse acted as a trigger. Reactions varied: she was ignored, told to be quiet, some attempted to calm her down and others provided her with more water. Reactions of other residents were consistently negative, urging her in the strongest terms to 'pipe down'.

Mrs S complained of nausea in order to 'seek attention'. She felt sick at the meal table and invariably had to leave halfway through. Her nausea was worse with difficult-to-digest foods. The other patients responded negatively and objected to being put off their own food, and although initially sympathetic the staff eventually became matter-of-fact in their approach. Medical investigations showed a partial oesophageal obstruction and so treatment plans were directed towards a special diet.

Two quite different situations and yet the same label 'attention seeking', illustrate the point that greater detail is necessary in order to avoid the consequences of what is undoubtedly pejorative terminology. Careful medical investigations are usually indicated when there are complaints of physical symptoms that may not appear to have a physical basis. Even when these are negative, it should be borne in mind that some studies have shown that the elderly patient's self-evaluation of health can be a better predictor of survival even than that of the doctor!

Finally, several studies have shown that there is very little staff–resident interaction in some long-term care environments. To those rebelling against routine and not being 'model' residents, the label of 'attention seeking' can be attached and natural independence can be stifled. To be a 'model' resident often seems to mean sitting quietly, asking for nothing and accepting without question. Rather than attempting to suppress the 'problem' by achieving an undesirable state of depersonalisation, such 'problems' should indicate a need for the environment to be modified. Attempts should be made to provide the residents with more scope for personal

contact, more choice, more individuality and more opportunities to be individuals in their own right with reasonable control over their own lives.

Listing needs rather than problems is a powerful way of developing ideas for care-plans. 'Incontinent' may become 'needs to go to the toilet when prompted', or perhaps, 'needs to learn the way to the toilet'. 'Cannot dress' may become 'needs to put clothes on in the correct sequence'. Detailed descriptions of exactly where the difficulties arise are required, and of what the person positively needs to do for the problem to be overcome.

4. Are there any behavioural inconsistencies?

This question should provide further clues as to capacity for change. It highlights aspects of behaviour that vary from situation to situation, or behaviour that depends on the presence of a certain staff member, or is inconsistent within an area of function.

An example of a situational variation in behaviour would be the person with dementia who sits alone and withdrawn in the lounge of an old people's home but in the pub becomes sociable and chatty (this precedes the ingestion of alcohol!), or the lady who is able to cook a meal at the day-centre but never at home. These variations demonstrate the retained capacity but suggest that some situations lack sufficient stimulus.

Different reactions to different staff are commonly observed. One nurse will say Mrs Brown cannot dress herself, another will say she can. Such inconsistent observations are extremely valuable and should not be concealed; they provide clues as to the best ways to help the lady concerned. On this occasion, perhaps one nurse may have stood back a little more, allowed Mrs Brown more time and managed to find the right way to help her. Other staff could then benefit from the discovery of the particular 'trick' in their own interactions with the lady.

It is in examining the inconsistencies of behaviour that 'excess disabilities' may be identified. These are deficits that seem worse than the person's level of actual impairment would suggest. Here multidisciplinary assessment is particularly valuable; some specific deficits, e.g. in dressing, eating, language and so on, may be related to damage to particular areas of the brain. Knowledge of these kinds of deficits will help staff understand the patient's difficulties, and enable suitable aids and adaptations to be provided and realistic goals to be set. Excess disabilities are identified where staff have some evidence to suggest that given the right conditions the person could perform a task which currently she does not. An example of this would be a person whose language functions are clearly intact, but who never initiates a conversation; or someone who has been observed to use a knife and fork once or twice, but who usually uses fingers.

5. Previous daily routines and social history

It is equally pertinent to enquire about the person's previous history and normal routines. Here the help of the social worker, neighbour, friend and relative is vital. So many apparently disruptive behaviours can be better understood with the help of such information. Was this person very independent, a bit of a hermit or socially very active? A professional client who has been accustomed to respect and responsibility could react forcibly to being addressed as 'Love', 'Johnny' or 'Maggie' by all and sundry. The person with minimal education and a simple job could be overwhelmed by close association with people whose past experience was broader. To be expected to participate in groups whose social and intellectual levels are totally different is unrealistic.

Some clients wander. They may be searching for lost freedom, friends of a similar background, or, commonly when there has been a recent bereavement, for a lost partner. A person who has lived a solitary life could be looking for the peace and quiet to which he or she is accustomed, as the noise and activity in the home or hospital is totally alien to him/her (Stokes 1986a).

Routines of many years are part of all our lives. Taking the dog out for an evening walk, having a late night cup of cocoa or even a glass of beer are common practices. Reading in bed, seeing the late-night film, having a sleep in the morning, tidying up before going to bed, putting the cat in or out are others. These simple routines can be severely disturbed by the policies and systems of a care-setting. However, to ignore them or not to be aware of their existence can lead to apparently disturbed responses from clients, resulting in misunderstandings all round. It is not too difficult to find measures to coincide with the old routines. If tea is served at night, those who prefer cocoa, or whatever they have usually, should be able to inform staff of their preference. Choice of bedtime is not a great upheaval and perhaps one of the staff has a dog that could enjoy taking Mr Jay for an evening stroll around the grounds!

The use of evaluation

Attempting to answer these five questions will certainly go some way towards meeting the first two possible purposes of assessment listed above. Finding retained abilities and isolating disabilities help to identify strengths and needs. Difficulties with speech, reading, writing and visuo-motor skills could be possible hindrances. Enjoyment of social interaction might be one of many factors which could prove of great value.

In using assessment for selection purposes, the most important issue is to match the person's abilities and needs with the demands and support of the group or treatments being considered. It could be detrimental, for instance, for a person to be included in a group that is too high powered, too demanding or too active for that individual. A group might be irrelevant to that person's needs, skills or interests resulting, at best, in boredom for that individual, at worst in them feeling insulted by the low level of activity offered. So in order to achieve, say, a well-matched group, some questions must be asked and some areas explored. Are the demands on the person's ability to understand too great, or too small? Are expectations of concentration greater than the person can sustain, or not high enough? Usually tests are of less use in this evaluation than careful observation of the person in particular situations. Equally important is a good all-round knowledge of the person's abilities and interests.

Monitoring change is essential to the individual care-plan. Plans should be reviewed regularly and progress, or lack of it, should be recorded. This not only helps you to see what is happening as a result of the plan, but it also provides feedback for the staff. Even going on a diet requires an initial weight to be recorded so that loss in a week can be measured and the person encouraged to continue. When working with clients, it is important to be clear about which areas of functioning are being monitored, and where change can be expected. There is little point, for instance, in assessing incontinence if the re-training programme is not directed at toileting skills. As emphasised in Chapter 3, evaluation of change also involves looking at changes in staff behaviour and attitudes, in relatives and in the environment as well as in the elderly people themselves.

How to assess?

Staff—trained and untrained—are observing and assessing patients continually. These assessments are based on the staff's perception of the patient and are coloured by their reactions and their attitudes to the patient. Most often they are 'stored' in the staff member's memory, to emerge in discussion and conversation. 'I'm sure Mrs Jones is more confused today' or 'Mr Smith didn't dress himself this morning—he usually does'. Problems arise when staff members use the same words to mean different things. 'I had to help Mrs Brown with her dinner' could mean anything from actually spoon-feeding Mrs Brown to helping her cook it, to take an extreme example. The introduction of the nursing process has facilitated recording and individual responsibility. Where this system is used, a member of staff takes on special responsibility for and interest in a particular patient. Aims, or targets, are agreed at weekly or daily meetings. Records are carefully kept, changes are noted and any misunder-

standings are referred back to the nurse in charge. Where this system has been established, it can work well and prove invaluable. It is important to ensure that targets are not too vague or set at too high an initial level. Relevant information about the person's previous lifestyle should be an essential part of these notes.

In carrying out Community Living Assessments, as required by the Community Care legislation in Britain, it is important that assessors are aware of the many factors that need to be taken into consideration in order to obtain a complete picture of the person's strengths and needs. The assessor needs to be able to, and know when to, call in other disciplines in order to assess the implications of specific or apparent difficulties, if a realistic package of care is to be set up.

In many residential settings, notes are kept but are limited in the information they provide. For instance, different staff place different emphasis on different aspects of behaviour and functioning, so that comparisons with previous behaviour and with other clients may prove difficult.

More formal assessment methods have been devised to overcome some of these difficulties. They provide a structure for the observations and ensure all the relevant areas are covered; they make more explicit how the person functions; they involve less subjective and potentially biased opinion from the staff member; they provide results that are easily compared over a period of time or with other patients. It is for these reasons that the use of formal assessment procedures is to be recommended. They do have their limitations and drawbacks, which will be pointed out, and they need to be used with common sense. They do not replace the care-worker's observations, but can enhance them by providing structure and the opportunity to highlight the problems of particular individuals.

What to assess?

Previous sections will have given some indications of important areas to cover. These would include:

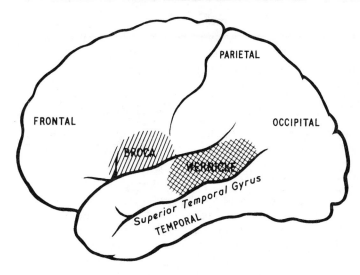

Figure 6.1 Main areas of the brain including speech centres.

of oral communication can result from nts not only in articulation but also in more of the following: respiration, resonance, volume, rate, voice quality, or rhythm. The use of word or onstruction may be correct, but, to the peech may sound indistinct.

or Wernicke's dysphasia

dysphasia occurs as a result of damage rt of the brain concerned with com- n, usually the Wernicke's area of the hemisphere where the temporal lobe the frontal and parietal lobes. This is posterior part of the superior temporal Fig. 6.1). In most right-handed people, nant hemisphere is the left side of the e situation is more uncertain in left- eople.

ient fails to understand what is being n/her. He/she has difficulty with verbal cations. Speech, superficially, may sound ut often there is a 'press of speech'— many words, bits of words, or even words; when this is put together speech unintelligible and is called 'jargon'. vith others is difficult or impossible. d problems can include difficulty in

naming objects and in reading and writing. With such difficulties, a person may even appear psy-chotic. However, the degree of impairment can vary from person to person, and because of ap-parently normal, though slow, speech the situation can be overlooked. Any doubts with regard to hearing should also include questions about the possibility of a receptive dysphasia.

Expressive or Broca's aphasia

This takes various forms. The damaged area is the posterior part of the dominant frontal lobe called the inferior frontal convolution of the temporal lobe (see Fig. 6.1). A stroke patient who is right-handed can have damage around this area of the brain, which causes a paralysis or weakness of the right side and produces an expressive aphasia. This impairment of speech can vary from complete loss to mild word-finding problems, grammatical errors, hesitancy and shortened sentences. Usually, understanding is preserved as are automatic phrases: 'one two three', or 'good morning'. Writing is affected, and reading and calculation may also suffer.

There are many other varieties of aphasia, including global aphasia, which affects all forms of language. For those who require a more detailed account a textbook such as Darley (1982),

1. History: what is known about the person's life, what did he or she do; successes, problems, family, etc.

2. Personality: what can relatives or friends say about the person's personality; was he/she nervous, outgoing, shy, confident, carefree, con-scientious, serious, short-tempered and so on?

3. Cognitive level: what is known about the person's previous level of functioning, educational attainment, etc; what is the person's current level of function, concentration, memory, orientation and so on?

4. The environment: what is the person's home or residential unit like; who else lives there, how good are relationships?

5. Attitudes: is the atmosphere around the person warm and supportive, or is the person devalued and invalidated as a person? How much strain are family care-givers experiencing, how is this affecting the relationship with the person with dementia?

6. How does the person feel: is she happy or sad, satisfied with life or depressed?

7. Physical health: what physical and sensory problems are there?

8. Neurological/neuropsychological difficult-ies: is there any evidence of speech impairments, visuo-motor deficits, etc?

9. Psychiatric problems: is there any sugges-tion of depression, paranoid ideation, halluci-nations, etc?

10. Is there any indication of the specific degenerative process occurring, e.g. frontal lobe dementia, vascular dementia, a type of Alzheimer's disease, etc. This may help ascertain which areas of function are relatively less impaired and assist in the setting up of appropriate interventions. For example, someone with vascular dementia may have a very slow response and will need patience and encouragement; someone with Parkinson's disease may have a communication difficulty out of proportion to any cognitive impairment and will need someone to take the time and trouble to listen to them; someone with a difficulty in initiating actions (perhaps arising from a frontal-type dementia) may benefit from distraction, so that he/she is not fully concentrating on the

task, allowing automatic processes to take over.

11. The person's general functioning and be-haviour: self-care, socialisation, activities and so on. What the person actually does.

Not all can be covered adequately immediately; assessment is often an on-going process. Some require specialised assessment, e.g. physical and mental health and diagnosis of a specific de-generative condition need medical input. Others, such as details of the person's history and per-sonality, are best collected fairly informally from discussions with relatives and friends. Here we will consider more fully the often neglected neuropsychological aspects and some formal ap-proaches to certain of the other areas, such as cognitive and environmental assessment, and assessment of general functional abilities.

As stated earlier, it is not our purpose to provide a comprehensive critique of test materials and specific assessment procedures, as this has been done elsewhere (e.g. Woods & Britton 1985, Gilleard 1984a,b, Holden 1988, Beech & Harding 1990).

COGNITIVE FUNCTIONING

In most cases, a simple mental status question-naire is most appropriate for a brief assessment. There are a considerable number of these avail-able. A frequently used example is included in the Clifton Assessment Procedures for the Elderly (CAPE) (Pattie & Gilleard 1979). A composite set of items devised by Woods (1979) covers much the same ground as the CAPE and the Blessed et al (1968) test: this is included in Appendix 1 as an example of the type of test in use. The items usually cover current orientation, personal information, current information, personal and non-personal memory. The frequently used Mini-Mental State Examination (MMSE—Folstein et al 1975) includes several other types of item, in-cluding tests of apraxia and language, and so is less purely a memory test than the other measures. The questions are asked in a one-to-one situation; no assistance is given to the patient, but usually it is permissible to re-phrase or repeat the ques-tion. Scoring usually presents few problems, answers are easily checked and if anything other than one point for each correct answer applies the criteria for two- or three-point responses are laid down. In short, these tests are intended to be objective and to produce a reliable score, regardless of the tester, which is indicative of the level of memory impairment.

If the aim of testing is monitoring change, then there is much to be said for devising a more personalised test, with questions relevant to the patient's family and circumstances. It is advisable to assess the person several times before the re-habilitation or re-training programme commences. Preferably the assessment should be at the same time of day, and should continue until the result is consistent from day to day, i.e. within two to three points at the most. If selection or identifi-cation of assets or deficits that will affect the care-plan is the aim, then the reason for any failure on the test should be examined thought-fully. A low score does not in every case indicate a severe dementia. Other factors that can lead to low scores are lifelong low intelligence, deafness, poor eyesight (for reading and writing tests), severe depression and/or anxiety leading to slowness of thought or distractability, and speech difficulties—expressive or receptive. Therefore, test scores need to be evaluated in the light of other information about the person. Specialist help for sensory deficits, and any possible amelioration, is a necessity. Likewise depression and extreme anxiety—if reassurance does not help—need appropriate treatment. Speech diffi-culties and their assessment are discussed in the next section. Lifelong low intellectual difficulty may be suspected from the person's educational or occupational history and from a low reading level that is not part of a visual or dysphasic problem. Reading level is a good predictor of previous intelligence, and the National Adult Reading Test is a useful tool to clarify this issue (Nelson & Willison 1991). It should be noted that the MMSE is particularly susceptible to the effects of low intellectual level (Orrell et al 1992). Of course, these factors can occur in com-bination, adding further complications! It is important to realise, therefore, that there may be multiple explanations for poor performance on

such tests. The converse occasionally happens also, and a person of superior intelligence, who has deteriorated from a previously very high level, scores so well that the true state is over-looked. Careful screening and re-testing are advisable in such cases.

More detailed cognitive testing may be in-dicated in certain circumstances, and should be carried out under the supervision of a clinical psychologist. Relatively brief batteries covering a wider range of areas than simply memory are now available, such as the CAMCOG (part of the CAMDEX diagnostic evaluation) (Roth et al 1988) and Middlesex Elderly Assessment of Mental State (MEAMS) (Golding 1989); used carefully by a trained assessor, they can be helpful in delineating the person's profile of cognitive abilities, without calling on the clinical psychologist's full armamentarium of detailed cognitive tests.

NEUROPSYCHOLOGICAL ASSESSMENTS

This could equally be entitled 'Misinterpreted behaviour'. When confronted with what appears to be unusual or disordered behaviour, the observer naturally interprets it according to per-sonal experience. If a person uses foul language, is socially objectionable or insulting in some way, it is not surprising to find he or she is labelled as 'psychopathic', coarse or socially un-acceptable. If a person looks much like anyone else, has no apparent disability and seems to be generally capable, the observer cannot be blamed for an inability to see inside that person's head. Brain injury and disease change behaviour. The behaviour may be an indication of brain disorder.

In practical terms, staff may see a patient eating only half a plate of food and will assume that the person is apathetic or has anorexia nervosa. Someone will walk into objects or trip over them and is regarded as forgetful, clumsy or going blind. Onlookers, or listeners, can believe that because a person has problems with words or reading he or she has completely deteriorated. Lack of recognition of objects or faces is classed as blindness or stupidity, and the inability to

perform a task on request has many impli-cations. The patient who is capable of dressing but who will not get dressed, no matter how often he or she is told to do so, is often viewed as a nuisance or attention seeking or unco-operative. The person who repeats words, phrases and gestures is seen as deliberately irritating family or staff. There are many behaviours which cause staff to conclude the worst about a person, and which, in practice, make life very hard for everyone.

Lack of knowledge about the relationships of brain and behaviour can also lead to the setting of inappropriate targets and the use of inappro-priate methods to obtain improvement. If some-one no longer knows how to speak, simply being praised for making a noise will not improve communication. Although even the very young who have sustained a closed head injury can suffer 'hidden' neuropsychological deficits, e.g. an outspoken teenager with frontal lobe damage ostracised by his old friends, some of the more subtle effects of brain injury and disease seem to be less likely to be identified and understood in older people.

It is important to appreciate that an apparently generalised dementia can be made up of a number of particular dysfunctions. Specific impairments do occur in dementing processes as well as in trauma (e.g. head injuries), stroke or physical disorders. In the early stages, these im-pairments may be minor, but as the deterio-ration in function becomes more severe, obviously, the problems become more apparent. Awareness of their implications and presence—for what-ever reason—can assist staff in planning manage-ment and treatment programmes in a realistic manner.

This is a complicated field, which we will attempt to simplify as far as possible. Abilities and functions are not necessarily linked to a particular location in the brain. Although certain major functions, such as speech, may be associ-ated with a specific location, other centres may also be involved in some way. These main centres will be mentioned, but it is the resulting behaviour which is of importance and which plays a vital role in management and treatment.

Readers are recommende (1987) for a more detaile psychology and Holden (ship of neuropsychology to

Disorientation

This is the most obvious tested problem. Disorient and person signifies some may occur with any illness any age. Tests of orienta mentioned above. In additi where he or she is, it i escorted around the ware spatial orientation is inta memory problems fill i memory, perhaps from a p plausible account *confabul* are and what others are d be convinced that the tin earlier than it really is, as in a previous phase of life injury or disease, e.g. Kor other amnesias, specifica memory and learning abil

Aphasia—speech di

Relatives and friends as staff are often under the disorders resulting from gressive deterioration ar able comprehension no l many forms of speech di many reasons. This is a mental divisions for gene

Dysarthria

This is often confused order. It is an impairm duction of speech caus upper or lower motor ne or in the cerebellum, wh paralysis or incoordin culature. The usual de describes dysarthria as

Prob impa one phon inton sente listen

Rece

Recep to the prehe domir joins called gyrus the do brain. hande The said to commu normal using made-u is ofte Contac Associa

1. History: what is known about the person's life, what did he or she do; successes, problems, family, etc.

2. Personality: what can relatives or friends say about the person's personality; was he/she nervous, outgoing, shy, confident, carefree, conscientious, serious, short-tempered and so on?

3. Cognitive level: what is known about the person's previous level of functioning, educational attainment, etc; what is the person's current level of function, concentration, memory, orientation and so on?

4. The environment: what is the person's home or residential unit like; who else lives there, how good are relationships?

5. Attitudes: is the atmosphere around the person warm and supportive, or is the person devalued and invalidated as a person? How much strain are family care-givers experiencing, how is this affecting the relationship with the person with dementia?

6. How does the person feel: is she happy or sad, satisfied with life or depressed?

7. Physical health: what physical and sensory problems are there?

8. Neurological/neuropsychological difficulties: is there any evidence of speech impairments, visuo-motor deficits, etc?

9. Psychiatric problems: is there any suggestion of depression, paranoid ideation, hallucinations, etc?

10. Is there any indication of the specific degenerative process occurring, e.g. frontal lobe dementia, vascular dementia, a type of Alzheimer's disease, etc. This may help ascertain which areas of function are relatively less impaired and assist in the setting up of appropriate interventions. For example, someone with vascular dementia may have a very slow response and will need patience and encouragement; someone with Parkinson's disease may have a communication difficulty out of proportion to any cognitive impairment and will need someone to take the time and trouble to listen to them; someone with a difficulty in initiating actions (perhaps arising from a frontal-type dementia) may benefit from distraction, so that he/she is not fully concentrating on the

task, allowing automatic processes to take over.

11. The person's general functioning and behaviour: self-care, socialisation, activities and so on. What the person actually does.

Not all can be covered adequately immediately; assessment is often an on-going process. Some require specialised assessment, e.g. physical and mental health and diagnosis of a specific degenerative condition need medical input. Others, such as details of the person's history and personality, are best collected fairly informally from discussions with relatives and friends. Here we will consider more fully the often neglected neuropsychological aspects and some formal approaches to certain of the other areas, such as cognitive and environmental assessment, and assessment of general functional abilities.

As stated earlier, it is not our purpose to provide a comprehensive critique of test materials and specific assessment procedures, as this has been done elsewhere (e.g. Woods & Britton 1985, Gilleard 1984a,b, Holden 1988, Beech & Harding 1990).

COGNITIVE FUNCTIONING

In most cases, a simple mental status questionnaire is most appropriate for a brief assessment. There are a considerable number of these available. A frequently used example is included in the Clifton Assessment Procedures for the Elderly (CAPE) (Pattie & Gilleard 1979). A composite set of items devised by Woods (1979) covers much the same ground as the CAPE and the Blessed et al (1968) test: this is included in Appendix 1 as an example of the type of test in use. The items usually cover current orientation, personal information, current information, personal and non-personal memory. The frequently used Mini-Mental State Examination (MMSE—Folstein et al 1975) includes several other types of item, including tests of apraxia and language, and so is less purely a memory test than the other measures. The questions are asked in a one-to-one situation; no assistance is given to the patient, but usually it is permissible to re-phrase or repeat the question. Scoring usually presents few problems, answers are easily checked and if anything other than one point for each correct answer applies the criteria for two- or three-point responses are laid down. In short, these tests are intended to be objective and to produce a reliable score, regardless of the tester, which is indicative of the level of memory impairment.

If the aim of testing is monitoring change, then there is much to be said for devising a more personalised test, with questions relevant to the patient's family and circumstances. It is advisable to assess the person several times before the re-habilitation or re-training programme commences. Preferably the assessment should be at the same time of day, and should continue until the result is consistent from day to day, i.e. within two to three points at the most. If selection or identification of assets or deficits that will affect the care-plan is the aim, then the reason for any failure on the test should be examined thoughtfully. A low score does not in every case indicate a severe dementia. Other factors that can lead to low scores are lifelong low intelligence, deafness, poor eyesight (for reading and writing tests), severe depression and/or anxiety leading to slowness of thought or distractability, and speech difficulties—expressive or receptive. Therefore, test scores need to be evaluated in the light of other information about the person. Specialist help for sensory deficits, and any possible amelioration, is a necessity. Likewise depression and extreme anxiety—if reassurance does not help—need appropriate treatment. Speech difficulties and their assessment are discussed in the next section. Lifelong low intellectual difficulty may be suspected from the person's educational or occupational history and from a low reading level that is not part of a visual or dysphasic problem. Reading level is a good predictor of previous intelligence, and the National Adult Reading Test is a useful tool to clarify this issue (Nelson & Willison 1991). It should be noted that the MMSE is particularly susceptible to the effects of low intellectual level (Orrell et al 1992). Of course, these factors can occur in combination, adding further complications! It is important to realise, therefore, that there may be multiple explanations for poor performance on

such tests. The converse occasionally happens also, and a person of superior intelligence, who has deteriorated from a previously very high level, scores so well that the true state is over-looked. Careful screening and re-testing are advisable in such cases.

More detailed cognitive testing may be indicated in certain circumstances, and should be carried out under the supervision of a clinical psychologist. Relatively brief batteries covering a wider range of areas than simply memory are now available, such as the CAMCOG (part of the CAMDEX diagnostic evaluation) (Roth et al 1988) and Middlesex Elderly Assessment of Mental State (MEAMS) (Golding 1989); used carefully by a trained assessor, they can be helpful in delineating the person's profile of cognitive abilities, without calling on the clinical psychologist's full armamentarium of detailed cognitive tests.

NEUROPSYCHOLOGICAL ASSESSMENTS

This could equally be entitled 'Misinterpreted behaviour'. When confronted with what appears to be unusual or disordered behaviour, the observer naturally interprets it according to personal experience. If a person uses foul language, is socially objectionable or insulting in some way, it is not surprising to find he or she is labelled as 'psychopathic', coarse or socially unacceptable. If a person looks much like anyone else, has no apparent disability and seems to be generally capable, the observer cannot be blamed for an inability to see inside that person's head. Brain injury and disease change behaviour. The behaviour may be an indication of brain disorder.

In practical terms, staff may see a patient eating only half a plate of food and will assume that the person is apathetic or has anorexia nervosa. Someone will walk into objects or trip over them and is regarded as forgetful, clumsy or going blind. Onlookers, or listeners, can believe that because a person has problems with words or reading he or she has completely deteriorated. Lack of recognition of objects or faces is classed as blindness or stupidity, and the inability to perform a task on request has many impli-cations. The patient who is capable of dressing but who will not get dressed, no matter how often he or she is told to do so, is often viewed as a nuisance or attention seeking or unco-operative. The person who repeats words, phrases and gestures is seen as deliberately irritating family or staff. There are many behaviours which cause staff to conclude the worst about a person, and which, in practice, make life very hard for everyone.

Lack of knowledge about the relationships of brain and behaviour can also lead to the setting of inappropriate targets and the use of inappro-priate methods to obtain improvement. If some-one no longer knows how to speak, simply being praised for making a noise will not improve communication. Although even the very young who have sustained a closed head injury can suffer 'hidden' neuropsychological deficits, e.g. an outspoken teenager with frontal lobe damage ostracised by his old friends, some of the more subtle effects of brain injury and disease seem to be less likely to be identified and understood in older people.

It is important to appreciate that an apparently generalised dementia can be made up of a number of particular dysfunctions. Specific impairments do occur in dementing processes as well as in trauma (e.g. head injuries), stroke or physical disorders. In the early stages, these im-pairments may be minor, but as the deterio-ration in function becomes more severe, obviously, the problems become more apparent. Awareness of their implications and presence—for what-ever reason—can assist staff in planning manage-ment and treatment programmes in a realistic manner.

This is a complicated field, which we will attempt to simplify as far as possible. Abilities and functions are not necessarily linked to a particular location in the brain. Although certain major functions, such as speech, may be associ-ated with a specific location, other centres may also be involved in some way. These main centres will be mentioned, but it is the resulting behaviour which is of importance and which plays a vital role in management and treatment.

Readers are recommended to consult Walsh (1987) for a more detailed account of neuro-psychology and Holden (1988) for the relation-ship of neuropsychology to ageing.

Disorientation

This is the most obvious and most frequently tested problem. Disorientation for time, place and person signifies some degree of confusion. It may occur with any illness, with delirium and at any age. Tests of orientation and memory are mentioned above. In addition to asking the person where he or she is, it is worth asking to be escorted around the ward or home to check if spatial orientation is intact. Some people with memory problems fill in the gaps in their memory, perhaps from a past experience or some plausible account *confabulating* about where they are and what others are doing. The person may be convinced that the time is 10 or more years earlier than it really is, as if he or she were still in a previous phase of life. Some forms of brain injury or disease, e.g. Korsakoff's syndrome and other amnesias, specifically impair a person's memory and learning ability.

Aphasia—speech disorders

Relatives and friends as well as a number of staff are often under the impression that speech disorders resulting from strokes indicate a pro-gressive deterioration and assume that reason-able comprehension no longer exists. There are many forms of speech disorder, which occur for many reasons. This is an outline of the funda-mental divisions for general guidance.

Dysarthria

This is often confused with true language dis-order. It is an impairment in the actual pro-duction of speech caused by a lesion in the upper or lower motor neurones, the basal ganglia or in the cerebellum, which results in weakness, paralysis or incoordination of speech mus-culature. The usual definition in dictionaries describes dysarthria as 'imperfect articulation'.

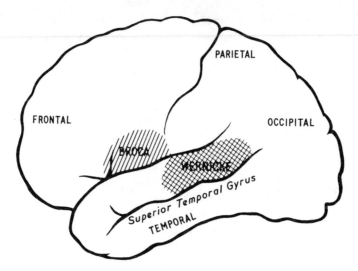

Figure 6.1   Main areas of the brain including speech centres.

Problems of oral communication can result from impairments not only in articulation but also in one or more of the following: respiration, phonation, resonance, volume, rate, voice quality, intonation or rhythm. The use of word or sentence construction may be correct, but, to the listener, speech may sound indistinct.

Receptive or Wernicke's dysphasia

Receptive dysphasia occurs as a result of damage to the part of the brain concerned with comprehension, usually the Wernicke's area of the dominant hemisphere where the temporal lobe joins into the frontal and parietal lobes. This is called the posterior part of the superior temporal gyrus (see Fig. 6.1). In most right-handed people, the dominant hemisphere is the left side of the brain. The situation is more uncertain in left-handed people.

The patient fails to understand what is being said to him/her. He/she has difficulty with verbal communications. Speech, superficially, may sound normal, but often there is a 'press of speech'—using too many words, bits of words,'or even made-up words; when this is put together speech is often unintelligible and is called 'jargon'. Contact with others is difficult or impossible. Associated problems can include difficulty in naming objects and in reading and writing. With such difficulties, a person may even appear psychotic. However, the degree of impairment can vary from person to person, and because of apparently normal, though slow, speech the situation can be overlooked. Any doubts with regard to hearing should also include questions about the possibility of a receptive dysphasia.

Expressive or Broca's aphasia

This takes various forms. The damaged area is the posterior part of the dominant frontal lobe called the inferior frontal convolution of the temporal lobe (see Fig. 6.1). A stroke patient who is right-handed can have damage around this area of the brain, which causes a paralysis or weakness of the right side and produces an expressive aphasia. This impairment of speech can vary from complete loss to mild word-finding problems, grammatical errors, hesitancy and shortened sentences. Usually, understanding is preserved as are automatic phrases: 'one two three', or 'good morning'. Writing is affected, and reading and calculation may also suffer.

There are many other varieties of aphasia, including global aphasia, which affects all forms of language. For those who require a more detailed account a textbook such as Darley (1982),

Albyn-Davis (1983) or—dealing specifically with older people—Ulatowska (1985) would be appropriate. The two forms of aphasia (or dysphasia; the two terms are often, if incorrectly, used interchangeably) mentioned do overlap in severe cases and so may be predominantly expressive or receptive. Guidance from speech therapists can enable relatives, friends and volunteers to assist in practice and in the constant encouragement that is required to obtain improvement. Special forms of therapy, such as melodic intonation therapy (a use of melody and rhythm), have been described and have proved successful in selected cases (Albert et al 1973, Sparks et al 1974) but require a great deal more development.

Apraxia

This is an impairment of voluntary and purposive movements that cannot be attributed to muscle weakness or defect, nor can it be attributed to lack of comprehension. Quite simply, the person is able to perform movements, knows what he/she wants to do, but if consciously trying to make a gesture or a required movement cannot organise and coordinate both the thought and the appropriate action. This disorder is fairly common and is often misinterpreted as uncooperativeness. Clumsiness, 'he's all fingers and thumbs' and 'she doesn't remember what to do with her fork' are usually noted. There are several forms of apraxia, the principal ones being constructional, ideomotor, ideational and dressing.

Constructional apraxia

This form of apraxia has been particularly in the province of neuropsychology as it is difficult to elicit clinically. Special tests are required to isolate it. Although movements are possible, the patient has difficulty in assembly, and the parts of an object cannot be put together correctly in order to achieve the whole. There is a defect in the transmission of information to the limbs concerned with the action. For example, a motor mechanic would develop problems in putting an engine back together. Arguments have arisen as

to whether the difficulty results from a motor impairment for complex, sequential activities or a defect in visuo-spatial perception (how one sees spatial relationships). Studies have shown that right hemisphere damage (parietal and tempero-parietal lobes) causes visuo-spatial perceptual defects, so that even with a model to copy the patient cannot construct or draw a simple geometric figure (Warrington et al 1966, Gazzaniga 1970, Dimond 1972). Patients with known damage in the left hemisphere (parietal or tempero-parietal lobes) can perform the tasks once supplied with visual clues and, furthermore, can improve with learning (Warrington et al 1966, Hecaen & Assal 1970). It is now accepted that left hemisphere lesions cause a motor defect—an inability to establish a programme for the required action—and right hemisphere lesions show visuo-spatial disturbances, which may even be aggravated by visual cues and learning situations (Hecaen & Albert 1978).

Constructional apraxia can be demonstrated quite simply by asking a patient to draw a star, a cube and a clock face. Construction of a star with sticks or matchsticks is also useful (Fig. 6.2). Even with a hemiplegia, it is possible to construct with the unimpaired hand. If the shapes produced are distorted or inaccurate, a model can be provided to copy. For less-educated patients, the cube might be too difficult, and drawing a house could be more appropriate (Moore & Wyke 1984). With elderly people, it is rarely necessary to provide a complicated and undesirable test battery, but with younger and fitter over-60s it may be possible to introduce the Block Design Test—or Koh's blocks—which provides more information (Walsh 1987).

Ideomotor apraxia

This condition is an inability to perform simple, single gestures. More complex gestures may be possible. Automatic or incidental gesture is performed perfectly. This may be thought of as a loss of memory for the pattern of the action—or engram. Although the pattern is preserved, it is not under voluntary control. A Catholic can go to mass, where she can make the sign of the

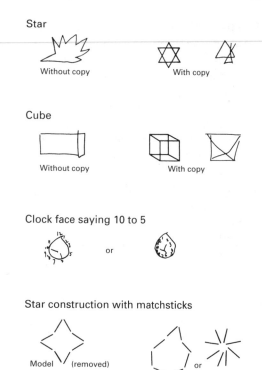

Figure 6.2 Drawing showing spatial or apraxic disturbances.

cross without any difficulty. When asked to repeat it in the clinic, she is totally unable to do so.

Simple gestures can be tested by asking the person to: wave goodbye, pretend to stir the tea, imitate a series of hand and arm poses (Christensen 1975). Responses to imitation are usually better. Generally, ideomotor apraxia results from bilateral brain damage.

Ideational apraxia

This is noticeable when a person attempts to carry out a complicated gesture or action. There is full understanding of what is to be done, and the physical capacity to perform the action is preserved, but there is a disruption in the order and sequence of the total action and in the ability to plan properly.

In ideomotor apraxia, the plan, or engram, is preserved, but the gesture is not. In ideational apraxia, the single gesture is preserved but the

overall plan is lost. The classical example is to ask the patient to take a match from a box, strike it and light a candle. The patient can repeat and understand the instructions but when responding becomes very confused. The match may be struck upside down, or on the candle, or the candle may be struck on the box. The correct, logical sequence cannot be performed. Once again, well-established and automatic actions can be normal, as they do not require conscious thought. However, once the patient has to think about the response, or there is some stress, errors are multiplied. Imitation is usually more successful.

With such a complicated disability, explanations can become equally complicated! Both ideomotor and ideational apraxia are associated with lesions in the dominant parietal and temporal regions, but there is still controversy about instances of bilateral or even diffuse damage causing such impairments. Practically speaking, the problem of location is irrelevant here. What is relevant is the need for an awareness of these disabilities as a sign of actual damage, so that suitable plans can be made for rehabilitation which will take the resultant behavioural problems into account. A detailed account of the apraxias can be found in Hecaen & Albert (1978).

Dressing apraxia

This seems to result from lesions in the non-dominant parietal and occipital areas. It is a visuo-spatial defect and the degree of impairment varies. Inability to dress, slowness, confusion as to which piece of clothing goes where, and inability to fasten buttons are all common complaints that can be related to a number of physical problems as well as to a dementing process—dressing apraxia is one of the more frequent reasons. The patient just cannot find the right gesture to associate the clothes with her body. The mental plan for an almost automatic action has been lost. Sometimes, when a patient suffers from one-side neglect (anosognosia) and actually ignores one side of the body (see p. 102), there will be difficulty in dressing that side. This form of apraxia is usually associated with damage to the right parietal and occipital areas.

There are a number of other forms of apraxia: for instance, buccofacial apraxia—the inability to perform voluntary movements such as sticking out the tongue; limb and gait disturbances; and even whole-body apraxia can occur. Apraxia for speech is a common disability in the speech therapist's day. A patient may be able to eat and swallow correctly, or even produce involuntary speech, but there is an inability to make the correct movements of the tongue and lips in order to produce voluntary speech. Once again there is no physical reason for this and comprehension is usually normal. The patient may produce the same automatic phrase when trying to speak, e.g. 'I don't know what to say, I don't know what to say' or 'Do, do, do, do'.

Treatment

Treatment of the apraxias varies; it is often based on using preserved function and adapting it to compensate for the loss, practice of a graded programme of related tasks or the use of rhythm. For instance, distraction can assist a patient to speak or complete an action normally. Concentration on a rhythm instead of the actual words can be enough to allow speech to come. Simple sentences like 'It's a ni—ce day' can be sung to a beat. The patient is amused, distracted from the real problem and then delighted to find that the words have been produced. Similarly with actions, by distracting attention from the movements the required action can be made. For instance, teeth brushing may be impossible until the chant of 'up, down' is used or a beat is tapped out. Grasp reflexes which will not release from a handshake can be resolved by distraction—stroking the back of the unwithdrawing hand. The graded programme could be used in re-training, for example, an apraxic hand. A series of large, medium and small beakers are of use. Aiding the person to grasp the largest beaker, and aiding movement in order to place, in it, another large beaker would be the first step. Encouragement to repeat this, then to try it alone would constitute the next phase. When this is

successful, the next size can be introduced, until, by practice, and with reinforcement by praise, the actions are re-learned. Tasks with meaning, e.g. helping with the washing-up, are usually the most successful.

Agnosia

This is an impairment in the accurate perception of objects that is not caused by a defect in the sensory systems, ignorance of the nature of the object, defective intelligence or confusion.

It is a condition which is generally unknown, almost impossible to elicit by clinical methods and the subject of much neuropsychological investigation. The commonest and best recognised form is visual agnosia, but there are a number of others.

Visual agnosia or object agnosia

This is an inability not only to name or demonstrate the use of an object, but also an inability to appreciate its character and meaning, or even to remember ever having seen it before. Obviously it is necessary to distinguish this from aphasia and visual memory loss. Other sensory input is required. Usually if another sense is used, the clues lead to recognition. A characteristic smell, noise or feel provide these clues. A patient while recognising the colour, shape and size of a lipstick remained unable to name it. She stated that the object was a maroon and gold container, cylindrical in shape and about 3 inches in length. Only when encouraged to remove the lid, smell the perfume and rub the contents across the back of her hand was she able to identify it. The problem appears to be associated with damage around the lateral ventricles extending into the occipital lobes. The Popplereuter's test (included in the Luria investigations, Christensen 1975) is useful in identifying this impairment. It comprises a set of pictures of mixed-up everyday objects—a jug apparently containing a paintbrush, an axe, and a pair of scissors is one example. Another test from the Luria investigations comprises series of photographs; an object is vague in the first picture and later becomes quite distinct.

Colour and auditory agnosia are other forms occasionally found, which can cause problems in treatment and management. Patients with auditory agnosia have word deafness. They cannot grasp normal conversation and become very distressed. Usually slow, distinct speech helps the problem considerably. With colour agnosia, colour not only cannot be named, but matching and association of colour are impaired.

Spatial agnosia

This disorder is fairly common and is a spatial disorientation—a defect in finding the way even in familiar surroundings. A young navigator who had a mild stroke was unable to understand maps that had been given to him as an amusement during recovery. This happens in older people too. There is loss of appreciation of right and left, and incapacity for drawing simple maps of the house or the ward. Recognition of individual objects in the environment is preserved, though localisation of them is disordered. Under this heading, there is the not uncommon phenomenon of autotopagnosia—a failure to recognise or localise parts of one's own body (related to parietal damage). Body agnosia is also associated with another, fairly common disorder, anosog-

nosia. One side of the body is neglected or denied. The patient may say the left hand does not belong to him/her or even that it belongs to someone else. It is not rare to hear that a patient believes that there is a strange hand in his/her bed, and he/she can require some persuasion to accept that hand as his/her own. Dressing the neglected part of the body is also a problem, and food on one side of the plate will not be touched. The affected side is almost invariably the left one. From a management viewpoint, it is important to be aware of this state. Simple measures can be instigated. At mealtimes the plate can be turned around so that a full meal is obtained. The 'wanderers' who get lost on the way to the toilet or who get into somebody else's bed could have this complaint. The toilet is invariably approached from the wrong direction and the bed is on the wrong side on return. A simple solution is to transfer beds to the most convenient side. A drawing of a clock face, or the assembly of one of the educational variety will easily demonstrate the problem, as will the drawing of a house. (Fig. 6.3).

Other tests for body agnosia are to ask the person to point to various parts of their body and to use the finger agnosia tests. After a demonstration of the task, the patient is asked to close their eyes or is blindfolded. The examiner

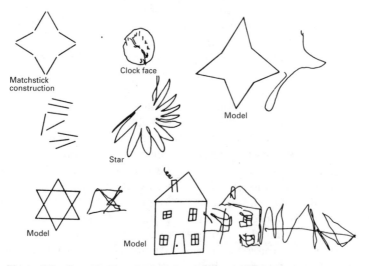

Figure 6.3 Reproduction of actual drawings by a 70-year-old lady with anosognosia, left-sided neglect.

presses one of the patient's fingers and requests the person to 'show' that finger on the other hand. There is a further test to see if the person can say how many fingers there are 'between that one and that one'. The examiner will press gently on, for instance, the forefinger and the little finger of a hand, and will expect to receive the answer 'two fingers' and so on.

As has been stated, unilateral spatial agnosia is almost exclusively related to the left half of space. Obvious exceptions would be people with right hemisphere dominance, usually left-handers. Other forms of agnosia include:

Tactile agnosia or astereognosia. This is discerned by requesting identification of objects, particularly coins, by the sense of touch alone.

Prosopagnosia: failure to recognise faces. Testing for this problem is through the use of photographs of familiar and unfamiliar faces. Occasionally, the person cannot even recognise self-reflection in a mirror.

Simultanagnosia. This is an inability to perceive a whole while being able to interpret the parts. If a picture of, for instance, a floral festival is presented and the person asked to supply a suitable name for the picture, the task will prove impossible. Each single flower will be pointed out, even each blade of grass, but the scene will be too difficult to grasp. There appears to be some association with reading problems, for although a sentence can be written correctly it can only be read back letter by letter.

Awareness of agnostic factors has very practical implications. To use 'left' and 'right' as meaningful concepts for someone with spatial problems is obviously inappropriate. Descriptive words either written or spoken—depending on the impairment—are more valuable to those with such difficulties. A picture above a bed, a name in large print and verbal directions using colour or some meaningful symbol are more useful in re-training than spatial directions.

Acquired knowledge

There are other factors which should be checked in any neuropsychological investigation. Impair-ment of acquired knowledge may have more implications than that of global deterioration.

Agraphia: an inability to write properly. This includes spelling, letter construction and word organisation and is related to aphasia and tempero-parietal problems.

Acalculia: difficulty with numbers. This also can be related to parietal lesions, reading difficulties (alexia) and spatial disorders.

Alexia or dyslexia: inability to read. A disturbance occurs in the relationship between visual and language functions, and can happen in association with a number of other conditions. From the management viewpoint, if someone cannot read it is hopeless to expect her to cope in situations where such ability is vital. Directions on medicine bottles, and street or directional signs will prove meaningless.

The magazine method of testing

A useful and unthreatening method of investigation is to use an ordinary, colourful magazine, which can provide a wealth of information without stress. Using a suitable selection of advertisements from the two open pages of a magazine it is possible to test for a number of functions (Fig. 6.4).

Reading. Can the person read, can only large letters be meaningful, can smaller ones be read or is reading impossible?

Comprehension. Can the implications and meaning of pictures be understood, as well as words? Are comments and memories produced, with encouragement, from the content?

Aphasia. Can the person use the right words and name the objects on the page with ease?

Agnosia. Has the person any difficulty in seeing the pictures and appreciating what they are? Is colour meaningful; can faces or parts of the body be noted? Can the whole of a picture convey meaning, or are only parts of the picture seen?

Anosognosia. By watching the person's way of reading and the initial direction of gaze, it is possible to tell if there is one-sided neglect. If the farthest column on the right-hand page is the first to be noticed there is a possibility of

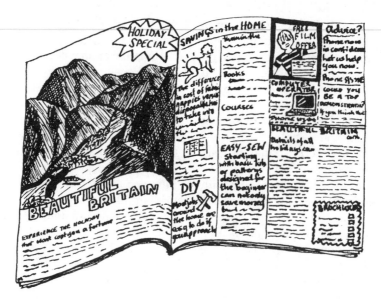

Figure 6.4 The magazine method. Using pages from a journal with clear, distinct pictures, words of varying size, columns, and colour in order to apply simple investigations of ability.

anosognosia. Check to see if there is difficulty in recognising the existence of a left-hand page and a column on the farthest left of that page.

Apraxia. This can be suggested by difficulties in turning pages and in pointing.

The 'magazine method' is by no means conclusive, but it is certainly very helpful and completely painless. It provides staff with information and useful interaction, and the patient with some stimulation. It is not vital to have strict assessment procedures with sick elderly people; what is important is to find out as gently as possible if there are impairments in certain functions. Using material from the natural surroundings provides a comfortable, unthreatening and easy way to screen for any possible difficulties which, if necessary, can be looked at in more detail later.

Frontal involvement

Though there are symptoms and signs associated with many locations in the brain and much to suggest that localisation is not complete, discussion of these aspects is not appropriate here. However, some of the personality changes and

function impairments associated with frontal lobe damage are of importance in understanding some of the behaviour frequently observed and are also helpful to the design of suitable therapeutic interventions. The frontal syndrome recognised in post-traumatic injuries usually shows some, if not all, of the following signs: impulsiveness, aggression or apathy, poor planning and logic, and an inability to monitor or control what is said or done. The person may not be able to end a letter or a conversation and may appear rather garrulous.

Emotional lability—inappropriate sudden crying and/or laughing—can be very upsetting to relatives and staff. It is often the result of a stroke or other neurological trauma. Euphoria, the use of undesirable language, sexual exhibitionism and erotic behaviour are disturbing and they are usually out of character. The mechanisms of control have been lost, emotions can run riot and inhibitions disappear. If the involuntary nature of this emotion is understood, it is easier to use distraction than inappropriate sympathy which aggravates the situation. Lack of initiative is another common feature. This is not caused by paralysis, apraxia or confusion but by an inability to voluntarily and spontaneously initiate a desired or automatic motor task. Recently it has been found that thought processes can also suffer from this inertia. Quite simply the victim cannot get going. There is a disorder of attention. Questions must be repeated over and over in order to elicit a response. This is linked to initiation difficulties. Similarly the patient forgets to remember. The information has not been forgotten, but the ability to start the necessary 'wheels' turning to make the memory process work is impaired.

Perseveration is common. On long-stay wards, patients can be heard repeating the same phrase all day or seen performing the same action again and again.

Writing and drawing show repetitions; for instance:

the girl has a nice hat can be reproduced as— the girl has has a has, or when asked to copy MNMNMNMN, MNNNNNNNN is produced.

This form of perseveration has a bearing on the difficulty in changing set, or in progressing from one idea to another. When asked to complete a series of sequential tasks, errors occur, such as the pattern in Figure 6.5.

Similarly a set of wooden or plastic shapes, which are also in sets of different colours, can only be sorted into either colour or shape groups; the alternative group cannot be found.

Luria (1963) has many suggestions for aiding rehabilitation programmes that are in difficulty because of this perseverative process. Though time-consuming they are effective. Distraction at the right moment is the key. The second an error in movement is commenced the action can be interrupted and distraction introduced. A com-ment on the weather or flowers or some nearby incident would be suitable. To ensure that the next movement in the task is correct, physical guidance is used. To make a stitch with a needle, for instance, a hand guiding a hand can ensure the correct path and so help to stop per-severation of an incorrect action. Phraseology can be interrupted in a similar manner and rein-forcement, usually praise and attention, can be given to non-repetitive talk. However, long-standing perseverations are very difficult to eradicate and early intervention is more successful.

Final comments

Understanding of some of the behaviour resulting from specific damage can improve the aims of programmes and rehabilitation. Relatives need to understand some of the changes that they see and cooperation from them can be increased. Examinations need not be threatening or stressful and positive approaches can play an important role in both assessment procedures and re-learning. If the person's problems are related to specific areas of damage to the brain, more appropriate measures of re-training can be used in conjunction with approaches such as RO and with the reinforcement of behaviour modifi-cation methods (Holden 1988, Fussey & Muir Giles 1988). Goals can be set at a suitable level, the right kind of attention and encouragement can be discussed and applied, and simple management measures introduced. Furthermore, such understanding will assist in better ap-preciation of behaviour patterns that have been incorrectly attributed to a dementia or to dis-ruptive or uncooperative personalities (Table 6.1).

$\triangle\triangle+\bigcirc\triangle\triangle+$ Please repeat across the page

The response might be, for example:

$\triangle\triangle\square\square\square++\bigcirc\bigcirc\bigcirc\bigcirc\bigcirc\bigcirc\bigcirc+++++++$

Figure 6.5 Sequential pattern completion. One of the tests to help in assessing frontal lobe, or operational thought, impairment.

Table 6.1   Neuropsychological disorders and their assessment

Neuropsychological deficits		Simple tests
Language problems		
Expressive dysphasia	Difficulty in conversation	Listen. Word finding, odd words and sentences, little speech, or complete rubbish
Receptive dysphasia	Comprehension difficulty	Lack of appropriate response to questions
Agraphia	Writing difficulty	Write a simple sentence
Acalculia	Difficulty with numbers	Write numbers, add, subtract, multiply and divide simple sums
Alexia	Reading difficulty	Read notice on ward, on TV or from a magazine
Apraxia		
Constructional	Difficulty in putting things together to make a whole	Use matchsticks to make a star. Draw a star or a cube. Also use model for copying
Ideomotor	Difficulty in making a single gesture	Ask to be shown hair brushing, waving, clenching teeth, etc.
Ideational	Difficulty in making complex gesture	Pretend to get out a cigarette, light it and start smoking
Dressing	Difficulty in dressing	Put on a coat, button it and take it off again
Agnosias		
Visual	Difficulty in appreciating meaning of objects	Use a letter or a number made up of other letters or numbers, e.g. a large 2 made of tiny 4s and see if both are recognised
Colour	Difficulty in appreciating colour	Naming, matching and association
Spatial	Difficulty in finding the way Unable to understand maps	Draw a plan of home
Autotopagnosia	Difficulty in recognising parts of own body, or another's	Point to parts of own body, and that of examiners
Anosognosia	Neglect of one side of body	Wash dinner plate Draw clock face or house
Astereognosis	Difficulty in recognising objects by touch	Name a selection of coins by touch alone
Prosopagnosia	Difficulty in recognising faces	Naming familiar and unfamiliar faces from photographs
Simultanagnosia	Difficulty in perceiving a whole	Name a picture with something suitable to describe its content
Frontal involvement		
	Personality change Euphoria or apathy Disinhibition Lack of initiative Perseveration Inability to plan	Watch Ask relatives about previous personality Use sequence of shapes or figures. Watch how games such as cards are played

ASSESSMENT OF GENERAL FUNCTIONING AND BEHAVIOUR

Three main approaches have been used with the elderly:

1. Rating scales, where staff who know the person well assess the person's functioning from their general unsystematic observations of them in their own environment.

2. Direct observation in a structured situation, where the person is requested to carry out particular tasks and then assessed on their performance.

3. Direct observation in natural settings, where a large number of systematic observations of the patient in their natural environment are made.

Rating scales

These have been the most frequently used form of behavioural assessment—perhaps because they are the most economical in terms of time. There are so many different scales that have been used with older people that their various advantages and drawbacks cannot be covered here. The interested reader is referred to Woods & Britton (1985, Ch. 6), Gilleard (1984b) and Applegate et al (1990) for reviews. Hall's (1980) review of rating scales in general use is also helpful for its advice on the development of new scales.

One of the major problems with rating scales, such as the commonly used Clifton Assessment Procedures for the Elderly (CAPE) Behaviour Rating Scale (see Pattie 1988) and the Crichton Royal Behaviour Rating Scale (Sixsmith et al 1993b) has been the difficulty in measuring small changes in behaviour. Most scales cover change in relatively large steps and are rarely sensitive to small changes or improvements. For instance, a person who is incontinent 10 times a day has made progress if the frequency drops to only five times a day. A scale which asks if incontinence occurs frequently, occasionally or never will not reflect such improvement. As a result, the ability to monitor fine change is limited and further assessment is normally required to identify specific targets in goal planning.

Some recent scales which have attempted to overcome this area of weakness by being more detailed and covering a broader range of function are the Behavioural Assessment Scale of Later Life (Brooker et al 1993) and the Brighton Clinic Adaptive Behaviour Scale (Ward et al 1991). The latter is particularly appropriate for people with more severe impairments in that it seeks to reflect more finely the real differences in function that do occur at this level and which are essential to identify in any care-planning process.

Most of the available behaviour rating scales focus on self-care skills and behavioural problems (such as aggression). Generally, raters tend to agree much more on the assessment of the person's physical function than on the occurrence and severity of difficult behaviour (see, for example, Ward et al 1991), although Patel & Hope (1992) have attempted to devise a procedure that more reliably assesses aggressive behaviour. Some scales include a very few items on communication and social behaviour, but the Holden Communication Scale (Appendix 2) has these areas as its focus. Despite its different emphasis, respectable correlations have been reported with the CAPE Behavioural Rating Scale and the CAPE cognitive scale (0.78 and 0.75, respectively, Merchant & Saxby 1981), supporting the validity of ratings on this scale. As a rough and ready guide, it has been suggested that scores above 25 indicate that the person may well do best in a group where expectations are at a fairly basic level; scores of 15–24 reflect a more moderate degree of impairment, and a probable response to a slightly more demanding group; scores of less than 15 suggest milder problems with less support and direction being needed in a group situation. As with all total scores where widely ranging areas of function are added together, these scores should only be treated as a general indication. The Holden Communication Scale is being widely used in RO and reminiscence programmes to good effect. Its content is more relevant to these approaches than other scales. It would, of course, be of little use in assessing progress in a self-care re-training programme!

In practice, how does one go about selecting

and using a rating scale? The first and most important consideration is to select a scale that is acceptable in the particular situation. It needs to be short enough so that time is available for it to be completed, rather than it being left half finished. It needs to be easy to use and understand, without difficult terminology. Scoring and interpretation should also be simple. It needs to be relevant to the situation; e.g. in many situations an item on 'regular work assignments' would be inappropriate. Item definitions must be clear and precise (Hall 1980). There must be no ambiguity or misunderstanding about the meaning of an item. Interpretation of behaviour reduces reliability; for example, different staff have different criteria for a term such as 'restlessness' unless it is defined more specifically. Items should have single definitions; items like 'misidentifies persons and surroundings but can find way about' cause problems for the person who cannot find their way about, and identifies people but not their surroundings! Where items are ordered the sequence needs to be carefully examined, so there are no anomalies. On one scale, a person who walks independently with a stick could receive a score of 2 or 4 on mobility depending on the staff member's interpretation of the item. Few scales have none of these faults; they are exceptionally difficult to avoid, particularly if a fresh scale is devised.

In using the scale, consideration needs to be given to who will make the ratings. The person who has most contact with the patient is the ideal choice; often trained staff members have less patient contact, so they may not be in the best position to carry out ratings. Training in the use of the rating scale should always be given. Making independent ratings of the same patients and then discussing reasons for any discrepancies is a useful exercise. The rating procedure needs to be clear; is the person rated as they are today, or has been over the past week, month? Can the rater only use his/her own observations, or can he/she make use of what others have observed? What is the procedure for commenting on aspects of behaviour not covered by the scale?

It can be seen that there are many problems inherent in reducing the whole range of behaviour of the elderly person into a brief rating. Added to these are the difficulties brought about by fluctuations in the person's behaviour, sometimes related to different staff. None of the scales available is perfect, but used with common sense and again in conjunction with other available information they can play a useful part in assessment.

Direct observation—structured setting

This is a well-established assessment method, where the person is asked to perform certain tasks in the presence of the assessor, who then rates their competence in this structured setting. A good example of this approach is the Performance Test of Activities of Daily Living (PADL), described by Kuriansky & Gurland (1976) and used extensively in studies of psychogeriatric patients in New York and London. This consists of 16 tasks, all easily demonstrated in an interview situation. These include drinking from a cup, combing hair, eating, making a telephone call, and so on. Most need 'props', e.g. a cup, comb, spoon with sweet, telephone, etc, and it is recommended that these be collected into a portable kit. Performance on each task is broken down into component parts and whether or not the person carries out each part is recorded. Simple tasks are given initially to reduce anxiety, and the whole test takes around 20 minutes to administer. The range of items is rather restricted with no coverage of socialisation or communication.

Independent ratings of patients' performance by the interviewer and an observer showed high inter-rater reliability (0.90). Evidence of validity—in its relation to physical health, mental state and prognosis—is presented by Kuriansky et al (1976). The test is reported to be generally acceptable to patients.

Several other procedures of this type are now available (Skurla et al 1988, Loewenstein et al 1989, Mahurin et al 1991), with tasks such as making a cup of coffee, 'shopping' for a simple item and financial skills such as counting change. These new scales extend the range of abilities covered, and tap into some of the more cognitive components of functional abilities (such as sequencing, keeping track of where you are in a task, simple arithmetic and so on) that scales assessing only basic functions tap less well. At the opposite end of the scale of impairment, the Guy's Advanced Dementia Schedule (Ward et al 1993) examines the person's response to common objects, recording the amount of prompting required for the person to take, name and show the use of the object. This is a very useful further attempt to delineate the differences in function even between patients with the severest level of impairment.

There are advantages to this approach, particularly in as far as the person's capabilities are revealed, whereas in the ward/home setting opportunities for some skills might not be available or necessary. In developing an individual plan, such tests might be useful if they revealed more ability than shown normally, providing potential areas to encourage and work on. However, this possible discrepancy between daily life and test situation renders this approach less useful for monitoring changes in the ward or at home. Discrepancy between everyday and test performance is also possible where the structured situation fails to elicit the person's best performance, which may occur more easily in some cases in a natural setting. Comprehension difficulties could lead to this, as could anxiety and insufficient motivation. Reasons for failure need to be explored carefully; the person may not have grasped what they are intended to do or may be too anxious or apathetic to carry out the task correctly; alternatively, specific dysfunctions, particularly apraxias and agnosias, may obscure other areas of preserved ability.

These tests may be useful for selection of patients, establishing a dependency level and for monitoring of some programmes focusing on specific aspects of the person's functioning. They could be utilised alongside ratings of the person's functioning in the same areas in everyday life.

Direct observation—natural setting

This is where the patient's actual behaviour on the ward, old people's home or day-centre is observed and recorded. On the face of it, if the aim is to change the person's performance within this setting, this should be the assessment method. It has been used extensively with children and people with learning difficulties and to some extent in behavioural studies with the elderly.

Two initial issues concerning direct observation relate to producing manageable data from a potentially massive amount of observation. Firstly, some method of sampling the person's behaviour must be chosen. By time sampling, a snap-shot picture of the person's behaviour over a longer time period is obtained. Thus, observations might be made of the person every 3 minutes or every 10 minutes or every 30 minutes and so on, depending on the frequency of the behaviours being observed. A further decision must be taken as to whether to record over a short period (e.g. 10–30 seconds) all the behaviours the person exhibits, or only to record what is happening at the exact moment of sampling (see Murphy & Goodall (1980) for a discussion of the merits of these various options). If a very frequent discrete behaviour (smoking and shouting can be examples of this) is being observed, then all the occurrences in a certain time period (e.g. 15 or 30 minutes) might be counted at different times of the day.

The second issue is to decide on what areas of functioning to observe, and at what level of precision. Often social behaviours or other readily accessible areas are chosen. The range of precision extends from the relatively crude categorisation of a person's behaviour as 'engaged' or 'disengaged' to the level of fine analysis of behaviour, for example, recording the person's direction and duration of gaze.

Some complex problems can arise. Readers are referred to Hutt & Hutt (1970) for a full exposition of direct observation. If it is desired to monitor a range of behaviours, the problem of the observer having to use too long and detailed an observation schedule will have to be faced. If behaviours occur infrequently, say once or twice a day, then they may be missed entirely by most time-sampling methods; direct frequency counts are preferable here. The observer needs to fit unobtrusively into the surroundings, so that his/her influence on the patients' behaviour is minimised. An adaptation period is needed for staff as well as patients. Staff may either keep well clear or arrange special events, which bias the picture obtained. Behaviours to be observed need to be defined carefully, without ambiguity, and a second observer making observations simultaneously, but independently, is helpful in ensuring this has been achieved. Time sampling is easiest when all patients are together in one place and very difficult if they are scattered throughout a number of rooms.

The simpler the observation method used the more reliable results will be. Jenkins et al (1977) used the concept of 'engagement' in their study of activity in old people's homes. Residents are said to be engaged if they are interacting with people or materials; non-engaged if they are doing nothing; a detailed manual is available with full definitions. The method is to enter the room where patients are being observed, count the number of people who are engaged and then count the total number of people present. A percentage is then calculated of the proportion of those present who are engaged. This is then a group method, which may be useful where changes throughout the home or ward are being monitored. McFadyen et al (1980) and McFadyen (1984) have extended the method by recording engagement for individuals and by breaking the types of engagement and non-engagement down slightly. The definitions of Jenkins et al (1977) are given in such a way as to make this analysis quite straightforward. McFadyen et al made observations on each patient every half-hour over a $2\frac{1}{2}$ day period. They found greater than 90% inter-rater agreement on simultaneous observations of 20 patients. Other systems for observing activity and interaction have been described, for example, by Macdonald et al (1985). Bowie & Mountain (1993b) report a system using a hand-held computer, which allows accurate recording of the onset, relationship and duration of the seven categories of behaviour they identified; this obviates the need for time sampling, allows multiple behaviours to be recorded simultaneously and may allow easier analysis of the data obtained. However, the categorisation is fairly crude; for

example, it does not allow interactions with other residents to be distinguished from those with care-givers. A more detailed schedule covering a wider range of behaviour was used with people with severe dementia by Ward et al (1992), but the frequency of many behaviours (including behavioural disturbance) was so low that the procedure was felt not to be worthwhile in terms of the amount of time involved. However, in settings where there is more activity, a more detailed approach such as this might be of more use.

Observations that look only at engagement and interaction are reasonably manageable and can be useful in monitoring treatment programmes. For example, Head et al (1990) monitored the effects of a reminiscence group by direct observation of interactions in the group. Morton & Bleathman (1991) used a similar technique in evaluating the impact of their validation groups. It makes possible the monitoring of staff–patient interactions, which are the main vehicle for change in most positive approaches. The necessity for ensuring changes do occur at this level has already been emphasised. This method would enable elderly people to be identified who have low levels of engagement or social activity; the reason for this could then be explored. It has been suggested that engagement is an indication of the 'quality of life' in an institution; if this is so then this method could help to identify the need for environmental changes of every kind in institutions for the elderly and help to monitor them. Lindesay et al (1991) and Dean et al (1993a) have used Macdonald and co-workers' (1985) Short Observation Method to evaluate changes in activity and engagement associated with the development of 'domus' units, small special care units for people with dementia.

There has been a recognition that simply counting the number of interactions or measuring the level of activity is insufficient to ensure that the quality of the care environment has improved. Interactions can be devaluing, activities can be demeaning, and this must be reflected in our assessment. This has led to the development of direct observation methods that incorporate a value judgment regarding the care-giving inter-action, e.g. the Quality of Interactions Schedule (QUIS) (Dean et al 1993b) where interactions are rated as positive social, positive care, negative protective, negative restrictive or neutral; Dementia Care Mapping (DCM) (Kitwood 1992b, Kitwood & Bredin 1992) similarly is a direct observation method, where the person's activity and the care-value of what is happening (positive or negative) are recorded. In addition, in keeping with Kitwood's important emphasis on the personhood of the person with dementia (see Ch. 5), instances of the care given that detracts from this are noted. The method is intended to be part of a quality assurance cycle, with the results fed back to staff in order to help them improve the standard of care, and it is intended to have a strong subjective element, which may reduce its reliability as a measurement tool but not necessarily its utility as a vehicle for change (Wilkinson 1993). A slightly different approach is adopted by Adelson et al (1982) in their Health Professional–Geriatric Patient Interaction Behaviour Rating Code. Here the value judgment is embodied in the instrument, which involves rating factors deemed by experts to contribute towards a positive interacting style.

Direct observation can be a time-consuming method, producing a great deal of data that at times may simply seem to confirm an evident lack of activity and interaction; however, there can be few better ways of discovering what life is really like for the person with dementia than to take one step back, to look and to listen, as the extracts from the observer's diary, published by Bowie & Mountain (1993a) clearly illustrate.

ASSESSMENT OF THE PERSON'S AFFECTIVE STATE

So often, it seems that the last people to be asked about the effects of treatment programmes are the elderly people themselves. A very few studies of RO and reminiscence have included a measure of the effects of treatment on the person's feelings; Baines et al (1987) used a Life Satis-faction Index; Goldwasser et al (1987) used the Beck Depression Inventory. The difficulty with these and other similar measures is that they are based on the person's own responses to ques-tions about their mood and feelings. Their validity is doubtful in more severely demented patients, who may not be able to comprehend the self-report format or be able, in any case, to have a clear sense of their mood over time (Feher et al 1992).

For patients who are less deteriorated and can complete a brief questionnaire, a number of mood, morale and life-satisfaction scales are available. Gilleard et al (1981) and Woods & Britton (1985) review many of these.

An alternative strategy is for an observer to rate the person's apparent mood or level of depression. Katona & Aldridge (1985) describe such a scale, which has been widely used with people with dementia including those with a more severe impairment. It includes a number of features associated with low mood, although further work is still required to establish which are the best indicators; for example, poor appetite may be a good indicator of depression when there is no cognitive impairment, but there may be other factors in a person with severe dementia. Folstein (1991) reviews the use of rating scales for depression in cognitively impaired patients.

STAFF ATTITUDES AND ASSESSMENT OF THE INSTITUTION

It was thought that attitude changes had been measured successfully in earlier studies. How-ever, when an attempt was made to measure staff changes in attitude after training in the use of RO, using an adaptation of the Oberleder Attitude Scale (Oberleder 1962), Bailey et al (1986) found that the scale proved of little value despite the staff's agreement about improved morale.

This is one of the most difficult areas to assess and monitor. It may be possible to create an atmosphere for change (see Ch. 10), but to evaluate and monitor how this is achieved and maintained is a considerable challenge. Staff responses to attitude scales, where the expected 'positive' answer is fairly obvious, may not relate well to actual staff behaviour (Saxby & Jeffery 1983). Accordingly, the approach of some workers, such as Adelson et al (1982), has been to look for behavioural changes reflecting the underlying attitude. Direct observation of care-giving interactions is becoming the primary method of assessing the staff approach.

Environmental rating scales, such as the MEAP (see p. 113) do throw light on some aspects to the extent that they look in depth at the en-forcement of rules, policies and practices in institutions. The degree of tolerance and leeway allowed to residents can be estimated. MEAP provides some indication of a particular insti-tution's concern for its staff, but it does not throw light on their feelings, their conception of their role, how they spend their time, where priorities lie or on factors such as attitudes to age or job satisfaction (although the last area is included in the scales used by Willcocks et al (1987)).

Most training centres are becoming increasingly aware of the problems of staff 'burn-out' (Quattrochi-Tubin et al 1982). The implications of this state of exhaustion and demoralisation are obvious and probably most common in isolated, unsupported homes and hospitals where encouragement, relief, staff and resources are at a minimum. Staff turnover and sickness rates will be high. It is probably even more common with caring relatives, alone in what can be a demanding and stressful situation. However, the concern may well lead to improved assess-ment procedures for morale and job satisfaction in the near future. A number of scales evalu-ating stress and strain in carers are already available (Greene et al 1982, Gilleard 1984c, Morris et al 1988).

The environment, as discussed in Chapter 7, plays an essential role in influencing indepen-dence, stimulation levels, maintenance of personal identity and needs. An environment in which a person can exercise no control will encourage institutionalisation. It, therefore, becomes im-portant to be able to evaluate an environment, and the questions of how this can be done, what should be examined and how changes can be monitored all require an answer. It is necessary to look at both the physical and psychological environments in order to obtain as full a picture as possible.

Psychological environment

Here we would be assessing level of activity, the degree of choice, interaction between client and client, and client and staff and considering the amount of engagement. Meeting individual needs, privacy, preservation of dignity and self-respect, retained abilities that are being used, help being available when required and the en-couragement to achieve goals are all areas which are too rarely assessed. Some could be covered by life satisfaction indices, but such ratings require a greater ability to judge, respond and be critical than most people with dementia retain. The direct observation methods mentioned above could be relevant, employing an individual re-cording system and breaking down the definitions of engagement into the component parts of self-care, social activities and the inter-actions between clients and between staff and clients. Using such methods, it is possible to obtain some insight into the quality of life provided, but there are many aspects about which more should be known. In measuring activity levels, for example, it is also important to know the amount of choice residents have; are they allowed *not* to participate! How relevant are the activities to the person's interests? How much does each person value the activities in which he or she takes part? Similarly, with interaction, *quality* is as important as *quantity*. Thus, the development of direct observation systems—such as Dementia Care Mapping—that make judg-ments regarding the quality of the care-giving interaction is particularly important.

Another approach is that adopted by Ager (1990) in the Life Experiences Checklist. Here, someone who knows the person well identifies to what extent the person takes part in a variety of situations and roles that are often valued in ordinary life, in several domains. The person's scores may be compared with those of the popu-lation at large, to identify to what extent the environment allows the person to live as normal a life as possible.

Several of the environmental assessment procedures now available do assess aspects of the psychological environment: collecting data through interviews with staff and managers and observation. For example, the scales developed by Bowie et al (1992) include one focused on the restrictiveness of the ward environment; Willcocks et al (1987) have scales indicating the degree to which the setting is resident-orientated rather than organised around the staff, and the amount of choice, privacy and involvement offered to residents. Inevitably most assessments pay little attention to what goes on outside of the daytime. The Night Scale (Holden 1991) does recognise the importance of privacy and normal routines later in the day and overnight. Noise levels, lights on all night and the lack of personalised bed areas are factors which may disturb an individual unused to invasion of normal privacy; the habitual routines of putting out the cat, checking the doors, having a bath at a set time and having a particular bedtime drink can all be lost in an environment with different rules from those to which the person is accustomed.

Physical environment

The effects an environment can have on an individual have been recognised for many years, and various attempts have been made to develop checklists to evaluate whether the architecture and internal layout provide relevant facilities and meet reasonable standards. In recent years, there has been an increase of interest in this area, particularly for people with learning difficulties and elderly people. Lemke and Moos (1980, 1986) have developed the Multiphasic Environmental Assessment Procedure (MEAP) for the elderly (Moos & Lemke 1980). Although standardised in the USA, it has been used in several British studies (e.g. Benjamin & Spector 1990, Netten 1993, Dean et al 1993a). The environment is broken down into five specific areas, each part forming a sub-scale of its own. Each of these parts can be assessed and scored separately, with a total score to provide an overall picture. The MEAP covers architectural and physical features of the building and surroundings; the policies and programmes; information about staff and clients; as a rating scale, which is useful in

that it covers the living environment in detail and looks carefully at the grooming of the clients, their clothing and activity levels, at staff interaction with them, and it also examines organisation and possible conflicts. The Sheltered Care Environment Scale forms the final part. This is in a simple 'yes' and 'no' format designed to be completed by both staff and patients. It is open to the criticism that the 'right' answer is obvious to staff, and clients may respond with caution, doubt or may not even understand or be capable of completing it.

The whole MEAP takes an age to complete! However, components of it can be used separately. At times it poses problems as to who is responsible for completing it. It takes a careful and thorough investigator to obtain valid responses. Undoubtedly, it provides a very useful overview and can highlight problem areas. It has especial value in comparisons between units, in setting up new centres and in finding targets for change. Additionally, it provides a system for re-evaluation. It is, of course, impossible to change or improve everything—buildings are hard to move and additions are sometimes hard to supply! An old unit can be modernised, but the fabric will be the same.

When examining the MEAP in detail there are many omissions—despite its length—and, for many, the time required to complete it is daunting. A shorter version which could be used as a screening device for most institutions or units was devised by Holden (1984c). The Orientation Facilities Checklist (ORIF) concentrates on some of the more salient features of internal planning, sensory stimulation and facilities to encourage independence. It is divided into two parts: architectural and sensory stimulation. Each part has 20 questions which are scored on a four-point scale. As with the MEAP, each sub-scale has its own score and the combined scores provide an overall picture. An old setting may score low on the architectural aspects, but may be active and stimulating; the converse is also possible. The ORIF has been used in practice to good effect. Bailey et al (1986) showed that despite the age of the hospital unit, the changes made by the staff to the environment were clearly demonstrated by changes in the scores on the ORIF. In looking at residential homes and hospital wards, it is designed to draw attention to areas which could be improved and to monitor changes taking place.

Other scales which have been inspired by and adapted from the MEAP include those developed by Willcocks et al (1987) and Bowie et al (1992). The former were used in a national study of 100 residential homes for the elderly and produce a profile of the physical and psychological environment that can be compared with the 'average' home for elderly people. The latter study produced scales from evaluations of long-term care-wards in a hospital setting and include consideration of the extent of provision of RO aids and other facilities for social recreation. Netten (1993) has looked further at the influence of the complexity of the physical environment on the difficulty the person with dementia experiences in finding his/her way around the residential home environment.

Measures of the environment can provide a guide as to what to change and the success of change, can help to define the type of institution in reports of research studies and can, perhaps, clarify some of the conflicting results obtained in studies, which may be related to differences in institutional structure, policy and priorities.

CONCLUSION

In the use of assessments, it cannot be stressed too much that to employ any test requires that the examiner should have the individual, as a whole person, in mind. Anything which causes distress or is irrelevant is of little value and of a doubtful ethical standard. The person's needs, wishes, strengths and weaknesses are of prime importance. Not only is the individual to be considered, but also there should be investigation of those aspects of living which can affect his or her ability to live and function at an optimum level. So the people around, the staff and the relatives must be involved in the assessment, and the environment must be carefully observed and evaluated. The needs and feelings of those closely involved should also be considered. There are still several areas for which there is a dearth of appropriate measures—attitudes, for instance. There is an increasing awareness of the gaps in knowledge and much work has been done and is continuing to be done to improve our pool of information and resources.

7

The basic approach to the person with dementia

There is great beauty in old trees
Old streets and ruins old.
Why should not I as well as these
Grow lovely growing old.
                    (Seen in old churchyard in Cornwall)

POSITIVE INTERACTION

For most people with dementia, the greatest scope for enhancing the person's sense of well-being arises from the communication and interaction shared with those providing care. Developing ways of interacting positively with people with dementia is an important task. In essence, the methods are simple, obvious and practised automatically by many caring people, and so there is no reason, in principle, why everyone in contact with the person with dementia should not be part of this system of positive interaction. In this chapter the practical aspects of communicating with elderly people with dementia will be discussed. The approach described here has its roots in the informal, or 24 hour, component of reality orientation, but it should be emphasised that the primary aim here is to communicate and interact, rather than to orientate at the outset. This communication is a two-way process, requiring *listening* and *responding* as well as putting across what we want to say; in our experience, it is the listening aspect which is the most demanding and challenging, requiring just as much active concentration as the other aspects. In addition, this approach demands certain environmental changes, which will be described in this chapter together with techniques for making the most of the person's learning potential, however limited this may be.

It is likely that difficulty in communicating with elderly people with dementia is one factor in the frequent reactions of distaste, repugnance and rejection that occur in younger people faced with working with them. (The barriers to easy communication may be many; some, at least, are potentially soluble. If they can be overcome then care-providers will find their work more satisfying and enjoyable, and patients will feel less rejected, frustrated and distressed.)

Sensory deficits

The normal process of loss of acuity provides difficulties for staff, relatives and friends, as well as for those involved in the actual loss. Eyesight is not as keen, nor often is hearing. The skin is less elastic so gesture is limited. Ageing bones, joints and muscles cause a decrease in mobility, so fluency of action and movement change. As a result, social contact and communication change (Bromley 1978). Because they do not hear, see or move as easily as in earlier years, elderly people are often less aware of events occurring around them. A nurse can appear on the ward before breakfast and her general, cheerful 'Good morning' will elicit no response. Quite naturally she may feel upset and rejected. The patients may wonder why she becomes less friendly and helpful. A serious misunderstanding has occurred! The nurse was too far away, too impersonal and spoke too quickly and quietly. Even when standing fairly close to an individual, a greeting or question may not be observed. If relatives mistake this lack of response for mental deterioration they begin to talk to each other as though their ageing parent was not present. The reaction of many patients in such a situation is withdrawal. Another misunderstanding!

Severe sensory loss is easier for staff and relatives to accept and understand; efforts are always made to help the very deaf and blind. The normal loss of sensory acuity, coupled parti-cularly with any form of infirmity, is often overlooked. The attitudes of others caused by unawareness of the situation can lead to withdrawal, which together with sensory loss has serious psychological implications.

In Chapter 2, the possible role of sensory deprivation in increasing the degree of confusion in elderly people was discussed. Sensory deprivation is the loss of sensory input for any reason; loss of sensory acuity and withdrawal are two ways by which a person's sensory stimulation may be reduced.

Other processes by which withdrawal may be related to loss of acuity are probably common. First, some patients may feel embarrassed about their failing senses, and suffer loss of self-esteem. A reaction to this may be to cut off from potentially embarrassing social situations. Secondly, some environments for elderly people may lack interest for particular patients; if they have a loss of sensory acuity, 'shutting off' the unpleasant, boring situation is easy. Even where there is more interest, the amount of effort required to maintain attention when hearing or sight are impaired, even slightly, is often not appreciated; the person becomes fatigued and 'switches off' much more quickly than would otherwise be the case. In each instance further sensory deprivation, and probably increased confusion, will result.

To combat these problems, the barriers to communication should be attacked. Eyesight and hearing should be tested. When aids are required they should be used and checked regularly. Dentures should fit well, be comfortable and in their owner's mouth not in a glass or box! Thus the person's sensory and speech functions are aided as far as possible. Environmental help is also needed: lighting should be bright (but not glaring), extraneous noises damped down to a minimum. Staff need to remember that conversation should be at close range. It is better to be beneath the older person than to speak looking down at him. Slow, clearly enunciated speech is more appropriate than most quick-fire remarks. Shouting is usually unnecessary; clarity is more important. Ensure you have the person's attention before launching into the message you want to get across.

To avoid sensory deprivation, as many of the senses as possible should be stimulated in conversation; the person is encouraged to feel objects, smell them, and taste them where appropriate. Particularly where one of the senses is impaired, this sensory enrichment of the more intact senses is crucial in helping the person keep in touch with his or her surroundings.

Non-verbal communication

Non-verbal communication, or 'body language', is important in facilitating interaction. To join in a conversation, people will move forward, or move away if they wish to escape. Gestures are vital in some cultures and have their place in every language. Not only limbs, but eyes, eyebrows, lips and the head can be used to express emotions, reactions and other messages. Close relationships have their own private system which is completely meaningless to outsiders. The movement of an eyebrow can mean anything from 'That's good' to 'Let's go' or, 'What a funny man'. Eye contact can be used to encourage the shy, to embarrass or to console someone; it can imply concentration or interest or many other factors depending on individual ability and expressiveness.

Elderly people with sensory loss will be less sensitive to non-verbal communication; in normal conversation many of the signals given are subtle and easily missed if eyesight or hearing is impaired. Staff need then to make their non-verbal messages slightly more clear-cut than usual. Thus, a slow approach from in front of the patient is less likely to be misinterpreted as aggressive than suddenly appearing at the patient's side from behind. In face-to-face contact, a warm smile expresses friendliness; eye contact expresses the staff member's desire to interact and is useful in gaining and maintaining attention. Many (but not all) people will respond to the use of gentle touch, a hand over the other's hand, a reassuring arm around the person's shoulders. These and other gestures are warm, reassuring and imply concern and friendship; touch is also helpful in attracting and keeping the person's interest and concentration. If the nurse, by these means, appears to the patient as calm, warm and friendly, then the patient is more likely to respond and be relaxed and reassured. The nurse's aim is not to put on an act, but rather to express clearly, minimising the danger of misunderstanding, whatever he or she is trying to communicate. Remember that, although you may have known the person for some time, to them you may appear almost a complete stranger; with severe memory problems, the person may be living in a world where first impressions of people appear to be all they have to work from in making sense of what is happening around them. Body language is the key to the formation of our first impressions of other people; from our own experience, we appreciate it can often be misleading, as we get to know people better, below the surface. The person with dementia is less able to go readily beyond the surface 'here and now' level, and so the need for clear, accurate non-verbal expression from care-providers is all the greater. Ultimately, it can make all the difference between being perceived as a threat or a source of danger rather than as a possible source of support and safety; a grim-faced, brisk, stiff advance as opposed to an easy-paced, relaxed, smiling approach.

In listening to elderly people, attention must be given to the messages they give non-verbally, as well as to what they say. Here it must be remembered that the ability of elderly people to give out messages may be impaired as well as their capacity to receive them. This is caused by the decrease in mobility and dexterity mentioned above. However, as will be discussed later, the signals that are given can be important in making some sense of what the person says. It may take a little longer for the non-verbal signal to appear or to sink in—good reasons for adapting the pace of the interaction to the individual's speed. If the person seems to be having difficulty following what you are saying,

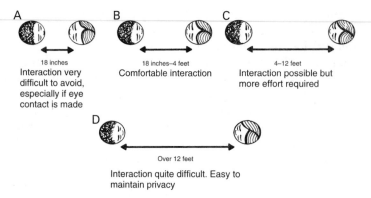

Figure 7.1   Effects on interaction of interpersonal distance.

slow down, give time for what you are saying to be processed and understood.

Personal distance

The distance between people affects interaction to some extent. This varies from culture to culture, from situation to situation and from person to person. Generally, total attention is required at a distance of about 18 inches; at 4 feet some communication is indicated and a distance of up to 12 feet still provides the possibilities of social interaction. Over 12 feet allows for public space, so it is possible to sit in a park, or on the beach or in a waiting-room and maintain privacy even in a crowd (Fig. 7.1). Sometimes, however, distance cannot be controlled and difficulties arise; for example, in a crowded lift or train, passengers maintain social distance by studiously avoiding eye contact. It can be difficult to cope with sharing the most personal zone of physical proximity with complete strangers.

Problems caused by the need to manipulate distance are fairly common. For instance, the train is late, the station is very cold; to the relief of the passenger there is a fire in the waiting-room. Before rushing to the only available seat, the passenger notices that it is adjacent to one occupied by an undesirable, objectionable being. The need for warmth is greater than scruples, but precautions are essential. Non-verbal communication provides the answer. A newspaper

is raised, a shoulder is turned to cut off direct view and any form of self-sufficiency is employed to illustrate the wish to preserve anonymity. How different the situation would be if both persons were attractive!

Elderly people can be lonely even in a residential home; the lounge can be like a waiting-room, with little interaction occurring and residents remaining strangers to each other. Staff need to bear in mind that some chair arrangements help and others hinder social interaction (see Ch. 2). It is difficult to converse side-by-side, it is much more comfortable to be facing the person (Fig. 7.2). A lounge with many people in it will inhibit interaction; it is difficult enough for younger people to get to know 25 or more people at once; the problem is immense for the person with memory problems whose awareness and recognition of others grows very slowly indeed. A smaller group will help the development of relationships and interaction, particularly if there are common interests and a shared task or activity. In this situation staff–resident interactions are made easier and more natural than when residents are dependent on staff for most opportunities for conversation. Staff do not have to search for topics of conversation as they are provided for them by what is happening in the group. This does not imply that all homes with large lounges have to be rebuilt; it is possible with room dividers, partitions and careful furniture arrangement to achieve a great deal in encouraging the development of

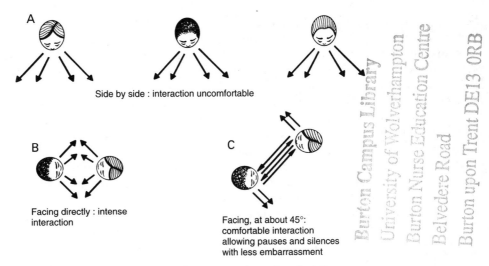

Figure 7.2   Effects on interaction of interpersonal angular orientation.

small groups (see Ch. 2 for references on and more details of the group-living concept). A number of practical steps can be recommended to aid communication:

- correct sensory deficits
- speak clearly
- use all the senses
- use eye contact and touch to gain and hold the person's attention
- be aware of the messages in your own and the person's body language
- arrange furniture to assist conversation
- reduce size of groups
- do not rush the person; slow down communication to suit his pace.

The whole person—basic attitudes

Far too often the need to treat the whole person is forgotten. Treatment programmes, either at home or in care, provide for the physical needs but ignore psychological and emotional needs. Staff attitudes need to develop certain aspects of the whole person:

- individuality as an adult
- dignity
- self-respect
- choice
- independence.

These attitudes underlie any positive approach. Without them any approach will fail at a human and emotional level.

Individuality

On hospital wards, individuals can become medical diagnoses and the physical cure pursued vigorously. It is as if the identity of the person is forgotten. The patient in bed 4 becomes a broken femur, the occupant of bed 10 a heart condition, instead of Mrs Anne Brown or Mr Peter White with their personal concerns relating to their rent, their possessions, their families or their own individual personalities. The use of the nursing process, with its emphasis on careful individual assessment, can help to ensure that patients are persons in their own right. If the staff, family and friends know how to communicate they will know more about the whole person and be able to meet his or her individual needs.

Elderly people have had longer to develop and perhaps are more different from each other than younger people. Their psychological needs can only be heeded if they are seen and treated as individuals. They have had adult status for 50 or 60 years or more; to be then treated as a child will be potentially deeply upsetting. Even elderly people who are extremely impaired may have an awareness at some level beyond that which they are capable of expressing. Interaction should then be attempted at an adult–adult level, however child-like the response may seem. Where it is obtainable, information about the person's background can illuminate present functioning and even help to make more sense of apparently random behaviour. Attempting to write a brief biography of the person can be a useful aid here. Compiling a scrapbook about the important experiences, events and people of the person's life, with the help of relatives as well as the person's own reminiscences, is a marvellous way of really getting to know the whole person.

Dignity and respect

Preservation of dignity and respect play a major role in assisting elderly people to cope with their problems. To lose independence suddenly as a result of hospitalisation or by being placed in a home is disturbing in itself. When dignity is further upset by total strangers, presuming (for instance) to use familiar first names, status is lost and self-esteem jeopardised. Some people do prefer to be addressed by their first names, but some do not. For example, a retired surgeon was taken ill and admitted to hospital where he became confused and difficult overnight. It was noticed that the staff were addressing him as 'Joey'; he was completely bewildered by a situation of unprecedented equality, as surgeons of the 'old school' were notorious for their concern for personal dignity and aloofness. Once the staff began to call him 'Sir' he promptly regained his composure: within a few days he began to order everyone about in his customary manner and was quickly discharged!

Similarly, a lady in her 80s was called 'Lavinia' by the staff. The younger nurses arranged her hair in pigtails and tied it up in pink ribbons. Until shortly before her illness she had been a very independent, arrogant spinster and a much feared and respected Justice of the Peace. In hospital she began by preserving her authoritarian demeanour but slowly lost her ability to dominate the scene. She stopped thinking for herself, lost independence, deteriorated into a confused, institutionalised, child-like waif and simply faded away.

There are innumerable situations in which dignity and self-respect can be stripped from a person, often by lack of thought. Examples are talking about a person in their presence as if they were not there ('she doesn't understand'); leaving toilet doors open while occupied; doing something to a person (combing their hair, lifting them and so on) without first explaining to the person what is about to happen. The reader will be able to add many more instances; in short, any situations where the person is to some extent made to feel small, worthless or is humiliated are to be avoided.

Dignity and respect *can* be maintained. The individual's experience, standing in the community, achievements, and knowledge of the past are all aspects that can be used to retain his or her self-esteem. Explanations of what is happening, or will happen, are necessary. Day-to-day events, from the immediate environment or from national and international news, should be discussed. A concern for privacy, personal likes and dislikes shows courtesy which is appreciated by all age groups and preserves self-respect. Politeness is noted and invariably merits a response, particularly from people who grew up in a culture which valued good manners.

The attitude involved here might at first glance be characterised as behaving as if the person were not impaired at all, as if the memory and behaviour problems did not exist. In fact, the approach is, first, to treat the person with dementia as a *person* and to recognise that because of this, dignity, respect, individuality and so on remain important. Secondly, however, the person must be accepted as he or she is now. This involves recognition of current limitations, but to see these as a starting point, as being possibly modifiable and not necessarily fixed. By doing this, expectations and demands can be sensitively set at a level which does not place the person in a position of failure, whilst at the same time they may be gradually increased if and when the person's functioning improves. Failure is avoided, as it leads to loss of self-respect, particularly when the tasks involved are still perceived as extremely simple. The avoidance of failure is not to be the passive 'if I don't do anything at all I can't possibly fail' variety. It is instead an active avoidance where those areas in which the person can succeed are emphasised. Too often the presence of dementia is unnecessarily demonstrated and made obvious by the use of direct questioning of memory, rather than allowing the patient to succeed by the skilful use of cues and prompts.

In summary, allowing dignity and self-respect is not achieved by pretending that any dementia is absent when it clearly is not; it is achieved by removing the focus from the disability onto preserved areas of functioning. This is, of course, exactly what happens with physical disabilities, and the same should apply to cognitive disabilities also.

Choice

Two further related aspects of the *whole person* need to be discussed, particularly in relation to the elderly person in institutional care. The first is choice; it is only too easy to remove choice and to place elderly people in a situation where they have little control over even the small—but nonetheless significant—features of daily living. For example, a cup of tea may be provided at breakfast-time when the patient had always been accustomed to coffee, or clothes may be laid out for the patient without any consultation about the selection. Complete freedom of choice is of, course, available to hardly anyone. In a communal setting inevitably there are restrictions; the approach here is to identify what choices can be made available and to present these to elderly patients. Encouragement may be needed to help them make their own choices, especially when they have become apathetic and accustomed to the staff deciding. This is an important part of being an adult, dignified, self-respecting individual. Choices need to be presented in a clear, tangible way, that does not overwhelm the person, bearing in mind the limitations on memory span. Thus, a choice between two meals which the person can see and smell might be more readily made than a much bigger choice from a menu card some time before the meal. Or two or three items of clothing might be offered for the person to choose from, rather than the choice being presented in a question, such as 'what would you like to wear today?', which relies on the person's ability to recall the contents of their wardrobe.

Independence

The final aspect to be encouraged and developed is independence. Again, no-one is ever truly independent; we are all interdependent to a greater or lesser degree, and, inevitably, in communal settings particularly it is more difficult to be less dependent on other people. Once more though, many instances occur of patients being more dependent on staff than is necessary; thus patients are sometimes completely dressed by staff for the sake of speed when the patient can manage slowly with much less help; or sugar is put in the patient's tea when they are capable of adding it themselves. Self-help is important to a patient's self-esteem; the success of doing something for oneself, albeit slowly, can be rewarding. Interdependence was mentioned above; a neglected aspect of the whole person is often the extent to which they can do things for other people, i.e. the extent to which other people can be dependent on the patient. By helping the patient to have a meaningful role, be it clearing the table, sweeping up, telling a story about the past, singing a song or whatever is appropriate and possible, again the patient's self-esteem is built up.

Privacy

The option of having privacy must be provided also. Hospitals and homes need to allow some space for privacy, plus the necessary arrangements to ensure it. Screens or curtains, the ability to display some personal items, personalisation of clothing, storage, thinking and entertaining space are vital to the quality of life.

It is no easy task to apply these attitudes. For instance, providing basic physical nursing care for a severely impaired person that preserves real dignity calls for a high level of skill, consideration and creativity. Using these aspects of the whole person as a yardstick to look at and evaluate our own practice will help in developing such qualities. Kitwood & Bredin (1992) provide many useful examples of how common care situations can enhance the person's well-being, rather than being experienced as devaluing and detracting from personhood, depending on the care-provider's approach.

These attitudes are a central feature of the normalisation approach, which is being applied increasingly in relation to other disabilities. This involves allowing the person access to experiences and lifestyles valued in society. Thus, a physically disabled person would work at a conventional job, despite being confined to a wheelchair; they might drive to work in a specially adapted (but otherwise conventional) car and live in an ordinary (but adapted) house. This is in contrast to a person living in an institution with other physically disabled people, driving an invalid carriage and working in a workshop for the disabled. Similarly, people with a learning difficulty are increasingly integrated into 'normal' society, rather than being placed out of sight and out of mind in a large country hospital.

We saw in Chapter 1 that 'normal' for elderly people is largely a continuation of previous patterns of living. If we apply this to the person with dementia, the implication is that independence in self-care should be encouraged. Previous activities and interests, social, recreational, domestic, occupational, etc, adapted where necessary, should be facilitated. Adaptations to the person's living arrangements so that previous lifestyles can be continued are entailed.

It is, of course, quality of life that is the prime concern. This rather nebulous concept in this context could be assessed by the extent to which the person's lifestyle can continue despite the dementia, memory difficulties and so on. If this seems a far cry from the average long-stay ward, the normalisation principle does have its implications there also. Personalised, rather than shared, clothing; choice of food from a menu; space for personal possessions; choice of activities and so on all help to form the fabric of an existence comprising more that is valued and generally agreed to be desirable.

Three commonly quoted implications of the normalisation approach (e.g. Woods 1987) are:

• People with dementia should be accorded full respect and dignity as people with human worth and rights.
• People with dementia should be treated appropriately to their actual age.
• People with dementia should be helped to participate in good social relationships in the ordinary community.

The first of these is clearly embodied in the attitudes discussed above. The second is an important consideration in selecting activities, recreational materials, etc, though, as Woods & Britton (1985, p. 273) discuss, this can be a complex issue. It is important to define 'age-appropriate' without accepting the devalued conception of elderly people and their activities prevalent in society. We should be guided by what was valued by each individual over their lifespan, rather than by what is seen as the 'norm' for elderly people. Attaining the third implication may be aided by the growth of positive approaches emphasising the assets, strengths and resources of the person rather than his weaknesses and deficits.

COMMUNICATION—CONTENT

Having covered barriers to communication, non-verbal communication and the attitudes underlying communication, the next section considers much more the content and form of communication with the elderly person. It is what the staff member actually says that is to be considered here. The guidelines are summarised in Box 7.1.

Presentation of communication

The aim is for each interaction that the elderly person has to be viewed as an opportunity for positive input, to help the person keep track of what is happening, as well as to help the person to experience a sense of being valued and respected. There are numerous opportunities during the day when even a short contact between the care-provider and the older person can be used to advantage. Waking people up, helping them to the toilet, serving meals are all natural situations for conversation.

Simple methods of varying the presentation of similar material—to allow it to be absorbed without undue repetition—and attention to everyday, simple matters such as the weather, the day and the month, and the time encourage awareness in the elderly person. This can be done by drawing attention to what is happening indoors and outside the window; all the senses can be involved, as for instance by remarking on the lovely smell of breakfast or the feel of cold hands just come in from the snow.

Some examples of simple interactions are as follows.

Hello, Mrs Smith; this place? It's called—Hospital; . . . yes, that's right—Hospital.
Mr Green, it's 12 o'clock now; time for lunch; that's right, the dining room is through that door there.
Your bath is ready for you, Mr Brown. Take off your jacket, then your shirt . . . ; when you've finished undressing, there's a nice hot bath for you.
My name is Jean; . . . yes, Jean. I'm a new nurse here at—Hospital. May I ask your name? . . . I'm pleased to meet you, Mr White. Have you seen what an awful day it is today? Come and look out the window . . . Yes, it's pouring with rain; I suppose we can't expect good weather in November. It's good to be indoors today. At least—Hospital is warm and dry, isn't it?

Note the frequent use of names (patients and staff) and the relatively short, simple statements and questions, which are intended to encourage a response, repetition wherever possible, and conversation aimed at *not* making the person fail. Opportunities for repetition are needed to enable the person with memory difficulties to process more fully what is happening and to give the opportunity for increased contact with their surroundings. Repetition should be disguised by varying its form, to avoid what is being said coming across as patronising.

There is a need to be aware of a short attention span or wavering concentration. In order to hold attention, a number of related items which stimulate the senses are useful. For example, when waking Mr Smith in the morning, one may say 'Good morning Mr Smith; it's eight o'clock, time to be getting up for breakfast'. After a short time a further comment on the time can be followed by 'Have you looked out the window yet? It is really spring-like today, the sun is out and it's quite warm for March.'

At breakfast this can be repeated, 'Look, we've daffodils on the table. It's almost spring, don't they smell nice?' Later in the day, the calendar can be pointed out, the day and the month indicated and further reference to spring can be made. Repeated presentation of information may sound like a broken record to staff, but to the person with memory problems it may be only vaguely familiar!

Communicating through reminiscence

The use of past experiences in comparison with the happenings of today allows reminiscence to play a vital role in a conversation (Fig. 7.3).

Elderly people know more about the past than their children or care-staff. To capitalise on their experience helps to provide an opening to talk about the present. Older people are aware of their superior knowledge and do not feel threatened by a possible exposure of inadequacies.

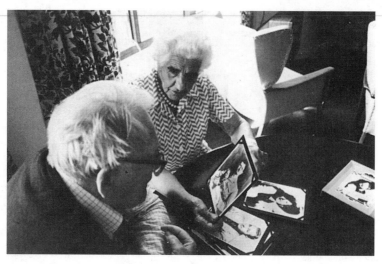

Figure 7.3   Using reminiscence as a means of developing communication.

Past experiences may be used to help the person become more aware of the present—contrasts and similarities can be emphasised. When talking about past events, a sense of perspective may be retained by the use of past tenses of verbs and so on, distinguishing the events from current reality. For example: 'You used to work in a coal mine didn't you, Mr Green?' or 'Before you came into hospital, you had lived in South Avenue for 30 years, hadn't you, Mr Brown?' One aspect of disorientation for time is that the person may have lost track of where in their life they are—Are they at school? Should they be at work? Where are the children? Gently helping the person keep track of the passage of the years can be helpful in reducing this type of disorientation.

Focusing communication

One difficulty in communicating with an elderly person suffering from some loss of memory function is the frequency of 'crossed wires' in a conversation. The staff member is continuing on one subject, the patient drifts on to another, perhaps related topic, until the two diverge completely. The problem of many conversations is that they rely on memory of the words that have just been spoken a few sentences ago; this is very difficult for most patients with dementia. A way around this is to have a focus for the conversation. Words are spoken and then have gone, but if both the participants in the conversation have their attention on something specific—a picture, an object, an odour, a view from the window, etc—then it is more likely that the patient will remain on the same topic as the staff member. Although inevitably there will be some repetition, at least both parties will be talking about the same thing! Avoidance of vagueness by the staff will also aid communication. Everyday contacts that are specific and concrete will be particularly valuable.

If a discussion of current events arose and one aspect, for example the prime minister, was chosen for discussion, rather than simply using words, relevant items could be employed as a focus. A picture, television programme or a book about him or her would help. If the time of day is the subject, a clock or a watch could be used. Conversations about relatives can be facilitated by the use of photographs from the past and present. Without such references the person could be talking about his/her daughter aged 3, but the staff could be discussing the 50-year-old lady whom they meet regularly!

Humour

Humour is to be encouraged. Laughing *with* the elderly person and never permitting the person to feel that he/she is being laughed *at* are vital aspects. Humour breaks the ice, helps the patient to relax and perhaps, makes it easier to cope with the reality of disability and impairment. No examples can be given, as what is funny depends on the situation, the people concerned and the timing. Its occurrence is a positive sign, especially when patients begin to initiate the humour and make gentle fun of the staff!

Conversation does not have to concentrate on major events; a straightforward comment on the day's happenings, however mundane they may seem, is important for the person who is having difficulty keeping in touch with reality. Physical care need never be given silently. Even if the patient is withdrawn and unresponsive, the nurse can still talk about what is happening. It is not a rare occurrence to see two people attending an old person and talking to each other as though there was no third party present. 'I was at a party the other night. The band was great'. The friend will ask 'What were they called?' The discussion will continue as a duet. The older member of the trio could be included quite simply by enquiring 'What kinds of music do you enjoy?', or whatever may be appropriate to extend the conversation. Normal conversation is not impossible!

To an extent what we are talking about here is normal, social behaviour, and the right of an elderly person living at home or in a care setting to be treated on equal terms. The fact is that older people generally are not treated equally, and accounts of younger people skilfully made up to look old who experience much less help and courtesy in carrying out normal daily tasks, such as shopping, boarding a bus, etc, confirm this powerfully. If this is how older people are treated 'normally', then how much worse the situation may be where confusion and impairment are also present. If all staff and visitors are encouraged to show courtesy and have the person's dignity in mind, then patients' well-learned social skills may re-emerge and they will function closer to their optimal level. The volunteers who bring the flowers to the wards could make sure that the residents see the arrangements and touch and smell them instead of simply placing them on a windowsill or an out-of-the-way table. Flowers are beautiful, colourful, seasonal and smell delightfully. These qualities should be remarked upon and appreciated. Senior staff should watch the attitudes of regularly visiting services, for example barbers, hairdressers and others, to ensure that dignity, choice and independence are preserved. No man should be shaved without being first consulted, and if he is being shaved he should be treated like any other customer and not as an object. Similarly relatives and junior staff need to be encouraged to include the elderly patients in their conversations.

Encouraging success

Finally, helping the person succeed is a major aim. In normal conversation, questions are often asked to draw a person into talking and to elicit a response. If a question is asked of a person with dementia and that person cannot answer, the disability will be exposed. Prompts should be given so that the patient is able to respond and join in the conversation. The amount of prompting and clues needed depends on the person; just sufficient to produce the response should be given. Answers can often be given in the original question, e.g. instead of asking 'What's the weather like today?', the staff member might say 'What a lot of wet, showery days we're having.' In other situations, it is appropriate to give the first few letters of the answer. For example, if conversing about a record, the younger person might ask 'Who's that singing? Isn't that Bing something—I think it begins with C . . . Yes, of course, Bing Crosby. What was that famous song of his, remind me, wasn't it White something or other . . . ?'

In this way, memories may be reawakened, the older person being unable to recall them freely without this help from the younger one. Often information is remembered by the elderly to some extent, but they are unable to recall it fully, or the memory is slightly vague. Therefore, many elderly patients are, for example, unable to name the current prime minister, but some recall the name if a special clue is given, or by using letters from the name, perhaps even by giving the first name. By using clues and prompts sensitively, the elderly patient's limited memory can be used to the fullest extent.

Night-time confusion is well known. A calm response full of simple, reassuring information is helpful. A statement such as 'Mr Jones, it's three in the morning. Look it's dark, everyone is asleep. What's wrong, couldn't you see the clock?' will help him to reorganise his thoughts without exposing his genuine confusion. Restoration of the missing information will assist his self-confidence and calm him. The effect of waking up in the dark on an elderly person with impaired functions may be compared to regaining consciousness after an anaesthetic when even personal identity is lost and short-lived total disorientation occurs. By providing the person with information, without questions which might expose the areas of difficulty and thus cause loss of face, confidence in the self and in the other person is restored.

Handling confused and rambling talk

People with dementia often talk in a way that does not make immediate sense to the listener. A person may chatter away talking apparent nonsense about where he is and what he is doing, or may seem to live in the past. 'Oh, I just baked a lovely tea for this picnic. We're in the park I used to play in as a child. That's my sister over there eating chicken.' This kind of statement is commonly heard in the midst of a ward and possibly in the midst of winter. The only thing in keeping with reality may be the fact that it is mealtime. Rambling talk like this shows that the person is mixing past events, experiences and present events indiscriminately. Sometimes it is described as 'confabulation', implying the person is inventing more or less plausible responses to the demands of the situation. Reactions can include impatience or sharp correction, acceptance of the remark as

indicative of a dementing mind, or agreements with the incorrect statement to 'humour' the elderly person.

It is sometimes thought that the RO approach always involves 'putting the person right', correcting the person in line with the staff member's view of reality. The important principle is to never agree with apparently confused talk; after this there is a choice of strategies depending on the person and the situation.

Do not agree with rambling and confused talk; instead:
- tactfully disagree (on less sensitive topics) *or*
- change the subject, discuss something concrete *or*
- acknowledge the feelings expressed but ignore the content.

The sensible use of tenses when responding to a statement such as 'I am a grocer and I must go and open up my shop' can preserve dignity, avoid contradiction and give recognition to the person's knowledge or skill. The reply could be: 'Oh, Mr Zee, you *used* to have a grocery didn't you? It *must have been* good to know all your customers personally: not like the supermarkets today. Did you pack all the dried fruit in blue bags? *Was* it hard to fold them up so neatly?' Mr Zee is only too pleased to explain how it was done and will almost always use the past tense too.

Gentle correction is possible, particularly in situations where sensitive topics are not involved. These corrections should be tactful, so that they can be accepted without loss of dignity. For example:

Actually it's Tuesday today—but one day does seem much like another here.
This is a hospital, in fact, but we like to think that it is as good as any hotel.
That's Jim Smith, one of the other nurses, perhaps he looks like your son, Bill.

Such statements could be possible corrections for confusions of day, place and person. Where more sensitive areas, such as a bereavement, are concerned, it is wise to first ascertain the type of response which occurs after correction to errors on a more general plane. If these responses are usually reasonable then it would be feasible to attempt open discussion about the more emotionally loaded situations. The important point is to choose appropriate occasions for correction, when the person is calm and there is time available. If a bereavement is to be discussed, it may appear fresh to an old person, almost as if it was new information. Therefore the same procedure should be followed as when it is necessary to break bad news to anyone. Time, also, should be allowed for this and for sitting with the person as he or she grieves. It is not such a terrible thing if the person cries—indeed it may be more abnormal not to cry in the circumstances.

It is seldom, if ever, useful to correct a person in such a way that a head-on confrontation ensues. Indeed, a direct confrontation may result in the person becoming *more* fixed in his or her mistaken belief, or agitation will become so intense that further information simply will not 'go in'. What are needed are ways to calm and reassure the person, without agreeing and colluding with the confused talk.

On many occasions—where time is limited or there is already some agitation or confusion and talk is vague and incoherent—it is better not to correct apparently confabulatory statements. Instead of emphatically denying that such a thing is possible, it is better to ignore the content of the rambling talk and use distraction. A gentle touch on the arm, eye contact and an attempt to attract attention by speaking in a firm, clear voice should be followed by a distracting statement. The use of an interesting item such as a flower accompanied by a suitable comment, 'Ellen, Ellen, what do you think of this?', will usually suffice to promote a definite response. Moving the person's focus of attention onto something in the surroundings is important in any attempt to change the subject of the conversation—everyday objects and pictures can be used to achieve this.

The final response option is relevant when it seems that a statement or remark is an attempt to express an underlying feeling. This feeling is hidden, perhaps simply because the appropriate words are not available. Possibly non-verbal methods are used to convey the message, e.g.

'I'm sorry, I must go home now and get my Dad's tea.' The lady is 84 years old, has been hospitalised for 3 years and her Dad died 20 years ago. Pointing out these facts to her would be inappropriate in many situations. The 'hidden' meaning may well be the simple one that she is expressing boredom or a feeling of insecurity for the moment and wishes to escape. The response is to acknowledge the feeling—but not the actual words. Here it might be 'We've done enough for today, haven't we, let's get a cup of tea on the ward', which allows the person to retire with dignity.

A further example would be 'My mother is coming soon', when the patient's mother had died several years previously. The response to this might be 'It must have been a good time of life when you were with your parents, and they were there to look after you.' The feeling communicated was again one of insecurity, a need to recall the time of life when the patient was very dependent but had her mother there to provide security for her. In the midst of the perplexity and insecurity of dementia, the need for feelings of safety, attachment and security—associated with parent-figures from early in life—is indeed powerful. The young child's first and probably most significant experience of being loved and safe is in the arms of their parents: running to them when a strange person or object appeared, holding on tightly to a parental hand in an unfamiliar place to avoid being lost, being enveloped in their arms when scared ... In dementia, a desire to return to the position of safety, of attachment to the figures who came to represent security and well-being, is understandable. Miesen (1992, 1993) shows how parent fixation—where the person with dementia talks about one or both parents a great deal and appears to believe they are alive—develops in some patients as their dementia progresses, as a form of attachment behaviour.

An interesting case of the 'hidden message' was an elderly lady who talked to her 'sister' in a mirror. She knew it was a mirror but had constructed a fantasy world where she was able to pass the time of day with her own reflection. Again responses like 'It's great to feel you have relatives nearby', seemed more appropriate than outright correction, which the patient resisted. The point may be reached where one can say 'You know it is a mirror and I know it's a mirror, but if you want to say you're talking to your sister, that's fine.' However, in situations like this, the possibility of involving the person in activities and interests that were previously enjoyed should also be seriously considered.

A refusal to cooperate often indicates a reaction to stress and an avoidance of a situation which might be threatening to self-esteem. Sudden deafness is an example of this! By smiling broadly and remaining silent, by being inattentive or by confabulating, anxiety is avoided. 'I don't want to answer any more questions' is an attempt to control a situation; once control is achieved cooperation usually follows. Older people may buy time in order to think, to control and to make sure that they understand the implications of a situation. 'Oh, I've forgotten my glasses' or 'I must go to the toilet' can be useful excuses to allow a delay. The importance of helping the person succeed, by not making demands or asking questions that will lead to failure, is clear. Helping the person to feel reassured, relaxed, and self-confident can thus also reduce the amount of apparently confused and rambling talk.

Attempting to tune in to the person's feelings in this way has been developed by Feil (1982) as 'validation'. Feil provides many valuable insights and techniques for facilitating communication with the person with dementia and particularly develops the notion that the person may be expressing feelings relating to unresolved conflicts and difficulties earlier in life (Feil 1993). The validation approach is adapted for people at different stages of dementia, but the key technique is, as suggested here, to listen carefully to the emotions behind the speech and to respond empathically to these, rather than to the words (Feil 1982):

The Validation worker is always honest. The worker always tries to recognise and be aware of feelings. Acknowledge with words and physical movements that the person's feelings are true. Share out loud the need to return to universal longings in times of stress. Validate the feelings. Forget facts.

Three basic human needs are identified (Feil 1992). These reflect needs for love and safety, a need for a sense of usefulness, related to work and identity, and a need to express strong, raw, basic emotions to someone who will listen and seek to understand. Needs for love and security are often related particularly to parent-figures, as suggested above. The need to be useful may be shown in the person's behaviour, wiping tables over and over, folding cloths or tissues, trying to clean windows in the corridor, for example. The raw emotions—of anger, frustration and despair—may not be hidden but, Feil suggests, do need someone who will listen without rejecting in order for the person to feel understood and less isolated in the midst of the powerful feelings being experienced.

Feil tends to emphasise the importance of unresolved past experiences emerging in what the person with dementia is trying to communicate now. However, not all communications have such a 'deep' hidden meaning, and attention should be given to what the person is experiencing now as they struggle to cope with what must often seem an alien environment. The key element is not to simply write off what the person is saying as 'confabulation' or 'confusion', but to engage in a real effort to listen to the words and the feelings. By seeking to stand alongside the person with dementia, to see the world from their perspective, a deeper level of communication may open up, reaching more of the whole person of the dementia sufferer, which is so often obscured by the effects of the dementia and our own limitations in comprehension, sensitivity and time.

ENVIRONMENTAL ASPECTS
Physical environment

An important aspect of any positive approach is to provide the means whereby clients can be as independent as possible and pursue their normal existence to the best of their ability. This can be better achieved if staff, and all those working with the elderly, can understand more about the impact of the environment on all of us.

Our home, our work, our friends, interests and possessions are all part of our environment. We choose our homes, or at least change them, to suit our purposes and needs. We organise our possessions so that we know where they are and so we can make the best use of them. We choose the colours with which we feel happiest; we place things in frequent use to hand and those of less importance we put away. Our home must run smoothly and fit in with our activities. Why else is it only the unwary who offer to 'put away' instead of 'help to wash up'?

If we recall our initial move to our present home, we can remember the chaos, the priorities for unpacking and the difficulties encountered in finding our way about the unfamiliar neighbourhood. It was vital to locate the right signs and cues ... the pink house on the corner, the name of the pub, the big tree before we turned left ... which, in time would all become automatic. Those first few days or even weeks in the new situation were filled with trauma and aggravation, trying to turn the key in the lock, reaching for a light switch that was not there and trying to decide how welcoming the neighbours were. All of this, no matter how difficult, was within our control, our choice, and the decision for change, organisation and inclusion were ours also.

Imagine what it is like for a person who has lived in the same place for many years to suddenly find him or herself in totally alien surroundings. Everything is under someone else's control. There are no personal possessions, no familiar things, routines or even faces: a place where wall and curtain colours are distasteful, which lacks privacy, contains too many strangers, has too much noise or horrendous hush, and is all unfriendly. There is no way to tell where things are, no personal chair, no familiar kitchen, no place to put anything and nothing to put there anyway. The culture shock, the realisation of the loss of control, the feeling of isolation or even imprisonment must be a devastating experience: one which need not be so traumatic if only it had been more carefully planned. Any move should be preceded by a few visits to get acquainted, although, of course, hospitalisation rarely permits this.

If the physical environment is designed to reduce disorientation and all the accompanying difficulties and traumas, an admission could prove less painful, and this is where environmental aspects of 24 hour RO have an important role. Simple, commonsense measures could help. In the first place a guide is essential. Someone, perhaps an able resident, should be responsible for a guided tour. Even if the person is bedridden, some explanation of where and what could help. One tour or explanation is not enough. Attention and concentration will be stretched, the person needs to be told a number of times. Parrot-like repetitions are not necessary, or desirable, but opportunities—like returning from a trip to the bathroom—will offer a chance to say again, 'Look, there is a notice saying where the diningroom is', or the toilet, daily information board, or whatever.

There is a need to supply orientation aids. These will do little good if no one points them out, but with the help of a guide they can prove invaluable aids to independence. Some basic, but helpful aids are indicated in Box 7.2. The aids must be large and clear enough for the elderly person to see; above all they must be accurate, or confusion will be increased! Getting these details right is an important—and inexpensive—part of RO.

Box 7.2 Environmental aids: use of orienting cues in the person's environment		
Clocks	*Ensure that they are*	
Calendars		Large
Signs		Clear
Pictures		Accurate

Patients may need to be taught where the signs and aids are and encouraged to make use of them. This initial effort is well worthwhile in view of the time saved later.

Colour plays a large role in creating an atmosphere. Bright covers on beds assist identification as well as looking pretty, and toilet doors are easier to find if they are painted a special colour as well as bearing a printed notice. Attractive curtains and tablecloths, interesting pictures, the tasteful use of wallpaper and colourful crockery provide a varied environment with plenty of landmarks to aid orientation. The staff are helped by the memory aids too! They act as a reminder to use interactions positively. Here as well as clocks and calendars, boards with clearly written information about the day, month and weather, colourful pictures or collages of food, national leaders, places, children, seasons, occupations, maps, etc, should also be on view. A daily newspaper and journals of particular interest should be easily available. There is always time in the day for comments on these, and they are valuable aids to communication, providing a visual reminder to the patient of the topic. Care should be taken not to overload boards with information; if there is too much the person will not be able to extract anything from the morass of conflicting messages.

Common sense will dictate the important aspects of the environment that require emphasis. Why are toilet doors always so hard to find or identify? Why do they look like any other door so that the chance of finding the right one is limited and the chance of being labelled incontinent is so much greater. Why are corridors so long and threatening? Some indication of where the corridor leads might lessen the confusion and make the trip along it worthwhile. Signs at right angles to the wall which the person can see whilst walking down the corridor are helpful in this respect. If individual bedrooms or areas had some significant picture, photograph or personal item on the door or bedside table, owners could locate them so much more easily and unaided.

A home or ward should be concerned to encourage independence and the continuation of normal living as far as possible, but rarely is there a room for simple laundry purposes, or a kitchen in which basic cooking can be done. If it is normal to have only a cup of tea and a piece of toast for breakfast, why cannot the person do it for themselves and get up at their chosen time? Not everybody will be capable of doing this, but are there other residents or patients who might enjoy helping?

Public space is necessary, but private space is equally important. Possessions, items recalling past experiences and successes, family souvenirs

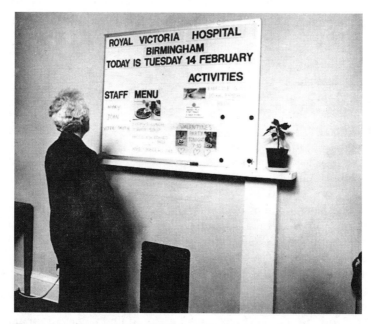

Figure 7.4 Signs, calendars and information boards can be extremely valuable in supplementing 24 hour RO.

and personal mementoes are part of a person's private world. Interests can be pursued; letters and books can be read. Programmes on TV or radio which do not appeal to others can be seen or heard in private. Sometimes just to sit and look outside can be a pleasant relief from the activity on the ward or in the home. Everyone needs some personal space.

Lighting can often cause problems which are unnoticed by staff. Not only is it important to ensure that elderly people can see properly in order to read or write, but strange illusions can be caused by faulty lighting. One lady was thought to be deluded as she would insist that she could not leave her room at certain hours of the day because 'the hall is on fire'. Only when someone sat beside her did it become apparent that reflections from the lights produced a line across the floor that looked as though there really was a fire!

Only those who have had the experience of picking their way around on crutches can fully appreciate the importance of flooring! Anything that looks slippery, uneven or hazardous in any way can arouse anxiety. Too many floors seem to be problematic and often this too is caused by poor lighting, shadows and reflections. Contrasting colours of vinyl flooring meeting on a corridor may appear like a step to some patients. This has occasionally been a problem with the use of coloured lines on the floor leading the way to the toilets. This same sort of line is not helpful in encouraging older people to walk upright and to look ahead. A line drawn along the wall, or clear signposting is preferable.

The evening and night-time

Previously when environmental influences have been considered, most of the emphasis has been on the daytime, with evenings and night-time virtually ignored, despite the good intentions behind the term '24 hour RO'. In understanding and evaluating behaviour and seeking to meet the needs of people with dementia, the whole 24-hour span must be considered.

Often at home, the evening is a time for change; the working day is over and these hours are used for relaxation and enjoyment, according to individual taste and circumstances. The theatre, sport, visiting friends, going out to a pub, watching a favourite TV programme or even doing household chores may all be different activities from those of the daytime, yet in care situations there often seems to be little difference. Many 'odd' behaviours may have an explanation in relation to this. Agitation can increase; Mr Turner can begin to pace around a ward, Mrs Blake can wander looking and calling for the family—could it be that they are trying to pursue their normal routine, gathering with the family at the end of the working day? It is accepted that activity is necessary in daylight hours, but it is also important that something different should occur in the evening. Apart from well-established habits, some activity in the early evening followed by a more peaceful or routine activity is thought necessary to evoke satisfactory sleep (Morgan 1987, Morgan & Gledhill 1991). Sleep charts can identify a problem; if a person sleeps for most of the 24 hours or sleeps at inappropriate times, the reason for this must be sought and appropriate changes made to minimise daytime dozing in order to stabilise the sleep/wake pattern. Perhaps there is not sufficient stimulation or activity, or perhaps depression is a problem, with dozing the only available option.

An abnormal bedroom environment can cause further problems (Holden 1991). Is the noise level high, is lighting interfering with sleep, are the toilets nearby, is there sufficient privacy, is heating at a correct level for the individual, can beds be readily identified, are they too close? These and many other questions need to be asked and proper assessments of both the physical and psychological environments should be made and added to those made in the daytime.

Staff needs at night-time should also be considered. If morale is low, if their needs are overlooked and if the necessary facilities and support are not available for them, their ability to provide quality care will be diminished. Night staff require training, contact with other professionals and managerial staff just as much as those working by day, yet often this seems to be forgotten. Programmes may be set up and established without any discussion with, or comment from, night staff. Perhaps this helps explain why some care-plans fail: if staff have not been informed or had the opportunity for discussion and clarification, or if something occurring overnight has been omitted. Increasingly, night cover is being provided by the 'day staff' on rotation, and this certainly seems a positive way of achieving a more consistent 24 hour approach.

Psychological environment

Anything which creates a feeling of worth or well-being is relevant here. Sensory stimulation should always be considered. Colours, good views from the windows, pleasant surroundings, peace and activity levels to meet the needs of each individual are all important. Information about orientation, forthcoming events, newspapers and journals should all be available. A simple library, relevant games, reminiscence aids, such as pictures of the old town and area, historical aspects of the locality, Then and Now books, royalty, anything to prompt memories; these are all very useful for personal and group perusal. Just as important is some personal collection of photos and mementoes. Outings are an added stimulation and, again, may spark off personal memories—the church where the person was married, the annual fete, the new buildings replacing the old shop or workplace.

Group sessions are important as a means to increase engagement, interaction and the establishment of good relationships with other clients or with staff. Understanding can grow. Visits from members of the local community and schools provide a link with local affairs. If the carers know their clients well, abilities, skills and experiences become more obvious and can be used to increase independence and confidence.

Lack of control over the environment coupled with lack of knowledge about clients can result in deprivation of many needs. For instance, Mrs T was an opera lover but was in bed every time an opera was shown on TV. The radio blasted out pop music all day, so there was never an opportunity to hear the classical music that she loved. Possibly others suffered from sounds and sights they did not appreciate either. This could have been rectified by installing a radio in her room, providing a tape recorder or by ensuring that she could stay up and watch the programme in a quiet corner. There were many possibilities, but no one had bothered to find out about her interests and so no one knew that she was suffering.

There are so many aspects of living where the person loses control, from the room temperature to being able to lock away personal possessions. Helping the person exercise some control over their lifestyle must be a major aim of a home or ward, offering realistic choices appropriate to the person's abilities and interests. In some homes, with more able and articulate residents, Residents' Committees have been formed. Often they are rendered impotent by lack of attention to their requests and criticisms. Where they do have a say in policy and planning events they appear to be a responsive, lively group who make the staff's work much more stimulating. Independence does mean having opportunity to express opinions and make suggestions which are put to use.

Finally, there are some practices which, despite the growth of positive approaches, still appear to operate in some units. In assessing the good and bad points of environments, consideration should be given to whether there are any environmental features which, used routinely, may cause acute distress and hasten the process of withdrawal. The use of cot sides is still, unfortunately, a common example of this. Restless patients, elderly stroke cases and others could wake up to a world cut off by bars. This must confirm feelings of rejection. If the patient wishes to use the toilet and no one is around he/she either attempts to climb over the bars—and has the accident the bars were meant to prevent—or is incontinent. Dignity and independence are lost, perhaps permanently. Similar problems are caused by the *routine* use of geriatric chairs, or even beds that are too high from the ground, or large open spaces offering no aids to mobility.

A rich environment

The aim is to create an environment to which it is worthwhile to be orientated, where withdrawal is not the only option. The environment requires careful consideration and evaluation—of both physical and psychological aspects—in order to ensure that it provides facilities and features which will encourage the person to live as independently as possible. Such aids would include activity levels which are neither too low nor too high for each individual, personalisation of clothing and possessions, and the opportunity to continue to cater for the self as far as possible. It also recognises the need for a group identity, by providing either a form of group living or some degree of group activity, neither of which interfere with individual choice or need for privacy.

While a positive approach is urged, disabilities do exist. They too require aids and efforts so that the person can adapt to the deficits. Emphasis should be on regaining confidence by the continued use of retained abilities and skills, but the disabilities cannot be ignored. The retained functions can aid in re-training the lost ones or be used in adapting to difficulties arising from the loss of function.

COMMUNICATING WITH DYSPHASIC PATIENTS OR THOSE WITH SPEECH PROBLEMS

People who have had a stroke, head injury or some neurological disorder resulting in damage to the parts of the brain responsible for speech will suffer from some form of speech disorder. This is a complex field; fuller definitions are given in Chapter 6; here three major types of speech problems will be indicated.

1. Dysarthria. Here it is the actual production of speech that is affected; words and sentence construction may be correct, but the articulation is poor. The listener finds the speech indistinct and difficult to understand. Temporary dysarthria is familiar after a substantial consumption of alcohol!

2. Expressive dysphasia. This takes various forms; essentially the person's ability to express him or herself is impaired and the words and sentences do not come out correctly. There may be difficulties in finding the right word, leading to a high frequency of 'thingumajigs', 'whatsits', etc, or to long-winded or circumlocutory speech when, for example, the person says 'a small piece for fastening articles that people wear' instead of 'button'. Words may be invented, reversed or omitted. There may be difficulty in reading, writing and calculation. Automatic speech such as 'Monday, Tuesday, Wednesday . . . ' or 'one, two, three . . . ' may be possible, as may be singing; these do not represent the overall level of functioning as they are so well known to the person. The person may well feel frustrated at this inability to make others understand; such insight is distressing.

3. Receptive dysphasia. Here the patient has difficulty in appreciating what is being said. There is incomplete or even no understanding of conversation, directions or questions, which leads to a considerable degree of isolation. Some associated problems include reading, writing, calculation and spelling. The person is placed in a world which seems meaningless and is likely to be bewildered, perplexed and frightened. The nature of the difficulties of comprehension is such that the person is also often unable to express him or herself clearly; a person's own speech is continually monitored by the receptive system, so expression is also likely to be affected by receptive difficulties.

Communication

Wherever possible a speech therapist should be consulted to guide, advise and treat. However, there is a great deal that can be done by care-staff, as the success of 'stroke clubs' and volunteer 'speech after stroke' schemes has demonstrated.

The first step with these—and other—impairments is to recognise and accept that they are not within the person's control, that the impairment arises however hard the person tries to overcome it. Secondly, speech impairments may make people appear more deteriorated and confused than in fact they are. Thirdly, no two people have the same problem; even if the site of the damaged area of the brain is the same, each person is different, with experience, intellect and personality which will influence the problems in a variety of ways. Here the basic positive approach of not writing anybody off but continuing to treat them as a person is of great value. Fourthly, particularly where a stroke has led to the impairment, improvement may well be possible. Where the speech problem is a feature of a dementing illness, more restricted aims will be appropriate.

More specifically, the problem of communicating with individuals with receptive dysphasia is the most challenging of all. They should not be included in group settings and communication should be on a one-to-one basis. The group situation aggravates their sense of worthlessness and frustration. Others appear to be enjoying themselves, but they do not understand what is so pleasing to the others in the group.

On a one-to-one basis, communication must be simplified as much as possible. Remember that although the *language* centre is damaged, the brain's non-verbal communication centre is probably perfectly intact. In other words, the person may comprehend tone, rhythm, emphasis gesture and all non-verbal language. Non-verbal signals are then very important; sudden movements or an approach from behind may be misinterpreted as threatening and lead to aggressive lashing out. Gentle touch, an open and warm approach and voice tone should be employed to encourage a feeling of security and acceptance. Verbal messages must be simplified, avoiding complex concepts; sentences must be short and involve one idea at a time only. Words should be backed up with demonstrations, gestures, pictures, etc. Every possible effort to understand the person's attempts at communication must be made; again non-verbal signals and gestures are important in making sense of what the person says. Any communication abilities the person does retain should be capitalised on, whether it be reading, writing, mime, etc. With interaction being so difficult, there is a tendency to avoid such patients; if only some feeling of warmth and acceptance is conveyed then something will have been achieved. Conversely, if others use pejorative tones, dismissive gestures and critical remarks, these aspects will also be understood, with detrimental effects.

Individual situations

Patients with expressive dysphasia or dysarthria respond well to a positive approach both in groups and in informal interaction.

Mr D, a 79-year-old who had a right-sided hemiplegia and severe expressive dysphasia resulting from a stroke, could say an occasional word, but more frequently said 'Five, five, five' or 'Go to Hell! '. He was incontinent, negativistic, a little aggressive and cut himself off by burying his head in his arms. Though included in an RO group, he remained isolated for 2 weeks. Suddenly he began to write with his left hand and made several meaningful and distinct drawings. Gestures, eye contact and interest in the materials used in the session began to increase. As his gestures and the therapist's understanding of them improved, his needs could be interpreted. He showed his delight by increasing his efforts and warmth of response. His drawings became so meaningful that it was possible for him to give an account of himself and his past life. His intelligence was put to use in finding ways to tell his new friends about his experiences. His improvement was dramatic and his family were pleased for him to be discharged home.

Mrs V had a severe form of receptive dysphasia as a result of a stroke. She was extremely depressed and weepy, but there was little that could be done to communicate with her. Initially, before the problem was clear, she was included in a group. It soon became apparent that there were many problems and the situation was becoming intolerable for her. Individual therapy was instigated. Using warmth, information from her past, much respect and by introducing items that she recognised, it was possible to build up a happy relationship between her and the staff. Simple things, as for example bringing her a posy of the flowers with a similar name to hers, pictures of places she had visited and the use of gentle touch, all aided in at least improving her life on the ward. It also encouraged her to attempt to express herself non-verbally, so that the staff were able to learn more about the things which pleased or interested her.

Mrs F had a mild stroke one evening and in the morning was unable to speak properly. She was frightened and disturbed and the staff were anxious. By using sentences which required the minimum of response—initially 'yes' and 'no'—it was possible to calm her and to gradually increase the span of response. For example, 'Would you like some tea?' would become 'Would you like some tea or coffee?' Later, perhaps in a day or two, as she improved, a calm voice would enquire 'Would you like to get dressed this morning? What would you like to wear?' This permitted the use of 'yes' and 'no', but also allowed longer responses. These were aided by 'What about this?' or 'Do you like the pink jumper?' In an atmosphere of calm and of minimal demand on speech, confidence can return and normal processes of recovery can be aided, with the minimum of stress.

These are some of many examples of how positive approaches can be used to help those with speech problems. Special allowances must be made for them. Patience is vital and the person should be given time and encouragement in order to appreciate that others are willing to help. The atmosphere should be one in which the clients do not feel that heavy demands are being made on them to express themselves, whilst being friendly and inclusive. The person's disability is not to be exposed and demonstrated once more, but again help is given for the person to find success. He or she should be greeted, and materials used by others should be shown, brought near or left in reach. Reactions such as eye contact or gestures should be noted and a response made to them. Again non-verbal responses are useful—touch, warmth, gesture and so on; but in expressive dysphasia there is more scope for verbal responses and reassurance. A reaction should not be forced, but any effort, however small, should be greeted with interest and attention. Too fulsome a response could be inappropriate, but warmth and moderated praise are indicated. 'What do you think of that, it's nice isn't it?' or 'You can do a lot with that left hand can't you? I like your drawing.' Lack of speech does not mean lack of intellectual ability, but it does mean that everyone has to try harder to understand and be understood.

Where some speech is retained but there is perhaps a word-finding difficulty, then the patient may be able to indicate a choice from several alternatives; naming may prove difficult or impossible, but matching with an identical object or picture might be possible. Any communicative ability at all should be capitalised on, and the speech therapist may indicate certain aspects that are less impaired. The dysarthric patient may need to be taught to talk more slowly and precisely, and to use non-verbal means to provide a context for the verbal message. Words are easier to understand if the listeners knows roughly what is likely to be said. In all cases, isolation and withdrawal are possible consequences of the speech impairment; the aim here is to ensure this does not happen, by helping the person feel accepted and to some extent understood, and—importantly—unpressured.

HELPING THE PERSON LEARN

People with dementia have considerable difficulty in learning, but, as we have discussed in Chapter 2, learning is not impossible. Here we present some basic techniques for encouraging learning of new skills, re-training old skills, maintaining retained skills and for dealing with some of the problem behaviours that arise.

Reward

The fundamental principle in encouraging change is the use of a reward for desirable behaviour and no reward for inappropriate behaviour. A 'reward' consists of something enjoyed by the patient. As individual tastes and values vary enormously, it is vital to know what the patient's likes or dislikes include. Undoubtedly, elderly people most appreciate staff approval and attention, so good interpersonal relationships have a strong motivational force. The word 'behavioural' is often mistakenly equated with 'mechanical', but warm and affectionate relationships are of prime importance and preclude the possibility of mechanical and automatic responses being the rule in relationships. Apart from approval, other practical rewards might include a favourite drink or food, a special event or outing, even cigarettes, any of which could be used to encourage new behaviour initially. Some studies have used tokens as a reward. The token can later be exchanged for rewards of the patient's choice. Token giving structures staff approval. If it is difficult for the elderly person to remember or to perform the necessary actions to exchange the token, it is probably only a useful reward system for them in as much as it reminds staff to give their attention appropriately.

The use and relevance of rewards should be considered. It is illogical to reward a full stomach with food; a cigarette for a patient with a packet in his pocket is like taking coals to Newcastle; if someone wants to sleep he is not impressed by extra attention.

To delay a reward is to lose an opportunity. A very confused person forgets quickly and might not connect the praise with their own response: it is also advisable to make clear what is so pleasing. In the initial stages, the rewards should be given virtually every time the desired behaviour occurs. If the behaviour becomes well established they can be slowly decreased, though continued, if only infrequently.

If rewarding the behaviour of elderly patients appears difficult and artificial it should be borne in mind that people are rewarding and failing to reward each other all the time, often without being aware of it. We all smile at those we like, listen attentively to what they say, yet ignore those to whom we are indifferent; these are examples of reward and lack of reward in everyday life. What is being advocated here is the use of these everyday phenomena in a planned, structured way to bring about specific changes in a patient's behaviour. Praise and encouragement are part of all good training programmes, and where the elderly are concerned, many of the skills were previously in their possession and only require re-learning.

One problem in using a reward system is to ensure that the behaviour to be rewarded actually occurs in the first place. For instance, if a patient never goes to the toilet without prompting, how can they be taught to go on their own? There is nothing to reward. Clearly the behaviour must be elicited before it can be rewarded. Several strategies are possible. One method is to increase the probability of it occurring. The environment can be adapted so that the patient sits nearer to the facilities instead of a long way from them. The patient could be taken for a walk in the vicinity so that when the toilet is seen he might feel disposed to make use of it while close at hand. If social interaction is the target, a patient could be invited to join a small group in order to play a game or have a drink in company. In such circumstances, the desired behaviour becomes more probable, so then it can be immediately rewarded. Three other possible strategies are discussed in the succeeding sections.

Modelling

A second approach is to demonstrate, or model, the required behaviour. To increase recreational involvement, an actual game can be shown; mime can be employed to show how to get dressed, how to wash, or how to eat correctly. A group already engaged in discussion can demonstrate to a withdrawn patient that by conversing they can have an enjoyable time with each other and the staff.

Shaping

Here successively closer approximations to the target behaviour are rewarded, and as each stage is achieved the demands become a little stricter. If, for instance, the normal use of a fork and knife is the target the reward system could commence at a very low level:

1. any sort of self-feeding, even with the fingers
2. reward only for an attempt to use a utensil
3. reward only when a fork is used
4. finally, reward only when the correct use of utensils is observed.

Similarly if the target is to be self-initiated toiletting:

1. a visit to the toilet even when accompanied
2. managing with less and less help in getting up and walking there
3. only response to verbal reminders is rewarded
4. fading of verbal cues into non-verbal cues: initially a mime, eventually perhaps a simple nod of the head
5. finally, the only reward to be given is for self-initiated toiletting.

The entire procedure would consist of initial response to guidance, response to a verbal reminder, then a non-verbal prompt and finally no reminder at all.

Consistent use by the staff of the minimum prompt needed to begin or continue the behaviour in question is very important. When dressing a patient, for example, if verbal prompting does not get a response the patient's arm might be placed gradually in the sleeve of his shirt with firm pressure until he begins to continue the movement, when the pressure is relaxed and the patient praised. As soon as the patient stops the required movement, the guiding hand of the nurse becomes firmer until he takes over again and can be praised once more. Thus small amounts of dressing behaviour can be reinforced and become more likely to occur again in the future.

Shaping involves the setting of intermediate goals in order to achieve the main one. If aims are set realistically it will enable the patient to obtain encouragement along the way and so increase the likelihood of complete success. Breaking goals down into small attainable parts is necessary in order to progress. If goals seem a long way off, they discourage both patient and staff.

Backward chaining

The final related technique to be mentioned is backward chaining. Many target behaviours, in fact, consist of a sequence of smaller behaviours, for example, toiletting includes:

1. get up from seat in lounge
2. walk to toilet
3. remove clothing as necessary
4. urinate in appropriate receptacle
5. adjust clothing.

As the term implies, backward chaining involves starting at the end of the sequence, establishing that behaviour and then going on to work on the preceding link in the chain, again establishing that before going on to the next part of the sequence.

Thus, in the case of toiletting, the person's dressing ability should be checked, perhaps arranging for any necessary adaptations to clothing, and practice in dressing skills should be provided so that these parts of the chain can be performed. Next, there is a need to ascertain if the person connects urination with being at the toilet. If when on the toilet urine is not passed, then this part of the chain requires assistance until the person reliably uses the toilet area (experience with adults with learning difficulties suggests that increased fluids and very frequent supervised visits to the toilet are useful at this stage). Then comes the 'approach response', which is the actual decision to go to the toilet, finding the way to it, walking to it and so on. As with any skill, the component skills of toiletting or dressing, etc, may be learned (or here re-learned) by repeated practice with rewards of praise for success.

In the case of a person who has lost the skill of self-feeding, backward chaining might involve initially praising the person for mouth-opening to allow the spoon in, then letting the person help to carry the spoon the last inch or so into the mouth, then giving encouragement and praise when the person gradually takes over more of the complete sequence of actions that constitute independent feeding. The importance of backward chaining is that the completion of the chain has in it the reward of fulfilment—in this case food. This acts best on those responses closest to it, until these are well-established and can then be extended to include appropriate preceding responses.

Maintenance of re-learned skills

The previous sections have concentrated on procedures for bringing about behavioural change, building up new behaviours and re-establishing old ones. What must be understood, however, is that for change to be lasting the person's environment must maintain the new or re-established behaviour. When targets are set, maintenance of the targets must be considered. For instance, if we teach Mrs Jones to make a cup of tea for herself, will she continue to do so when there are six cups of tea provided daily in the home? If we help Mr Smith to use the toilet independently, will he continue to do so if most of his fellow patients are incontinent and so receive extra staff attention? Will Mrs Brown continue to dress herself if being dressed had been one way of obtaining staff attention? Having taught Mrs White to cook her own meals at home, will she continue to do so when her neighbour provides her with a meal on most days? Although the emphasis may have appeared to have been on changing the individual's behaviour, behaviour–environment interactions are always present. How the environment must be modified to maintain the changed behaviour is as important as the actual change.

Reactions to problem behaviours

Sometimes the behavioural approach is characterised as 'reward good behaviour and punish (or ignore) bad behaviour'. The saying 'ignore it and it will go away' is only true in so far as the behaviour can be completely and consistently ignored: if it is rewarded at all, even infrequently, it will persist for a long, long time. To ignore a problem behaviour is usually an extremely difficult task for residents, relatives and staff. We are advocating an approach where the focus is rather on building up compatible behaviours to take the place of those that are inappropriate. The first step in this process is to seek to understand more about the person and his behaviour, and to identify the factors both within the person and within the environment (including the responses of others) that are related to it.

Punishment is used in one form or another in everyday life, and not just with children. Everyone does or says things other people will not like, to get revenge for some real or imagined wrong. Withdrawal and moodiness may be used as punishments.

However, on ethical grounds, we would not wish to see the development of programmes for the elderly (or anyone else for that matter) based on punishment. Care-staff have—whether they realise it or not—a great deal of power over those in their homes or wards; power to use wisely but also power that can damage, hurt and even destroy. The great majority of care-staff use this power sensitively, responsibly and constructively. Inevitably, there are those who do not; in institutions under pressure from poor facilities and resources, experience in other fields has shown that systems using punishment have lent themselves too readily to abuse. Too quickly, the aims of treatment are forgotten and punishment has become a way of running a ward or home for the convenience of the hard-pressed staff. In fact, punishment has been shown to be a rather ineffective way of changing behaviour, in comparison with reward systems.

How can problem behaviours be treated if they arise before alternative positive responses have been established? What reaction is appropriate if one patient literally throws another onto the floor because she has taken the chair she usually sits in? Obviously this would be difficult to ignore; clearly, if the offending patient reclaims 'her' chair, she will have succeeded and may continue forcibly ejecting 'intruders'. One possibility would be to take the offender to one side (having ensured that help is being given to the patient on the floor) and reiterate in a firm, clear, calm voice, looking at her directly, face to face, that violence to other patients is unacceptable. A good way of calming the situation might be to take her out of the lounge, or to her own room. There it may be possible to discuss calmly with her what happened; what did she feel, what made her angry, what exactly was amiss? However, the plan must not stop there. Positive preventive measures are required. In this instance, a decision must be made on the contentious issue of ownership of chairs! If it is held that chairs are common property, then patients should be encouraged to sit in chairs in different parts of the lounge; the pros and cons of each chair could be discussed—position, view and comfort, for instance. A wider field of interpersonal relationships could be encouraged so that a number of chairs would be attractive alternatives. On the other hand, if patients' needs for their own space and territory is to be reflected in allowing 'ownership' of chairs, the 'owner's' name could be attached as an indication to others that this is 'reserved'. The patients could be encouraged to practise asking others, politely, to move and be allowed to call the staff for assistance if the chair was not vacated.

A second example could be the case of an elderly man who is incontinent of urine, but who is otherwise fairly good at self-care. His wetness cannot be ignored, some reaction is inevitable whilst his clothing is being changed. In this situation it is easy to make a critical remark that will only add to the humiliation of the whole event for the patient. The situation should be dealt with calmly in a matter-of-fact manner, so the patient is not given a lot of positive attention which might reward his being wet. The patient is prompted to get changed—as far as possible independently—and to take responsibility for the event, perhaps rinsing through the underwear, taking his trousers to the laundry room, or mopping up the puddle, as far as he is able. After this, a member of staff might spend time discussing the problem with him, establishing his concern, if any; what he feels might help; and how the staff plan to help him. This does not constitute a plan for controlling incontinence and it is still necessary to train the person to visit the toilet, as has previously been described. The desirable behaviour has to be established if the problem of incontinence is to decrease; the person is less likely to be incontinent if the toilet is used correctly.

It must be ensured that inappropriate behaviour is not rewarded, however unwittingly. The example of the person obtaining attention for being wet is clear, but in some situations a more subtle reward system might operate. Aggressive acts may be greeted by severe and critical responses which may prove to be rewarding enough to encourage further aggression. Even removing the aggressors to their own rooms may be rewarding for some patients; the accompanied walk, the peace and quiet of the room, the change of scene may be perceived as pleasant consequences of the aggressive act.

This area is one of great complexity and illustrates why problem behaviours can prove resistant to change. Considering the consequences for the particular event only and ignoring the totality of individual functioning can lead to errors. For any problem behaviour, it is necessary to bear in mind that reactions to it may be encouraging its recurrence; in each case a consistent, humane response which minimises this should be planned.

The individual planning approach illustrated in Chapter 5 together with the assessment process detailed in Chapter 6 offer a coherent framework for managing difficult behaviour within the context of the person's overall strengths and needs; the emphasis is on an individualised approach that seeks an understanding of the person's actions: two patients may both be 'aggressive', but quite different reasons may be discerned; one may be acting to ward off a perceived threat, acting in 'self-defence'; the other may be responding to frustration, having failed to carry out a task. Indeed Stokes (1989) lists 10 examples of types of aggressive behaviour in dementia, and the list is probably far from comprehensive. Such an understanding assists in developing more creative and effective ways of responding to difficult needs, but no technique will work all the time in all situations and it is important to regularly review what is happening, to refine our understanding of the person and their behaviour and to continue to creatively find constructive ways of preventing or diverting the difficult behaviour.

CONCLUSION

A positive approach which recognises the individual as a person with intelligence, experience, feelings, needs and interests, as well as with difficulties and deficits, should be consciously used by all those in contact with elderly people. There is a need to be aware of dangers; sensory deprivation, neglect of the whole person, poor environment, poor communication and lack of understanding of individual problems are the main concerns. Awareness of these leads to better planning, more stimulation and an increase in the quality of life. It is vital to preserve dignity, self-esteem and an interest in life. Volunteers, friends, relatives and caring staff should use every opportunity to reassure and encourage elderly people with dementia by drawing their attention to everyday events. The use of simple forms of sensory stimulation— such as flowers, pictures, seasonal items—can be employed even by grandchildren. The past, old experiences and knowledge, with comparisons from the present, are valuable aids to conversation and the re-awakening of interest in the self and the environment. Social contact is equally important.

Efforts to understand the person's words and actions should be made: do they suggest anxiety or insecurity? Do they make sense in view of their previous personality, interests, occupations, etc? Is the person wandering along the corridor opening each door in turn really behaving aimlessly; perhaps he is looking for something that seems familiar (as many people do when lost); with a severe memory deficit everything looks new and fresh, nothing is familiar, unless known to the person before the memory problems began. Alternatively the person may be searching for the toilet!

Encourage and praise all the person's efforts to behave normally; all successes and achievements; appropriate conversations and attempts to cooperate in activities. Praise and staff attention are powerful motivators where staff develop warm relationships with the elderly patients. The staff can help define the tenet that appropriate non-confused functioning is the aim for the ward or home by reversing the common trend for most attention to be given to inappropriate, confused behaviour.

Above all, never write off the elderly person as a *person*: by getting to know and understand older people and all that has brought them to where they are now, communication on a person-to-person level becomes possible.

8

Group work with people with dementia

If you really want to hear about it, the first thing you will probably want to know is where I was born, and what my lousy childhood was like, and how my parents were occupied and all before they had me, and all that David Copperfield kind of crap, but I don't feel like going into it.

J D Salinger

INTRODUCTION

Group work with older people with dementia requires careful consideration and planning. There are a number of issues that need to be addressed before getting underway. These include:

- the level of ability of the members
- the time available for the group, for each session and overall
- the approach, techniques and methods to be used
- the aims of the group
- who is to lead the group
- the equipment, aids and resources required
- organisational aspects, holidays, rotas, other meetings and groups

Although a 24-hour approach is of prime importance, a group session can provide the opportunity to focus on specific problems and assists staff and client to get to know each other better, encourages social responses and relationships and helps to create a more natural atmosphere in a care setting.

Intensive stimulation, guidance and re-training

are made available, but also it becomes possible to learn more about a person's history, personality, individual characteristics, likes and dislikes. This knowledge greatly assists staff in relating to the older person, to the benefit of both parties. Mutual understanding grows and generalises to contacts outside the group setting. Even apparently 'difficult' patients can become easier to handle because of this increasing awareness, understanding and greater insight which has developed. It becomes possible to appreciate and 'tune in' to the feelings and emotions of the older person, so often obscured by the severity of cognitive impairment.

Therapists become aware of the patients' capabilities and the older people feel more secure and closer to those who care for them. A bond is developed which can greatly aid rehabilitation.

This chapter will describe how to lead such groups. The organisation of staff training and support, patient selection, programme coordination and feedback are considered in Chapter 10. In Chapter 6 assessment was discussed, and Chapter 9 includes many examples of possible equipment and aids to be used. However, first we will outline some of the reasons why group work can be valuable for all concerned and suggest ways to achieve a suitable overall atmosphere.

GROUPS

There are at least two excellent reasons for developing group work with elderly people with dementia. First, it enables people who are unable easily themselves to develop relationships with others to feel some sense of belonging to a group, of *group identity*. Secondly, a group can provide a structured situation in which staff can directly help people to re-learn or adapt to difficulties and impairments, or to use their retained skills effectively.

Group identity

It is easy to forget how important belonging to groups is for people of all ages. Although a person may have grown old as a solitary individual, a

hermit even, it does not mean that this need does not exist. From birth to death we are all members of some group. Initially, the family provides sustenance, guidance, support, structure and rules. As we grow up, other groups have an influence; the people in the locality, neighbours, friends and relatives are among the first. School—with its rules, sanctions and rewards—is the second major group we encounter. From then on our identities are further developed by a variety of groups: interest, sport, political, religious, occupational and so on. Even apparently distant agencies, like the law, government and unions, play their part in our lives.

All these bodies of people demand something of us and give us something in return. Our behaviour can change from group to group and the demands made on us are equally varied. Occasionally these demands do not meet with our approval, or fit with our values and principles. Then we are in conflict with the group. We can leave the group, 'fight' for our beliefs or needs, or give way and submit to the group.

A move or other event leading to isolation from the groups of our choice can cause a loss of part of ourselves. Most of us have experienced to some degree the ensuing feeling of loss, and lack of support, consolation or encouragement which is normally taken for granted. This sense of isolation continues until new bonds are formed and we re-build our lives, or return to the groups concerned. If a person lives in complete isolation, she will develop other ways of adapting to the new situation.

When one group is particularly strong, it can enforce its will on its membership and, even more dangerously, on weaker external groups or individuals. Group conformity can at times weaken or threaten the opinions of even the strongest personality. Being ostracised can be a painful and confusing experience. Being overwhelmed by another group can be equally traumatic.

Institutions can form staff groups where the needs of staff become paramount to the service they are supposed to be offering. There is a reality in the idea that a new hospital with all its fine resources and highly qualified staff can be run like clockwork until patients are admitted! Staff can forget the reason for their employment. Without a customer there is no sale and no need for a salesperson. Hospital or institutional policy gets priority and the customer—resident or patient—becomes a cog, seen only as a part of the machinery of performing a job. The staff group, with its clear-cut role, its routine, the things to be done and the time in which to do them, is the efficient, powerful group of prime importance. Policy dictates that dinners are served at set times, that clients must be washed, dressed, watered and medicated, all according to the clock. The individual is lost and within a short time those who fit in well without complaint become the 'good' patients (no trouble, but well institutionalised!) and those who fight back and insist on recognition become the nuisances, the recalcitrants.

Patients and residents have a right to be part of a group too. They are in a weak position, faced by a strong staff group with clear-cut rules, strategies and aims. How can they survive the onslaught without support? Until staff appreciate how easily they can—perhaps unwittingly—manipulate their patients or residents into total dependency, they will find it hard to understand the responses of their clients and their tendency to become rebellious or sullenly unresponsive. It should be a recognised duty of staff to ensure that their clients do have the opportunity of some form of group experience, of peer support, where their position can be strengthened and their identity defended.

Creating a group

If a person is impaired, fragile or limited in ability, help will be needed for a group to form. From the staff's point of view, a group opens up many avenues for help, stimulation and self-care. It provides interest, livens up the day and allows people to get to know each other, staff included! In such a situation, it is possible to find out what the clients want to do and what they can do. A useful guide to setting up groups has been produced by Bender & Norris (1987). In this book they suggest ways in which staff can consider

their own skills, what they can offer, what realistic aims could be set and what kinds of groups would be possible.

It is too often the case that group work is set up on an ad hoc basis. Support from senior staff is not sought, careful planning is not undertaken and false expectations arise (see Ch. 10). Without careful planning projects are in great danger of floundering.

Clients do not always 'cooperate' and refusals do occur. Are the group sessions attractive and rewarding enough? Could more positive experiences be included—outings, tea-parties, etc? Are staff being supportive enough? Whatever the cause, attendance in the end must be voluntary, though the genuine degree of refusal needs probing carefully. It is surprising how factors like shyness, lack of confidence or reluctance to move from a comfortable chair can all prove the reason for a refusal, and evaporate after a little gentle persuasion! To miss something interesting or to be left out are both strong enticements and usually prevail.

Problems that are common to group work need to be recognised, and strategies planned to counter them. The garrulous person, the domineering member, the person who never speaks are frequently encountered and need to be handled with thoughtful leadership. It is important to have knowledge of the skills and experiences of group members so that they can be incorporated into activities. Very often these can provide strategies for helping the quiet person to become established.

Social atmosphere

A basic aim must always be to help the elderly person succeed; their dementia brings so many experiences of failure that every opportunity must be grasped to reverse this damaging trend. For this to happen he/she needs to feel relaxed and unpressured. It is important to consider cultural patterns and personal likes and dislikes when choosing a setting for group work. For instance, in the USA many RO programmes use a classroom format, with the leader acting as a teacher, and possibly having 'graduation'

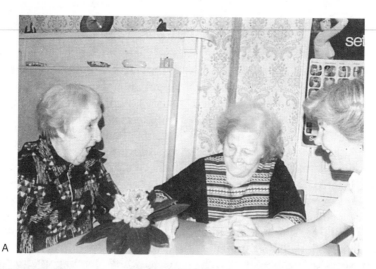

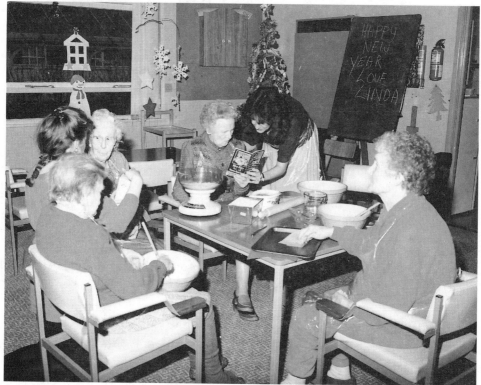

Figure 8.1 Good interaction using (**A**) humour and (**B**) established skills.

ceremonies when progress is made to a higher class. In the UK, this would generally be perceived as anxiety-provoking and demeaning; the cultural belief is that school is for children. Clearly much depends on the cultural background of those involved; if adult education becomes more widespread the classroom may become more attractive!

Where should the session take place? Ideally, a special room should be used. The atmosphere should be colourful, warm, sunny and relaxed and should be designed to stimulate interest and response. Large external windows are an asset. The ward atmosphere is not conducive to concentration or relaxation. It is associated with ideas of hospital, authority, routine and medical treatment. Even in community homes, the idea of a club or social activity room implies a change from routine and the possibility of being amused and diverted (Fig. 8.1).

In the room, a social atmosphere can be created with comfortable chairs, interesting and bright pictures and posters, small tables, flowers and plants, colourful curtains and so on. More elaborate settings can be devised. In Leeds, for example, RO rooms were established with a 'pub' atmosphere, reflecting the most popular British meeting place. In this situation people relax, amuse each other and talk freely. There are inevitably those who take the drinking aspect too seriously, but the vast majority go for the company and some may only sip at an alcoholic drink or simply stick to fruit juice. In former years, when current elderly patients were in their youth, most pubs tended to be male preserves. However when female patients were asked if they would prefer a tearoom they unanimously chose the pub, perhaps feeling slightly wicked in so doing!

To produce a simulated pub at low cost is comparatively easy. It is often possible to find old cupboards with the correct elbow height. Beer advertisements are on posters, ashtrays and labels. Help may be obtained from a kind local brewery. The hospital furniture store may have an old barrel and cash register. In everyone's home rests an object or two which would prove invaluable to such a setting. Enthusiasm and imagination on the part of the staff can work wonders! As most hospitals and residential homes have a little-used supply of beer, sherry and fruit juice for their elderly, there is generally no problem in finding the stock for the bar. It is more appropriate to have a drink in the right surroundings than by a bedside or simply at a meal table. Certainly it is more stimulating.

There are, of course, other kinds of suitable surroundings. One group in London were fortunate enough to have access to a swimming pool for their hemiplegic patients. They instigated an RO-type situation beside the pool where they could sit, relax and talk while not actually taking part in the water therapy.

Another ideal situation is an old-fashioned livingroom. The comfortable armchairs, old sideboard, table and dining chairs together with a real or simulated focal point fireplace provide a useful scene to stimulate social response. A family sittingroom demanded social response to visitors, required politeness and involvement in conversation and the playing of 'host and hostess'. It necessitated the need to entertain and produce tea and some form of refreshment. Old well-learned reactions are allies to positive approaches and in a livingroom such learned social behaviours are much more likely. A small female unit in Leeds used such a room imaginatively. Apart from employing it for formal sessions, each patient had the opportunity of occupying it at least once a week. This resulted in a greater awareness of the day of the week as each lady awaited her turn with eagerness. Once in occupation—usually in threes—each patient took over her chair, produced her crockery and utensils and adapted the room to suit her purpose and needs. Independence, interest and interpersonal relationships developed.

All is not lost, however, if a special room simply is not available. Group sessions can be carried out in a quiet corner of the dayroom or in the diningroom; the use of screens can partially remove any excessive distractions. If a special room is used, the distance from the dayroom is important as a great deal of time and effort can be expended simply getting the patient to the room if the distance is too great.

A further aid to a social atmosphere that should be considered is the avoidance of staff wearing uniforms in group sessions. Uniforms, so often a sign of authority, can be changed or disguised suitably before a session. However, more deteriorated patients may find uniforms useful aids initially to the identity of staff members; any change into everyday clothes should not change the staff member's appearance so much that he cannot be recognised as the same person by the patients! Removal of uniform does not, of course, necessarily remove authoritarian attitudes; we cannot emphasise too strongly that all positive approaches, group and individual, must be firmly based on the attitudes described in Chapter 7.

Levels of group sessions

It has been argued that to divide people into levels of functioning for group membership is both patronising and demeaning. However, in practice the concern has to be for the individual. Many programmes fail because the mix of extremes of ability is too great. It is much more effective and caring to ensure that a person is not stressed by members who are either much more capable, or very much less able. A person with a severe impairment needs to gain confidence and awareness in the group session, without feeling she is inferior to the other members. Equally, a mildly impaired individual would lose confidence in a group where others did not, say, know their own names and might, at worst deteriorate, at best become bored. It is appropriate to consider group membership carefully so that each group is more or less matched for level of ability, culture and possibly experience. This is the case no matter which approach is to be used.

GROUP APPROACHES

A number of approaches to group work with older people with dementia have been described. Three of these, RO-based groups, reminiscence groups and validation groups will be described here, before mention is made of groups with an emphasis on re-training. In addition, there are many examples of groups focusing on a particular activity, such as physical exercise, music, art or other activity. These will not be specifically described, but many elements of the communication methods described for the other approaches will be of relevance whatever the activity. Chapter 9 gives many examples of possible activities for group work with people with dementia.

RO sessions

Previously, we have described three levels of group: basic, standard and advanced (e.g. Holden & Woods 1988). Now that other forms of group work have become more common, it makes more sense simply to describe the first two levels where the RO input is most explicit; the advanced group was much more concerned with ensuring there was a good level of stimulation, of enjoyable activities shared with others in the environment, with members having choice and control over the programme. In fact even the standard group goes way beyond the focus on day and date that has become the stereotype of the practice of RO and incorporates a range of activities and topics.

Helping the elderly person achieve success—and thereby greater self-esteem and confidence—is the aim of the social atmosphere and of the methods used at all levels. Dementia so often is associated with failure at activities that were previously routine and automatic; helping the person to experience achievement by the careful choice of tasks and the judicious use of prompts can give a major boost to someone who is feeling defeated and who is reluctant to expose themself to further failure. This process is helped by using those skills and abilities that are retained and preserved rather than focusing on the person's areas of deficit and impairment. RO also brings people into contact with reality, by helping them be aware of what is happening around them, and by re-awakening interest and involvement in the environment. The groups differ in the scope of awareness that is covered, but all attempt to do this; all recognise that current reality makes sense only in relation to the past, so all use the person's store of past memories to a considerable degree; this means there is an overlap with reminiscence-based approaches. Finally, each level combats withdrawal, a process by which elderly people with dementia may appear much more impaired than in fact they are. At each level, communication is encouraged, with the leaders and with other group members. Conditions are created where this can take place. These aims can be summarised as helping the elderly person to:

- succeed
- use retained abilities and skills
- communicate
- know what is happening.

Basic group

Membership consists of those whose intellectual impairment is severe; they may be showing little response to or interest in their surroundings or in other people; attention and concentration are limited. The group needs to meet frequently, at least five times a week, for sessions of about 30 minutes, with only two or three members per member of staff. The aim is a simple one: to break through the withdrawal, using simple information on names, day, date, weather and so on in order to establish a rapport and a relationship, and to use repetition to aid re-learning or re-awakening. It is essential to reinforce even minor successes, to hold the person's attention and to avoid criticism or contradiction. After a week or two, the content of the group should be extended as in the next level of group.

During the first few days, the therapist must break through withdrawal with gentleness and courtesy, whilst encouraging trust and response. A situation in which failure might occur must be avoided carefully, so the aims are simple. A routine is established during which basic information such as names, days, months and the weather are discussed. At this stage, repetition is an essential aid to the re-learning process. Repetition is more useful and interesting if a variety of methods are used. The session is commenced by a handshake and a personal greeting: 'Hello, my name is …'. After the initial introductions it is appropriate to return to each individual with a further extended comment on names.

'Have I written your name properly? How would you like to be addressed, Mrs Jones, or would you prefer Mary? Can you say my name?' If the therapist's name has been forgotten, write it down and ask for it to be read. Simply writing the name, showing it and saying 'Look, this is how you spell my name' usually suffices. Large clear name badges can be useful in a small group, so that there is a visual reminder of group members' names. If errors in reading occur, further repetition is required. Names can be a useful means of reaching out to the group. Discussing other people with similar names reinforces the learning process and provides added interest.

The staff in groups at this basic level are extremely active in presenting information, directing the subject matter of the group and in sustaining the patients' attention. A board of some description is essential for the visual presentation of information. This can be fixed or portable, depending on the setting. If it is fixed, it should be clearly in the view of group members; writing on it should be large enough to be seen by all. A simple whiteboard will suffice; magnetic letters and names are widely available for such boards. Avoid the temptation to overload the board with information.

As part of the routine, this board can be completed during the session. The participants are asked what day it is, usually individually. If the response is wrong, the reply should be sufficiently gentle so there is no loss of face. 'Well, it is almost the weekend. It is Friday today', or 'Yesterday was Tuesday, so today it is Wednesday'. If the answer is correct, praise is given. Reading the correct day from the board reinforces this process. Prompts and cues are useful here; the day can be written letter by letter until someone guesses the answer. If no one guesses, the group can read the complete name, so whatever happens the correct response will be achieved. The clue of the first few letters could be given verbally of course. If the board is completed before the session then members can be encouraged to take their cue directly from the board, and so again be spared the risk of a wrong answer. A similar pattern is followed for the remaining information: month, year, date, whereabouts of the hospital or old people's home and weather are basics. In considering the month, help can be obtained from the view through the window. The introduction of seasonal flowers and fruit or calendar-like pictures can also be of assistance. The members are encouraged to look outside, to notice the sky and the state of growth of trees and plants. The look and smell of a spring or summer bouquet of flowers or a collection of fallen autumn leaves emphasises the season.

If answers to questions are vague, slow, unforthcoming or consistently incorrect the right answer is supplied gently and conversationally. Direct criticism or contradiction should be avoided as confidence could be destroyed. 'I just told you that' or 'No, that's wrong' are destructive remarks.

Once these areas of information have been covered, the whole board is re-read by group members, with the therapist prompting those with reading or speech problems. Diaries are commonly used in RO for those without reading or writing difficulties. Some people enjoy keeping a diary and complete it in detail; at least the simple routine facts may be recorded. This adds variety to the repetition, and members can read out their diary entries to the others. Large letter cards can be used by patients who have lost the fine motor control required for writing; they can be given the letters needed to spell their name or a short word and asked to put them in the right order.

A further aspect of information to be given is time. Initially this may be in terms of morning, afternoon and evening, but where appropriate a large clock with adjustable hands can be used to show current time, time of meals and so on.

This level of group is quite demanding on the staff, as they have to maintain the group members' attention throughout because their concentration span is usually exceedingly short. Preferably there should be two members of staff to support each other.

The group is made up of adults not children. To patronise or talk down to older people is to guarantee that they will remain withdrawn or become agitated or resentful. Friendliness and courtesy create the right atmosphere for response. The session should always start and end with handshakes, hellos and farewells. Interruptions and 'observers' who do not participate are not helpful. In order to establish rapport with this level of group, the subject matter may seem low level. As long as the therapist is gentle and

unthreatening, this initial period is necessary in order to establish a relationship of trust and expectation. As soon as the person is able to cope in a relaxed fashion with this level it is imperative that the simple aim be changed and the group member moved on to the next stage. In Box 8.1 the features of this level of group are summarised.

Box 8.1 Features of the basic group (for the most severely disorientated and withdrawn patients)

- Two to three patients per therapist
- Daily sessions, 30 minutes, social setting
- Emphasis on basic information, presented and repeated
- Repetition varied, reading from board, writing in diary, etc; many clues provided to guarantee successful response
- Use of RO board and other aids: calendar, large letter cards (for those unable to write) a teaching clock, etc
- Therapists extremely active in sustaining attention, directing group, presenting information
- Patients move on to standard group as soon as possible.

Standard group

The standard group is appropriate for patients who are responsive to some degree and who can take a little interest in people and things. The programme should be flexible, according to group members' needs, interests and skills. Rigidity in the programme will be demonstrated by complaints from individuals about being treated as though they were in school, or a refusal to attend because of boredom. The approach must be adapted to the group not vice versa. As soon as there is some evidence of improved response, the aim, scope and methods are broadened.

Introductions, names and warm greetings remain the natural starting point for the session. Again the RO board is used to discuss basic information, but this is achieved more quickly in this group. The information too may be in more depth and detail. Diaries are likely to be particularly useful here.

Following the brief, basic information part of the session, a wide variety of activities is possible. The type of activity and the equipment needed

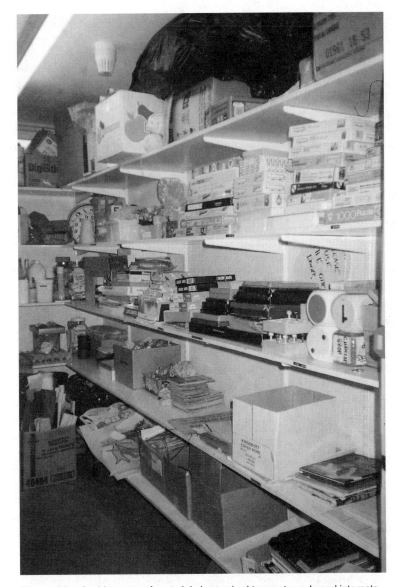

Figure 8.2   A wide range of materials is required to meet needs and interests.

(Fig. 8.2) are described in Chapter 9. The aims here are to:

- foster interpersonal relationships, social awareness and interest
- connect and compare past and present, capitalising on the person's previous experiences
- stimulate the person's senses.

Sessions are slightly less directed, and therapists will use the responses of group members to develop a theme or to change tack entirely! Thus, pictures of food may have been intended to start a discussion on shopping, prices, etc, but may elicit more response on cooking and favourite foods.

It is important to have knowledge of individual histories, experiences and interests. More personal orientation is encouraged: age, date of birth, names and whereabouts of family members, previous occupations and interests, places where the person has lived are among the items that might be covered over a number of sessions. Staff need to know this information themselves so they can reinforce the person appropriately. A separate index card with these details on it for each group member is of great value for this purpose.

Although the therapists are slightly less directive, their role is still demanding. Before sessions they need to plan topics and collect relevant materials. They need to guide discussion, encourage social interaction, gently praise appropriate responses, watch for patients who are bored, through the level being either too basic or too advanced, and modify the methods used accordingly. Group sessions can last for up to an hour, where staff time permits.

In encouraging social relationships, common backgrounds, occupations, interests and experiences are important. Topics that are likely to establish such links include old and new pictures and maps of the area where patients used to live, common occupations and industries of the area, and everyday items from the past.

For each topic, a tangible focus is essential: a picture, an object, a newspaper, slides, a short film, materials, and even a collection of smells. Everyday objects, such as fruit or even a cup and saucer, can lead to consideration of colour, shape, taste, smell, texture, preferences (in the case of fruit) or material (bone china or plastic!), design, texture, function, and then lead naturally on to memories of tea parties (in the case of a cup and saucer). That discussion would end, of course, with a cup of tea for the group!

The group does not have to be static. If mobility and weather permit, why not make a collection of autumn leaves. If the topic is the hospital or home why not have a tour, with members pointing out 'landmarks': the lounge, dining-room, their own sleeping area, etc.

At this level, as at the others, where gaps occur in members' memories, cues and prompts are given so that the person does not fail. The strategies for responding to things the person says which are apparently 'confused' or 'rambling' were discussed in Chapter 7.

Humour is important; a group where laughter is frequent is likely to be much more useful and effective than an over-serious group. For example, one 93-year-old man caused a stir by describing how he had made his wife *walk* several hundred miles to meet his family. Female group members castigated him for his irresponsible behaviour, and he, with a broad grin, responded by adding more outrageous detail, to the delight of all concerned.

In another group, a series of everyday objects was being named; one was a woollen tea-pot cover which one group member then put on as a hat and proceeded to dance a jig around the room, whilst everyone collapsed with laughter.

Reality is not, of course, constant happiness; the whole range of emotions may arise in the group. Topics should not be banned in order to 'protect' the elderly people. A moving group session was stimulated by a poppy, reminding participants of the 1914–1918 war and the awful loss of young men there.

Rather than banning religion and politics, the topics can be usefully employed to arouse active response and healthy emotion.

Sex, love and marriage should not be taboo either. Relationships between the sexes can do a great deal to combat withdrawal, and the group should be mixed for this reason. Their attitude towards sex is often humorous and teasing and they can turn the tables to tease the therapist when so inclined. Some useful and most amusing sessions can develop as a result of open discussion on their attitudes to sex and members of the opposite sex.

Death too is something that is too frequently a taboo subject. If one of the group should fall sick, or there should be a death on the ward or in the home there is no reason to fear open discussion. Those in contact with the elderly often underestimate their ability to cope with natural emotion and become over-protective.

The main features of this standard group are given in Box 8.2 and Chapter 9 should be referred to for detailed ideas for sessions.

Box 8.2 Features of the standard group (for the majority of moderately disorientated patients)

- Two to three patients per therapist
- Daily sessions, 30–60 minutes; social setting
- Begin with basic information, follow with wide variety of activities, topics for discussion, etc
- Stimulate all senses, with a variety of sensorial aids
- Encourage social awareness and interest
- Use the past as a bridge to the present
- Prompts, clues used as necessary: reminders of the past, money, pictures, everyday objects, food, newspapers, fresh fruit, etc
- Therapist needs to plan, collect relevant materials, watch for boredom, guide discussion
- Extend activities: outings, wide range of topics
- Encourage members' suggestions.

Reminiscence groups

Group work based on reminiscence approaches has become increasingly popular; with a small group of people with dementia at ease with each other and with the group leader(s), such groups can be a most enjoyable and rewarding experience. The knowledge and expertise of the older people can prove fascinating for all involved and, with more able participants, the simplest of prompts will elicit a response: 'What was it like to grow up in … town?' 'What sort of holidays did you have?' 'What did you manage to cook when food was rationed?' Others will need a greater level of prompting. All manner of tangible aids to reminiscence work are available: contemporary photographs of everyday life, newsreel video-tapes, reproductions of newspaper front-pages depicting major events ranging from coronations to airship crashes, photographs of famous people and events, audiotapes of music and radio broadcasts, and objects associated with a particular period, such as a ration book, gas mask and so on. These are of great assistance but should be seen as a starting point for developing further, more local reminiscence-based resources. Local libraries, museums of everyday life and even old people's attics are worth exploring in building up a collection of materials. Every area has its own peculiar stories and folklore, its landmarks and its major events that will prove stimulating in a reminiscence group.

The majority of older people enjoy reminiscing (as do younger people, hence the huge demand for instant nostalgia in TV and books); however, a word of caution is necessary, as there are some people who prefer not to think about the past, perhaps because of some painful memories or, in some cases, because reflecting on a happy past acts as a reminder of all that has been lost in the present (see Coleman 1986). It is important then to be sensitive to the individual's preferences in this regard. Participants will also differ in how much they wish to speak about personal matters in a group setting, and members should not be pressured or even strongly prompted to do so; those who feel sufficiently comfortable will offer more personal experiences when they are ready to do so. Preparation is required by group leaders, who should ensure they know enough about the person's life to ensure any potentially painful areas are handled sensitively and with tact. This is not to say that the discussion must always be 'safe' and bland, but rather that group members must have the choice of steering off more sensitive topics or of discussing them, and that group leaders must avoid prising personal information from a group member who wishes to remain quiet. For example, a group session may be discussing children and raising a family; the group leader might have a quiet word with a member who lost a child as a baby beforehand and ask whether she would prefer to sit out of the group today. Sometimes, despite such preparation, a particular memory quite un-predictably strikes a nerve in a group member, who perhaps starts to cry. The group leader's role here is clear: to ensure the person is supported by leaders and other members, has the oppor-tunity to say anything they wish to (without being pressured to reveal all), and that the support continues after the group session. It should not be seen as a failure if some tears are shed from time to time; life experiences are not all jolly and cheerful, and part of being human is to have the range of emotions; good cinema films may make people laugh *or* cry (or both)! The point here is that it is the shared sadnesses that the remi-niscence group should properly elicit rather than the deeply personal tragedies.

The aim of the group should *not* then be seen as helping members resolve problems from the past in order to improve their current adjustment; this requires self-evaluation and appraisal of the person's memories with the help of a trained therapist, is usually conducted on a one-to-one basis, and is properly described as life review therapy (see, for example, Garland 1994, Haight & Burnside 1992). As yet, its applicability to people with dementia is not known. This should be distinguished from life-history work, which aims to produce a factual account of the person's life without the necessity for the memories and events to be evaluated by the older person. Such life-history work greatly enhances reminiscence work, building up a fuller picture of the whole person. Enjoyment, sharing, interaction, building up relationships (with other members and with staff) are the proper, attainable aims of reminiscence groups with older people.

A number of useful descriptions of the practicalities of running reminiscence groups is available (e.g. Norris 1986, Haight & Burnside 1992, Bender 1994, Gibson 1994, Woods & McKiernan 1994), together with accounts of generally applicable group-work principles (e.g. Bender & Norris 1987). Careful preparation and planning is essential; it is not enough to take a few old photographs into the lounge of a residential home and see if they stimulate a discussion. Factors that should be considered in running reminiscence groups are outlined in Box 8.3.

Validation groups

Like RO and reminiscence, validation has individual as well as group applications, and the primary validation technique—of validating the person's feelings—is described in Chapter 7. Feil (1993) describes in detail the formation and operation of validation groups. She argues that for some patients such groups have benefits over one-to-one work in that they enhance the person's attention span, foster a sense of self-worth and involve the person in a natural social context. Validation groups aim to stimulate verbal and non-verbal interaction and to increase members' feelings of well-being in a setting where

---

Box 8.3 Factors of importance in reminiscence groups

- The group should be fairly small; four to six members with one or two leaders; where impairment is greater there should be at least one member of staff to every two older people.
- Level of ability should be similar among group members.
- Leaders require sufficient information about participants' backgrounds.
- There should be plenty of appropriate materials to aid reminiscence: pictures, books, music, photographs, objects, etc.
- About an hour should be allowed for the session, including refreshments.
- The group should meet in a quiet, undisturbed room, where members can feel comfortable and relaxed.
- Be aware of individual needs; only include those who wish to reminisce; do not push the discussion onto personal topics; let group members dictate how much personal material is shared.
- Move the discussion on if participants are becoming bored; use music and topics such as entertainment to balance some of the weightier discussions.
- As in all groups, be aware of the effects of members' sensory difficulties and attempt to minimise these through attention to seating arrangements, use of hearing aids, using aids from more than one modality (e.g. music *and* pictures *and* objects) and so on.
- All good stories gain a little extra in the telling, and reminiscence groups are certainly not intended to be history lessons; staff should not be over-concerned with how accurate the memories being discussed are and should not seek to 'correct' the person's account.
- Plan a theme for each session—childhood, school, work, holidays, etc—with appropriate prompts available; be ready to deviate when the flow of memories takes over!
- When it is appropriate, encourage the group to go beyond discussion, e.g. to sing a favourite song together, to dance, or to demonstrate a childhood game or how a particular job was carried out. Sometimes actions speak louder than words!
- A poster display showing aspects of what has been discussed, e.g. pictures of the different jobs that members used to do, makes a tangible reminder of the session. If put up in a prominent position it will interest older people not in the group and other staff, and members may enjoy pointing out their contribution.

---

social controls may be developed, with members taking on social roles within the group. Feil (1993) describes a number of features of validation groups, which have been incorporated to a large extent in the group described by Bleathman & Morton (1992).

Ritual. There is a clear ritual to the group, a structure to provide familiarity and security for the members. A consistent time and place for the group is important, but the pattern of the group is also ritualised, with a beginning, middle and end.

• The leader greets everyone formally and with overt politeness; everyone is invited to hold hands throughout the meeting.
• The 'welcomer' is invited to welcome everyone to the group.
• The 'song leader' is asked to begin the opening song; this may be followed by a prayer or poem.
• The leader introduces the topic for the day.
• The 'dance leader' or 'rhythm band leader' is asked to lead the movement and rhythm section.
• The 'song leader' is asked to begin the closing song.
• The 'host/hostess' is asked to pass the refreshments.
• The 'welcomer' is asked to thank everyone for coming and to look forward to the next meeting.
• The 'song leader' may lead another song.
• The leader says goodbye individually to each member.

The meeting lasts from 20 minutes to an hour, and participants should meet at least once a week.

Roles. As can be seen, a number of roles for members are envisaged: welcomer, song leader, host/hostess and so on. The person retains the same role throughout the life of the group. The role is intended to reflect the person's background, or it may arise from the individual's current needs; thus, Feil suggests that a man who acts out sexually might become the dance leader, with the opportunity to touch women in a socially acceptable fashion.

Leader's role. The leader has a demanding role and benefits from having a co-worker, to assist with observation and evaluation. The leader's key task is to facilitate interaction and to enable group members to help each other.

Music. Music has an important role in the group, being used to match the topic and mood of the meeting. Familiar love songs, marching songs and lullabies are recommended. Rhythm instruments, bells and cymbals may be used while singing.

Movement. Feil describes movement activities as an important element of the group, in encouraging interaction. She gives as examples dancing (Fig 8.3), throwing a bean bag, passing a soft ball, art and craft projects, finger painting, kneading dough and indoor gardening.

Topics. The topics selected for discussion in the group are intended to reflect universal human needs, such as affection, purpose, attachment and identity. The intention is to draw on the intuitive wisdom of the group in tackling these issues. This may be approached by calling on the person's experience of life: 'What advice would you give a young couple thinking of getting married?'; 'What makes people happy/sad?' Feil also uses more direct questions, such as 'Do you miss your parents/home/job?' New group leaders would be well advised to make use of more general questions, letting the person give a more personal answer if he/she chooses.

Food. Sharing food is seen as nurturing for the members; refreshments should be selected so that they can be passed easily without spillage, so as not to embarrass the host/hostess.

Comfort. The room should be comfortable, with chairs in a circle and any tables required for refreshments and activities outside the circle. The co-worker should sit next to any member who requires continual physical contact.

Security. The group is intended to be a safe place to express feelings, including anger, openly. Often these will be shown non-verbally, perhaps in ways upsetting to other members. The group leader seeks to help the person express the feeling verbally by directly commenting on it: 'Mrs Jones, you don't want to sit down; you seem really upset', or by mirroring the person's movements; for example, if the person is shaking their fist, the group leader copies him/them. The aim is to help the person be aware of their behaviour, and to indicate that a person's feelings are accepted in the group.

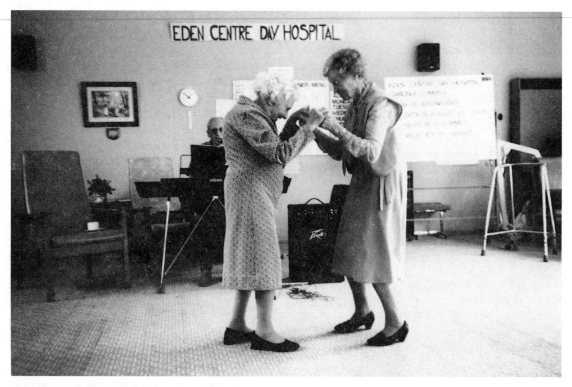

Figure 8.3 Music and movement serve many needs—exercise and pleasure among them.

Suitable participants. Feil recommends careful selection of participants for validation groups, and gives a lengthy list of exclusion criteria. Feil has a rather complex system for categorising people with dementia, and readers are referred to Feil (1993) for a full exposition of this. Essentially, the severely impaired, with very limited response, are thought to require an individual approach; among the more mildly impaired, those who have the tendency to blame others for any problems, adamantly denying any impairment in themselves, are said not to respond well to the group setting.

Workload. It is fair to say that carrying out validation work successfully is demanding and draining; we would recommend that new workers gain experience initially with other forms of group and develop skills in individual validation. When considering setting up a validation group, it is wise to seek advice, support and supervision from someone with more experience of the approach. Feil recommends training and certification for

validation workers and this reflects that this type of work requires special skills and experience, and on-going supervision; it is not to be undertaken lightly.

Re-training groups

The cognitive rehabilitation of patients with specific brain damage is an extensive topic (see Craine 1987 for a full coverage). However, as awareness grows of the contribution of particular areas of difficulty (see Ch. 6) caused by strokes or particular degenerative conditions, increasingly direct attention will be given to these difficulties, which, when unrecognised, can cause so much frustration to older people and staff. At times, special groups based around a shared difficulty will be formed and a re-training programme designed specially to meet this specific need.

People with language deficits will be helped by group activities which do not use verbal language as the primary form of communication.

Non-verbal material is provided: pictures, sequenced drawings to explain what to do; gesture and games that do not require either the spoken or written word will prove useful.

Those with spatial difficulties will benefit from games and activities which re-train spatial organisation: 'Connect 4', drawing house plans and placing relevant furniture pictures in the right rooms, picking out photographs of objects relating to a large picture of, say, a supermarket, main street or station.

When staff are aware of agnosias they need to provide other sensory cues, avoiding the impaired sensory pathway, in order to aid recognition. When apraxia is present, they need to avoid telling the person what to do when a difficulty arises in performing tasks under voluntary control.

People who are neglecting one side of their bodies are given opportunities to be able to view important aspects of their environment with as much ease as possible and efforts are made to improve their awareness of the neglected side.

Examples of groups for those with specific memory difficulties (Wilson & Moffat 1984, Moffat 1989, Lincoln 1989) have been described, using memory games and exercises; these bear some resemblance to RO-type activities. Overall the aim is to ensure difficulties are not reinforced and to encourage the development of coping skills.

CONCLUSION

The atmosphere for group sessions must be relaxed and non-threatening. Therapists must approach the situation with an awareness of the individual and of the dangers of rigidity. Withdrawal can result from boredom, too fast a pace, or by setting aims too high; these factors are under the influence of the therapists. Too many questions can prove very threatening and unnatural in a social situation. Conversations are not one-sided or composed of questions and answers. Re-training needs to be subtle and hidden in conversation. An interrogation where questions are asked as quickly as the patient fails to answer them is not RO; telling someone that the old shop was pulled down years ago is not resolving feelings; loudly stating 'She won't be able to do that' is not recognising the person's existence as a human being. Failure must be avoided as it could prove disastrous to the patient's progress.

If the aims are low, initially success becomes more probable. As each step forward is achieved, praise is given and another simple aim set. Praise can be freely given for minor successes. Many elderly people with dementia have received very little praise because of their difficult behaviour. Aggressive, domineering people need to be encouraged to help the less forceful so that they do not receive more than their fair share of attention. Praise can prove too fulsome for the more independent and may sound patronising. In this situation, reinforcement can be satisfactorily achieved by a gentle, matter-of-fact comment of approval. Generally, the enjoyment of social interactions and achievement is reinforcing in itself.

Therapists need feedback as well as patients. The coordinator can ensure that results and progress are made available to the staff. The expectations of staff must be realistic. Changes may be very slow or only minimal in certain cases. Group sessions are hard work and demanding. Factors that have been discussed in this chapter that assist in producing successful groups are summarised in Box 8.4. Initially, the elderly patient may be too confused or unable to respond without considerable effort on the part of the therapist. It requires good planning, realistic aims, energy and imagination to obtain worthwhile reactions and progress.

Box 8.4 Summary of effective methods for group work

- Create atmosphere. A special room modified for use as a pub, livingroom or clubhouse is ideal. A social setting helps remotivation and resocialisation.
- Elderly people with dementia have a short attention and memory span. Constant stimulation is required to maintain interest and cooperation.
- Constant but varied repetition is necessary to aid re-learning.
- Praise and approval can reinforce re-learning.
- Patients may be confused and withdrawn, but are not children. Their knowledge and experience are buried and need restoring.
- Positive approaches should be available for 24 hours, not just 1 hour! Positive attitudes are reinforced by a positive environment.
- Friendliness, courtesy and knowledge about the individual are vital aids in re-establishing confidence.
- Therapists and clients should know and use each other's names; the formal title or the intimate first-name basis must be decided among them.
- Signs of authority do not help relationships. Uniforms can be changed or disguised.
- Rigidity is retarding. A re-learning programme once assimilated indicates the need to progress.
- As soon as possible, individuals should be involved in group activities as social interaction is important to rehabilitation processes. Interpersonal relationships can be encouraged even in the early stages of therapy.
- Sensorial stimulation should be used: interesting smells, tastes and the feel of things are as valuable as visual material.
- Clients must be placed in appropriate groups so that suitable levels can be provided and realistic aims set.
- Therapists need to be friendly, involved and capable of using imagination and initiative.
- Relatives can be included but need guidance and monitoring as family attitudes can cause reversal.
- Basic to the therapy is the capitalisation on clients' long-term memory stores. Their prime of life— roughly 1920–1950 for someone who is aged 60–90 in the 1990s—is the period they remember the best. They are secure in discussing this era. This makes it possible to direct their attention to the present and bring them up-to-date by comparisons between then and now.
- Patients can be helped to succeed by the use of clues and prompts, and by avoidance of exposure of disabilities.

9

101 ideas for group sessions

The greatest source of pleasure is variety.

Dr Johnson

MAKING A PROGRAMME

Frequently, it becomes difficult to think of a topic or to plan a day-to-day programme for group sessions. As a result, the session deteriorates into a time when the staff and patients/residents just sit about and talk vaguely and without purpose, and this becomes a negative experience for all concerned. This can also arise when the therapist is tired or has been too busy to have time to prepare topics. The following suggestions are intended to help in such situations. They are not exhaustive but illustrate the range of possibilities.

Many of the items listed in Appendix 3 as aids to RO and reminiscence, as well as the small pocket book *RO Reminders* (Holden 1984b), are additional sources of ideas for stimulating, purposeful activities and for extending the range of possible programmes. Leaders should select and adapt topics and ideas carefully to be appropriate for the abilities and interests of the particular group. From the ideas here, and others that can be added, a set of 20 or 30 different programmes suitable for group work for a particular setting, clientele and level of ability can be constructed and written out on separate cards. A card may then be chosen more or less at random and can be used to give structure to the session; also any equipment needed can be assembled just prior to the session. Example cards are shown in Table 9.1; these were used

Table 9.1   Examples of possible programme cards

A	B
1. Introductions—greet each other by name.	1. Introductions—greet each other by name.
2. Enter day, date, name of home on RO board; change calendar; copy into personal diaries.	2. Enter day; date, name of home on RO board; change calendar; copy into personal diaries.
3. Use spelling boards to rearrange mixed-up words and use longer words only when residents gain confidence.	3. Enter age, date of birth and place of birth in diary. Discuss who is oldest, youngest, etc.
4. Bring in common objects: cup, saucer, plate, spoon, comb, hat, pencil, key, umbrella, etc. Name the object and its colour. What shape is it? What does it feel like? Cold, warm, rough, smooth, hard, soft? Draw round the object.	4. Discuss weather using weather board. Is it as expected for time of year? Is it changeable? What weather is forecast? What clothes would be needed outside today? Find appropriate weather picture.
5. Prepare a menu of residents' favourite foods. Compare with actual menu!	5. Play picture dominoes; small prize for winner.
Equipment: Diaries Spelling boards and letters Common objects Pencils and paper	Equipment: Diaries and pens Weatherboard and pictures Picture dominoes Small prize

with a standard group in an old people's home where most residents suffered from some form of dementia. Use of such a system ensures variety in the sessions and helps when the therapist's creativity runs dry. They should be quickly ignored when a group leader has a new or better idea or if something emerges from the group. They are to fall back on rather than to be used rigidly.

A cupboard for accumulated items of interest is essential, preferably in the room where the group session takes place. An alternative approach to planning a topic is to start with a piece of equipment. A small box of cards in two sizes can be used as an index. Each piece of available equipment can be given a separate large card, e.g. MAPS, HERBS AND SPICES, CLOTH, etc. Under each of these headings, an appropriate letter or letters will indicate which of the smaller cards to consult. Placed in alphabetical order, the small cards supply suggested topics that may be relevant to the use of the equipment. For instance, under 'T' suggestions for topics could include Travel, Taste, Touch, Transport, Tailoring, etc. So in order to find suggestions for the use of a bag of cloth, the therapist would look up the card headed CLOTH and find, for instance, the letters TCOH. On consulting the smaller card 'C' appro-

priate topics would be Clothing, Cost, Colour; under 'T', Tailoring, Touch; under 'O', Occupations; and under 'H', Household jobs, Homecrafts, and so forth. Each provides a useful starting point for discussion and stimulation. The topics included depend entirely on the experience and imagination of the therapist which can, by this means, be used collectively. Cues are needed by staff as well as by the group members!

Ideas for sessions are best described by breaking them down into those suitable for each level of ability. The following ideas are not intended to inspire rigidity; they are simply suggestions. A group may have interests which require other avenues not included. There are differences in every group, and in people from every area and cultural background. After only a few meetings these differences are noticeable and should be recognised.

BASIC GROUP

The lowest level of ability presents the greatest danger of material that is intended to stimulate being perceived as threatening, patronising, insulting or boring. Be sensitive to the person's background, previous level of functioning and experience; use the ideas here as a starting point, but move on if the person is able; be guided by the person's enjoyment of and involvement with the activity—if it is not helping to open up communication go on to something else. Effective ideas fall into a number of groups.

1. Introductions. Always a good (and necessary) starting point. Shake hands, use large name labels so members can identify each other without the embarrassment of forgetting names.

2. Large weather board. This comprises a main board and a collection of smaller pieces which slot into or adhere magnetically to the board. On these are written the days, months, comments and pictures about the weather. They can be made or purchased (see Appendix 3) and are used to present relevant information and stimulate some discussion on this most talked-about topic.

3. Personal diaries. Those who retain writing skills can copy basic information into their diaries, providing further repetition. Also there is scope for personal entries about past, current and future events, which gives the person an on-going record to refer to. All members can have their own 'This is your life' book, including details of important events and people in the person's life. Wherever possible this should be illustrated with relevant photographs. Such a book helps the person show others more of what they have experienced and achieved in their life than they may now be able to communicate readily. If put together carefully with the help of relatives and friends, it also aids the group leader in responding accurately to the person's queries about their circumstances and helps them find the information for themselves. A suitable booklet is available (*The Memory Diary*, see Appendix 3), or it can be made from scrapbooks and photographs.

4. Letters. Large letters: on wooden squares, or on cards (as in 'Lexicon'), or plastic letters with magnets attached for use with metal spelling boards. All can be used to spell out simple items of basic information, particularly where group members have difficulty writing. For instance, as a guessing game, they could be used to spell out the day of the week, letter by letter, until someone calls out the correct answer.

5. Flowers. Fresh and seasonal flowers can be used to emphasise the time of year and stimulate sight, touch and smell. Also, fallen leaves in autumn are effective.

6. Fruit. Again used fresh to emphasise seasons and stimulate senses, including taste!

7. Food. Other items of food can be brought in where appropriate: cakes, sweets, raw ingredients—flour, salt, raisins, etc—vegetables, sandwiches and so on, to stimulate senses and discussion, once they have been identified.

8. Drink. Provide various beverages—tea, coffee, fruit drinks, sherry, wine, beer, etc—for taste, identification, smell and enjoyment!

9. Maps. Plastic or wood shapes of Great Britain, America, Australia, Europe, etc. Large, clear map of the local city or town. Maps help in orientation, discussion of 'where we are' and 'where we come from'. Several members may be from the same area, so the maps help to identify possible neighbours or common knowledge. In later stages, 'places we have visited' is another topic arising from maps.

10. Large clock face with movable hands. This should be as realistic as possible. The clock can be used to indicate present time, breakfast, dinner, and bedtime.

11. Whiteboard (and pens). These have many uses in repeating and reinforcing whatever is discussed. More able patients should be encouraged to write on the board for others.

12. Collages. These can be made in the group; members search through magazines looking for pictures that illustrate the particular theme, cut these out and stick them on a large piece of paper.

13. Collages of seasons. To aid discussion of the time of year.

14. Collages of food. These can emphasise time, by depicting different meals for different times of day. Also they can help discussion about preferences, ingredients, prices, etc.

15. Collages of children. Used to emphasise a sense of lifespan, memories of patients' own childhood and their own children, grandchildren, etc.

16. Collages of places. Local pictures or pictures depicting places further afield can be used in conjunction with maps. Reminders of the group's previous 'haunts'—the main street, shops, local landmarks and so on—assist in recreating a temporarily forgotten daily existence.

17. Picture cards illustrating occupations. Occupation cards (e.g. postman, window cleaner, miner, etc) can be useful in reminding people about everyday jobs which provide day-to-day contact in the environment. The postman, the butcher and the bus conductor are part of everyday reality.

STANDARD GROUP

By using visual and other stimulation and by encouraging reminiscences through related materials, the person may be drawn into contributing to the group. Here too, it is vitally important to match the activities to the person. Learning more about them as individuals with specific interests can assist in the search for suitable equipment and relevant approaches, all of which can be exploited in building up good relationships. The person's culture, specialised experience and knowledge may give indications as to retained skills, knowledge and abilities that may be given opportunity for expression. It will be helpful to seek the suggestions of others from a similar background or with similar interests or experiences.

18. 'Then' and 'now'. Most towns have produced a book full of photographs of places and familiar landmarks of 'then' and 'now'. These are invaluable for discussion, showing how the town has changed since group members were children. If such a book is not available then libraries, etc, often have collections of old photographs, copies or slides of which could be obtained, together with up-to-date comparisons. If there is an area where most of the group live, it is possible that they also had schools in common. They have memories of the buildings, streets and activities of the district and may well have mutual friends and acquaintances. They may have shopped in the same shopping centre, been married in the same church, etc. Finding such things in common can greatly help a group interact.

19. Old newspapers. National and local papers can, again, provide a stimulus to reminiscence. This can aid grasp of current reality as it is brought up-to-date into the present. Libraries often have collections of old newspapers.

20. Gardening. Pictures and books may elicit memories and knowledge of plants, flowers, vegetables, etc. Advanced groups could try indoor gardening—bulbs, plants, cress and so on—as a continuing activity.

21. Cookery. Pictures and recipe books are useful (as well as real food). Discuss favourite recipes, particularly for traditional foods. More advanced groups could carry out simple cookery; all can help mix ingredients for cakes and sweets as a group exercise (Fig. 9.1) and enjoy the smell of cooking, as well as sampling the finished product!

22. Clothes. Books and pictures of fashions over the years may prompt fascinating reminiscences; current fashions always produce interesting comments! If costumes from the patient's youth can be obtained these can be 'modelled'.

23. Occupations. In any given region or area, there are many employed in particular local industries or occupations and knowledge of these is valuable too. Any relevant material from such industries inspires discussion and reminiscences. It also provides therapists with opportunities to introduce present-day comparisons. Pictures of coalmines and miners in the 1920s and 1930s can bind a group together in a mining area, for instance. Many members of groups may have spent some time in domestic service. Local or national firms may prove helpful. Films can be hired, there may be a library or museum on the subject, and most homes have objects or materials which would prove invaluable—old typewriters, miner's lamps, models of ships, old tools, looms, etc. Things lying around the home for years unnoticed suddenly assume importance as they could provoke memories and experiences. It is equally important to have a supply of modern material to show how things have changed.

24. Royalty. In the UK, books and pictures of the Royal family past and present often stimulate interest; tracing the Royal family tree through the use of pictures gives the elderly

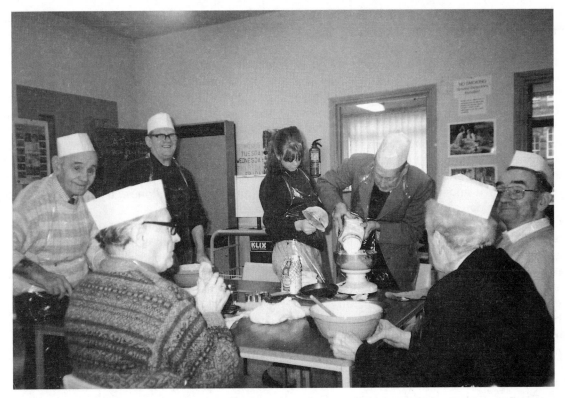

Figure 9.1   Men need and enjoy cooking skills as much as women.

person a sense of their own ageing and development.

25. Cars. Group members will have lived through massive changes in the motor car (and other forms of transport). Old and new pictures and models are useful here. Members may recall their first car, or their first journey.

26. Homecrafts. Members may have had previously interests in sewing, embroidery, knitting, crochet and so on. Discussion of these crafts, together with finished articles and pictures, may produce a number of memories, and may encourage members to attempt some tasks themselves.

27. Travel. A number of topics arise from this theme; members can describe their furthest travels, the method of travel, speed of journeys and so on. Pictures of places near and far will aid such a discussion.

28. Animals. Pictures would be the stimulus here. Have you ever seen a lion? Ever ridden a horse? Milked a cow? The questions draw on well-learned knowledge and may evoke memories, e.g. one old seaman vividly described his experiences with whales.

29. Pets. The real thing can be the stimulus here, as well as pictures. It can start a discussion of pets people have had and the sometimes harsh reality of not having them in the hospital or home. Different breeds of dogs and cats may also be a discussion topic, using relevant photographs.

30. Birds. This topic could be developed as above, with pet birds and wild birds being observed 'live' or in photographs. A bird table just outside the ward or home would facilitate this and provide a daily routine of feeding the birds.

31. Art. Interest in paintings, drawings and sculpture could be explored with the help of large colourful reproductions. Some popular paintings will be identified; others can be appreciated or in some cases can be the cause of group bewilderment! According to ability, a group art session of painting, drawing, modelling in clay, simple printing, sticking on of coloured shapes or whatever can be a good activity.

32. Stamps. Even if members have not been avid collectors, interest can be aroused by colourful stamps from around the world (use with a map) or using a range of stamps from the person's lifetime; the historical changes (and changes in price of sending a letter) can be a cause for comment.

33. Coins. Different value coins (and notes) can be identified and used to carry out simple arithmetic. The dates and heads on the coins are also worthy of discussion. Coins and notes from around the world could also be used; in the UK pre-decimal coins could evoke memories and comparisons.

34. Holidays. A rich source of discussion, prompted by picture postcards, brochures, etc. What sort of holiday: seaside, country; hotel, camping, boarding house; home or abroad? Where did members go on holiday? What did they do whilst on holiday? Where would they like to have gone?

35. Famous houses, castles, palaces. These are of interest, particularly if local. Pictures will help recall visits to such places.

36. Countryside. Pictures of local country areas may remind members of country walks, the rural life, the country year and so on.

37. Mountains. Pictures of grand mountain scenery provide another topic, with mountain sports and dangers being possibilities for discussion.

38. Racing. Pictures of famous horses and jockeys of the past, together with comparisons with the present scene will interest former racing followers.

39. Small antiques. Pieces of furniture or bric-a-brac brought into the group can promote discussion of the purpose of the items and whether group members had anything similar; what would be used now?

40. Old toys. Again, a comparison can be made, e.g. between lead and plastic soldiers, clockwork and electric trains, china dolls and dolls whose hair grows! Computer games defy comparison!

41. Traditional cards. Greetings cards and postcards were collected by many families, and make a fascinating contrast in materials and design with their modern counterparts.

42. Souvenirs. The small ornaments people brought back from holiday—often china miniatures—will again evoke memories of the time and places.

43. Jewellery. Compare old and new pieces; many group members will have some jewellery, a ring or brooch; does it have special significance? Naming precious stones, trying on necklaces, bracelets and so on.

44. Old kitchen equipment. Bring in the oldest kitchen utensils that can be found or borrowed: discuss all the gadgets and labour-saving devices of today, compare pictures of automatic washing machines with the 'dolly-tub' and so on.

45. War memories. Pictures of life during the World Wars; memories of air raids, women at work, fire-watching, friends who were lost in action, and so on. The Flanders poppy is an evocative visual aid around Remembrance Day.

46. Medals. What were they awarded for? Action in the First and Second World Wars; where were they stationed? What did they do? What was it really like? Memories of evacuation. Some will have pictures of themselves in uniform to show the group.

47. Ration books. And other reminders of the effects of war on life at home; how did members stretch the rations allowed—special recipes or menus? Comparison with present-day standards of food and clothing.

48. Mementoes of war-time leaders. Pictures, other mementoes of Churchill; the 'V' sign; a brief tape of his voice.

49. The Depression. Pictures of life in the 1930s; mass unemployment, huge marches and so on; how were group members affected? Comparison with present-day levels of poverty and state benefits.

50. Emigration. Did members consider emigrating, or have they actually emigrated? Any family abroad? Pictures and maps are useful here.

51. Prices. Pictures of food and other items: discuss current prices, prices in previous years, also the rise in wages. Make up a typical shopping basket for £1, £5, £10, then and now.

52. Religion. What beliefs do members have? Did they go to church because they had to or because they wanted to? Do they attend church now? What other beliefs are there?

53. Marriage. Were they (or are they) married? Where did they get married? What sort of wedding? (Photograph albums here are a great help.) What do they think of marriage now? What do they think of people living together—without being married?

54. Education. Where did they go to school? What age were they when they left? What was it like? What did they learn? Were there opportunities for further education? Were they trained for a particular job as an apprentice etc? Did they go to college? Would they have liked to?

55. Local festivities. Many towns have long-established traditions of annual fairs, festivals and celebrations. Pictorial comparisons of past and present will jog memories in the group about them.

56. Families. Using family photograph albums, each group member's family history can be pieced together pictorially: pictures of the person when young can be compared with ones taken as they are now; the development of their own children into adults and (possibly into elderly people themselves) can be seen.

57. The role of women. A brief illustrated article on 'women's lib' can stimulate a useful discussion about changing roles—particularly in a mixed group.

58. Sports. Old newspapers, magazines and illustrated books provide the material for a discussion of sporting interests; sporting heroes of the past—and what has become of them, teams supported by group members, changes in sports clothing, athletic ability, styles of play.

59. Local public transport. Use old pictures of trams, horse- and motor-drawn, trolley-buses, early buses and charabancs, together with modern counterparts. Fare prices might also be discussed.

60. Film-stars, singers and other celebrities. A scrap-book might be made of favourites from the group members' younger days, with pictures showing the stars in their prime, and also as they aged. Reminders of particular films, songs and catch-phrases would be relevant here.

61. Old-fashioned shop goods. Old tin boxes (which preceded packets) might be unearthed; old adverts from newspapers and magazines; 'then' and 'now' comparison.

62. Special events on TV. It is not always necessary to oversee viewing, particularly when the observers are deeply involved, but frequently the proceedings are meaningless to people with severe memory problems unless someone directs their attention to certain aspects of the programme. If a video machine is available, this could be used to repeat such events. In one day-centre a group regularly watches and discusses the lunchtime news bulletin on TV.

63. Music. Extremely useful in groups of all kinds. For enjoyment, it should be remembered that tastes differ widely. One use of music is to play a tape made up of brief extracts of singers well-known in the group members' younger days; this can be combined with pictures of the singers as in 60 above.

64. Music to reinforce orientation. A second use is in aiding the repetition of basic information; appropriate songs and rhymes are sung to back up the current information; e.g. 'April Showers', 'White Christmas', 'Easter Bonnet', 'Here we go gathering nuts in May', etc.

65. Music-making. A third use is as a co-ordinated group activity; simple rhythm instruments can be made in the group—shakers, blocks of wood to hit together, kazoos, and so on.

66. Movement to music. Simple, gentle group physical exercises are carried out to music; this can be done with group members seated; more active members may be able to stand and dance—like many automatic movements, this ability may be relatively well preserved.

67. Touch—hot and cold. The weather or the temperature can be stressed by a pair of cold hands just in from the snow or frost. The temperature of the room can be shown by the warm hands of the residents. Use a thermometer to show the temperature. Food and drink is hot or cold; bring in some ice! Parts of the world have different temperatures (use maps and pictures).

68. Touch—soft and hard, rough and smooth. Many things can be used to discuss these concepts: skin, fabrics, animal fur, surfaces, pumice stone, rock collections, scouring pads and powders, wallpapers, clothing, sand and tissue paper, fruit—apples, bananas, oranges, etc. Food can be examined to tell, by feel, if it is fresh, ripe or rotten.

69. Touch—dry and wet. Spills of liquid can be used. Travel cloths, sponges, mop heads, towels, washing.

70. Cloth. Provide a bag of pieces of material for the group to feel; they will reminisce about old fabrics such as chenille, flannel, tulle and cretonne. They will dismiss a piece of denim as something which is too 'rough' and be surprised by the cost of trousers made from it! Drip-dry fabrics will produce stories of difficult ironing problems. What would different types of material be used for? What colours and patterns go together?

71. Heating—old and new. Pictures of old-fashioned stoves and fires; discussion of the work they involved; pictures of modern heating systems—advantages and disadvantages.

72. Smell. Some elderly people, particularly men, appear to have lost their sense of smell, but generally this is a very rewarding sense to use. A box of smells made up with the help of a kindly pharmacist is needed. Little bottles containing, for example, attar of roses, lemon, peppermint, almonds, cinnamon, cloves, lavender, orange, menthol, cherries, Sloan's liniment. The bottled smell can be used as in a game, with clues and quick identification so as not to lose interest. The purpose is to arouse memories and excite discussion of use. For example, the smell of almond essence provokes thoughts of Easter and simnel cake, Christmas and Christmas cake.

73. Smell—herbs and spices. Discuss the smells and uses of collections of herbs and spices from the kitchen shelf, potpourri and collections of fresh herbs from the garden: thyme, sage, rosemary, mint, lavender, chives, marjoram. Uses in cooking, as air-fresheners and for keeping clothes fresh.

74. Smell—fruit and flowers. Fresh flowers: roses, carnations, sweet peas, lilac, daffodils, as available. Fresh fruit: tangerines, oranges, lemons, apples, bananas, strawberries, etc. Also discuss colours, likes, dislikes, of flowers and fruit.

75. Smells in the kitchen. Kitchen smells: coffee, soaps, moth balls, ammonia, cooking, polishes, etc. Compare carbolic and perfumed soap. Cooking smells can be introduced in an actual session by providing half-cooked bread from the supermarket. Old herbal remedies and medicines provoke memories that are often amusing and provide easy comparisons with today.

76. Smells. Perfume; compare various perfumes: lavender water, eau de cologne, etc. Use current toiletries: deodorants, aftershave, talc, etc.

77. Taste. This is closely associated with sense of smell. A game can be made of identifying foods and drinks from their taste, with eyes closed. Tea, coffee, beer, fruit, bread, cake, etc, can be used in this way.

78. Taste—sweet and sour. Contrast sweet and sour food, leading into discussion of preferences, etc. Lemon juice, vinegar, unsweetened cooking apples, rhubarb, etc, compared with sugar, jam, syrup, treacle, sweets, cakes and so on.

79. Tastes—unpleasant and disputed. Medicine, cod liver oil, taste of cigarettes, cold tea, stale food, disliked food, bitter aloes, alcohol, real versus instant coffee, tea bags versus tea leaves: all to stimulate discussion and response on food memories, preferences, current opportunities.

80. Tastes—hot. Peppers, spices, curry powder, radishes, raw onion, salad dressing, sauces, chilies and so on.

81. Menus—popular and unpopular food. Modern tastes. Wartime food—dehydrated eggs, milk, etc. Potatoes for flour in cakes. Funny recipes for icing sugar and almond paste. Wartime recipe books. Foods and tastes once enjoyed, now unobtainable. Food from other countries. Prepare typical menus from different times of members' lives, including the present. Discuss choices available—or lack of them.

82. Newspapers and journals. Placed on the table, these provide day-to-day current information that can be incorporated into discussions about current events. The TV pages stimulate discussions about favourite programmes and personalities; the horoscope encourages members to recall their birth-date; some groups have been seen to attempt a simple crossword.

83. Magazines. These are similarly a potentially rich source of discussion starters; a short paragraph from an article or a letter can be read out (perhaps from the problem page!); pictures accompanying articles and advertisements can also be used in this way—in addition to their use in collages mentioned above.

84. Current events. Local, national and world events can provide a continuing topic. An election, for example, could be the subject of a large poster with names and pictures of those involved, and the polling date clearly indicated. Reminiscences about previous elections, political argument and interest in the outcome could be stimulated. Posters of other continuing news stories could be made, e.g. royal tours, strikes, wars, etc.

85. Current events—politicians. Pictures of current leaders could be mounted on a poster or in a scrap-book with their names, parties and office. A montage of former prime ministers or presidents going back to the early years of this century, will allow comparisons and a historical perspective.

86. Current events—sports. Major sporting events: Olympic Games, soccer's World Cup or FA Cup Final, cricket test matches, tennis championships and so on can be discussed in advance, the outcome predicted and watched. Major horse races could form the basis for a sweepstake, depending on the interests of the group.

87. Everyday objects. Any common articles can be brought into the group, identified, and their use demonstrated; discussions of shape, colour and so on can be stimulated. Cups and saucers, knife, fork and spoon, shoes, hat, ball, light-bulb, umbrella, saucepan, key and padlock, purse and radio are among the sort of objects that could be used in this way.

88. Anagrams. Large letter cards or blocks can be used; a word is given in mixed-up order for the group member to rearrange into the correct order. The difficulty can be adjusted according to ability from two letters upward!

89. Word games. These can be played with letter cards—turning up, say, the letter 'E' and then naming a word beginning with 'E'. If the next card is 'T', thinking what word could be made from 'ET'...

90. Number games. Use a simple version of Bingo, with only the numbers 1–20 to bring the game within the person's reduced memory and attention span. Each person would have four numbers on a card to cover when they are called out; dominoes can also be used, with different colour spots for each number and large size dominoes. Small prizes for winners are essential.

91. Picture games. The picture equivalent of the above. In picture Bingo, each person has a card with four or five easily identifiable pictures on it; there could be 20 or so pictures altogether taken one at a time from a bag: the winner being the first to match all his pictures. Picture dominoes is another possibility, with pictures of common objects replacing the usual numbers. Again prizes should be given.

92. Shape puzzles. These are games where a number of plastic or wooden shapes are fitted into corresponding holes in a board. These can spark off discussion on shapes—squares, triangles, circles, etc—what else is a triangle? Point to the two squares and so on. Colours also can be used if the pieces have different colours: find another the same colour as this; what else is green? Has anyone any clothes the same colour as this? Use matching where naming is difficult for group members.

93. Jigsaw puzzles. These can be a useful activity if the number of pieces is small, the size of the pieces is large, and the finished picture is not childish. The completed picture can then be a topic for discussion.

94. Outings. These assist memory, reminiscence and socialisation. Relevant visits can be made to the home area, shopping area, churches where people were married; parks; picnic and beauty spots well remembered. Where physically possible, visits to shops and new supermarkets and shopping precincts are valuable. Local pub outings are always welcome.

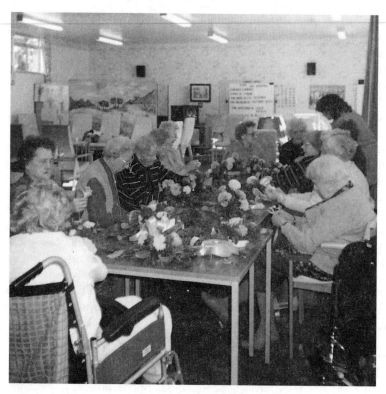

Figure 9.2 Flower arranging can interest a large group.

ADVANCED GROUP

Much of the material and techniques listed above would be relevant, suitably adapted to the ability level and interests of the group members. The group should be encouraged to initiate their own programmes and make their own decisions as far as possible, so the items listed here are more in the form of headings.

95. Events. A number of special events can be arranged; a fashion show, a brief film show, a school band or choir and so on, all can arouse interest.

96. Demonstration. By gardeners, beauticians, cookery experts, artists, local theatre, dance groups, handicraft experts and so on, may all be within the attention span of this group (Fig. 9.2).

97. Cooking. A complete group meal could be possible, with stronger members of the group helping and encouraging the more infirm.

98. Games. More complex card games and so on will be feasible; perhaps competitions can be organised. A number of suitable games are commercially available: memory and reminiscence games; spatial ability (e.g. 'Connect 4' and 'Space Lines'); visual recognition and logic games. Note that games should be appropriate for adults; the only exception would be when the group has been joined by visiting children, when the members take on the 'grandparent' role of playing them at their games.

99. Parties—with a special or relevant theme. Halloween, Christmas, Easter bonnet competitions, etc. The right food, the right decor, suitable entertainments can all be organised between the therapist and the group.

100. Making decorations. For parties at Christmas and for members' birthdays.

101. Reminiscence theatre. A local group putting on a show with music hall items and memories of life in previous years could be appreciated by this group. Making a reminiscence display, illustrating local history or group members' life experiences can be attempted. Volunteers, relatives, school children and local societies may help to track down appropriate items for display; local radio may help with an appeal for specific pictures or objects. The local library and museum may also be of assistance.

Each group can indicate where their interests and abilities lie and, with suitable support and imagination on the part of the therapist, can succeed in their aims and so increase their own self-esteem.

RECORD-KEEPING

Each day, immediately at the end of the session, a written record should be made of the group. A large book can be used with a page for each day. The record needs to include:

- group members present
- group leaders and other staff present
- times group began and ended
- topics discussed and equipment used
- a brief note about each group member's reaction
- anything discovered in the group about likes, dislikes, interests, abilities—things that should be developed
- things that should be avoided!
- general appraisal of the session.

10

Practical issues

In this chapter are discussed some of the key practical points that may arise when care-staff seek to introduce positive approaches into their work with elderly people.

PROGRAMME DEVELOPMENT

Intensity

How often should a technique, specific approach or method of re-training be employed? Can it be omitted when there is a staff shortage? Would sessions twice a day be more beneficial than one session a day?

At first sight it seems that these are important questions relating to the demands made on staff, with implications for the amount of staff involvement required in implementation. In fact, they reflect a total misconception of the basic principles by assuming that any approach is like a pill to be taken so many times a day after meals! They ignore the importance of the basic approach, of the relevance of every interaction between the care-giver and the elderly person, of that person's need to be recognised as an individual with emotions, abilities and needs. Positive approaches involve ways of working which need to be in operation for 24 hours a day, ingrained in the care environment.

In some 'care' settings, the environment is impoverished and staff–resident interactions are minimal; such situations can hardly be termed positive. Sometimes structured sessions, both individual and group, are perceived as an alternative to satisfactory interaction throughout the day. There is, however, no substitute for consistency in approach. Structured sessions provide a supplement and time to concentrate on specific problems. They allow staff and the patients or residents to get to know each other better, in a friendly, relaxed atmosphere, which will in turn facilitate the continuous daily contact.

The following points can be made regarding intensity:

• The amount of staff–resident contact needs to be increased as far as is possible, and encouragement given to use a positive approach such as RO in each of these contacts, ensuring that confusion is not reinforced, and/or using techniques such as resolution to understand better what the person is trying to convey. In some settings, talking with the residents is seen as avoiding real work; though in many senses, if it is done properly, it is perhaps more demanding than other more physical forms of work. Many of the routine physical tasks of the home or ward can be carried out whilst talking with a resident quite easily.

• Generally speaking, the more intensive a rehabilitative or re-learning programme can be, the more the resident will benefit from it. However, the elderly person must be allowed to respond to information supplied so that it can be absorbed gradually. Bombarding the person with information which cannot be assimilated, or pressurising the person to respond are *not* part of an intensive approach! A supportive, respectful approach that recognises the person's individual psychological needs at all times is the aim.

• The more confused and disorientated a person is the more intensive the intervention must be in order to stimulate learning. This may be reflected in the slower pace of learning and the much lower level of information required. A total of 2½ hours a week is hardly adequate to promote change. Even in a group, it is vital to provide individual attention, but the social atmosphere always proves a valuable aid. Very disturbed and restless, severely impaired patients may particularly benefit from individual contacts, if their concentration is too limited for a group session. The activity and atmosphere provided by a 24-hour active, interesting and normal living environment will prove helpful, as stimulation and aids to self-help and self-confidence will be available.

• There is relatively little benefit in having more than one group session per day, and the additional time could be utilised with briefer individual sessions. There are suggestions that not having group sessions at weekends may tend to detract from some of the gains previously made, and if at all feasible, group activities should be offered at weekends also.

Consistency

It is important that all members of staff work closely together. It is possible for inconsistencies to occur as the staff is made up of individuals. Each of them can perceive ward or home policies, and the way to implement those policies, in their own way. Furthermore, if team spirit is weak, understanding of such policies is limited. For example, in a situation where most staff members are employing a specific approach with a particular patient, their efforts to help her to, say, remember where she is could be destroyed by the faulty approach of a single staff member. Without appreciating the consequence, this nurse could seek to reassure the patient by telling her that this is a hotel at the coast! The effects of the care-plan would be weakened if messages received by patients were inconsistent. In effect they would reinforce confusion.

When team feeling exists and is encouraged, such problems will be minimised. The necessity for staff to feel involved in the programme must be emphasised rather than it being presented as another chore. Other staff who might not normally be included in a staff training programme (e.g. cleaners, domestics, orderlies, porters, etc) often have, in fact, a great deal of contact and interaction with patients. It may well be important, if a consistent approach is to be maintained, that they are at least informed of what is happening and the rationale behind it. Similarly, visitors to the ward, volunteers and most importantly relatives need guidance on how best to communicate with patients on the ward. A brief printed sheet may be helpful, giving details of the approach, but perhaps the best way of getting the approach across is by the care-staff being seen to put it into practice at all times themselves. In many ways an explicit, agreed approach could be a uniting force among staff, helping all to feel there is something useful that they can do, that they are important and valuable members of the care-team, whether or not they have degrees, qualifications or certificates. If these feelings can be nurtured—and they stand in marked contrast to the feelings of helplessness and uselessness so often experienced by staff working with elderly people with dementia—then the all-important consistency of approach is more likely to be achieved. It should be borne in mind, of course, that it is consistency of approach that is needed and not necessarily consistency of method. There are a variety of ways to put any positive approach into practice. For interactions to be enjoyable for all concerned, this variety is important. There is a great deal of scope for individual personalities, flair and imagination; every care-worker has a skill or an interest to offer.

Limited goals

However encouraging the results of studies of the various approaches might be, we have attempted to indicate that the gains have often been quite small and often not as clear in the person's general functioning as in specific areas targeted. These approaches are not a cure for dementia; severely impaired people will almost certainly not be discharged from long-stay hospital or nursing home care as a result of their use!

The potential lies in the nature of a degenerative condition such as dementia. Most of these conditions are currently regarded as irreversible (although it is as well to remember that there are some reversible conditions too). Figure 10.1 is a notional graph of self-care ability in dementia. Line (a) illustrates what generally seems to happen in dementia. Initially the person is independent but gradually needs more and more assistance as skills decline, until there is a need

for almost total physical nursing care. At this point, when the person is virtually being dressed, toiletted and washed, etc, it is difficult to see how any semblance of dignity can be retained, however caring and sympathetic the care-staff may be. Line (b) represents a stabilisation of self-care ability at a level where there is considerable independence; if a therapeutic approach could achieve this, then clearly this would be an acceptable aim as the stage of total nursing care is not reached. Line (c) represents a slowing down of the deterioration, with the person taking somewhat longer to reach the area of greatest indignity. Therefore, by comparison with line (a), we could say this person has overall a better quality of life as more skill has been retained and there has been more independence. Slowing down of deterioration can then be a worthwhile goal. In addition, total physical nursing care is costly in time and in the extra stress and burden for staff. However, there is a problem here; if slowing down deterioration is the aim, then the care-staff will continue to see their patients deteriorate despite their best endeavours to carry out a programme, and cannot know for certain that they are achieving anything. Untreated comparison groups are probably the best way to ascertain possible changes as a result of intervention. It is not always possible to use these, so it is often difficult to show that deterioration is being slowed down. Those using positive approaches need to be aware of the variability of deterioration in individuals and of the importance of close communication with patients in order to note even the smallest of changes in their behaviour, or in our interaction with them.

Aspiration levels should not be set so high that only dramatic changes are expected. Such expectations are courting disappointment and will lead to lack of confidence in the approach. While some patients can show impressive changes, the improvements of those with degenerative disorders may only be minimal. To miss small changes could prove disastrous to the programme as there would be no appreciation that a step forward had been achieved. A number of little steps can combine into a substantial one.

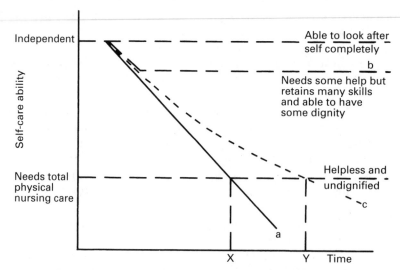

Figure 10.1   Schematic graph of self-care ability in dementia illustrating that halting or even slowing down deterioration can be useful aims. (a) 'Usual' deterioration in dementia; (b) stabilisation of self-care ability at an intermediate level; (c) a slowing down of deterioration resulting in a higher quality of life for (c) as compared with (a) for the period of time X–Y.

Realistic attitudes can help to analyse the progress and so permit staff to set or reset appropriate goals by lowering or raising them as is necessary.

Although the word 'therapy' is often employed in relation to one or other of the intervention programmes, it is probably inappropriate. The aim of therapy is to realise some level of improvement towards independence; this may be seen in relation to an intervention following some specific damage to the brain, such as a stroke. Where the person's condition is a degenerative one, the aim is to maintain function as close as possible to the limits imposed by the continuing damage to the brain; continued support is necessary to achieve this—interventions cannot be applied for a few months and then withdrawn. Various studies have shown that without some consistent input the effects of such approaches as RO and reminiscence will fade fairly quickly. It would seem that if an active, stimulating programme ceases to operate and the person is returned to a negative atmosphere lacking in encouragement, deterioration will quickly follow. In such an environment the gap between the person's actual and potential function widens. The person is actually under-functioning because their environment does not provide the opportunities or the stimulus to reach the level that their brain—damaged as it may be—could still sustain. What can be achieved is restricted by the person's neurological impairment; to reach this limit an appropriate form of input as a continuing part of the person's environment is required.

Staff attitudes

Attitudes underlie and colour so much of what we do or say, so no apology will be made for dealing with this topic at greater length, in this and succeeding sections, in view of its importance in work with people with dementia. If we have a negative approach to a task we will probably do it badly; if we have a negative attitude to a person then we may say pleasant, polite words to them, but our real attitude will probably be communicated in the way they are said. Conversely, positive attitudes are more likely to lead to enthusiasm and to convey warmth.

General attitudes to old age

What are our attitudes, firstly to elderly people in general, and secondly to those with a dementia, who are the focus of this book? If this question were asked of the general population, a wide variety of replies would be received. These could range from those who advocate euthanasia for all elderly people to those who would find it difficult to see elderly people as a group and would talk about attitudes to individuals who happen, by conventional arbitrary criteria, to be labelled 'elderly'. How do our attitudes to elderly people develop? One powerful learning experience may have been the way in which elderly people in our own family were treated when we were young. Were they revered and respected or were they despised? Were they frail, or were they strong and powerful? These types of consideration may lead to our first ideas about elderly people.

The attitude of society itself is another strong influence, as are the attitudes of those sub-groups of society to which we belong. Western society often seems to emphasise youthful qualities, like speed and productivity, and to devalue the mature contributions of experience, perspective and emotional stability. Staff from different cultures may have absorbed quite a different set of influences. They may be surprised that families do not provide all the care for older people, that older people are not universally respected and revered. An important factor in these expectations may be the proportion of older people in the population; in the Western developed countries this may be three or four times as great as in many less developed countries, where cultural norms about family care are only now beginning to have to adjust to large numbers of people surviving into old age.

A third major influence may well be our fantasies of what being old would be like, our projection of our own old age, which must have associated with it some of our feelings about death and dying. Given the various influences and learning experiences that each of us has undergone, it is hardly surprising that in any group of care-staff there will be a multiplicity of attitudes. There are even a number of different reasons for being involved in work with the elderly at all, from genuine interest to purely economic ones.

Staff awareness

It is important for all staff members to think about their own attitudes and to consider what experiences have led them to their current position; it is useful for staff to discuss their attitudes together, noting both agreements and differences. Attitudes cannot be changed overnight; what is necessary is a willingness to try alternative strategies of working with elderly people and not to reject these strategies out of hand. When elderly people previously considered to be confused and totally dependent actually respond in a group or one-to-one session, then attitudes begin to be modified. When the face of the elderly lady—who previously seemed rather ugly and unapproachable—lights up as an item from the past acts as an entry into communication with her and as we begin to see the person behind the 'geriatric patient' stereotype, once again we begin to change our ideas.

Not all staff are so willing to try new ideas, of course, and it is important that change proceeds at a rate that does not leave some staff feeling railroaded and coerced by others. It is important that staff at all levels really do communicate with each other, about their aims in their work and what they see as the means of achieving them. This may happen informally but is perhaps more likely to occur if there are regular, frequent meetings of the staff group. The introduction of the Nursing Process in the UK helped to structure meetings and is assisting nurses to look in more depth at these aspects (see Stockwell 1985). The recording and identification of target areas for each individual patient has greatly increased discussion and understanding.

Again the importance of all staff being involved must be emphasised. This is not only for reasons of consistency, but also because if a small group of staff is chosen to lead, say, RO sessions, tensions may result. The staff omitted may see RO as a higher level activity than the general chores and feel resentful. At the other extreme, RO may be seen as an officially recognised way of avoiding the 'real' (physical) work that needs to be done, so those leading the sessions will be regarded as idle when they laugh and chat with the elderly people! To allocate the work of therapist to certain staff members may seem satisfactory in delegation of responsibility, but in practice it is not to be recommended. The result can isolate the staff, be the cause of jealousy and feelings of strain, and, furthermore, will make consistency of approach from all staff impossible to obtain. The programme would be jeopardised by sick and holiday leave, not to mention staff changes. In 1980 in Leeds, seven people representing different disciplines acted as therapists in a 2-month study. Videotapes of the sessions suggested that it was not necessary to involve the same staff. The group related well to all the therapists and it is, in our view, the consistency of approach that is important.

Attitudes to dementia

The basic approach to working with people with dementia involves an awareness of the elderly person's psychological, as well as physical needs. In Chapter 5, we discussed Kitwood's description of a 'malignant social psychology' surrounding the person with dementia, which illustrates many of the pejorative situations so often confronting older people. In order to reduce the impact of this malignant social psychology, attitudes need to allow the elderly person individuality, dignity, self-respect and choice. There is a need to avoid the sort of caring that stifles the person's attempts at independence: 'Let me help you with that, it takes you such a long time on your own'; that treats the person as a child rather than as the adult they have been for 50-odd years: 'What you want is ... ' or 'Come along now, eat it up'; that treats the person as an object: staff member to visitor in front of resident, 'Now this man here is very confused and incontinent'; that misunderstands positive approaches: 'Why interfere, leave them alone, it

is our turn to do things for them'. The person needs to be nurtured; allowing as much independence of us as possible. As with the parent–teenager relationship, this can be a painful process. We must hold back, suppressing the desire to take over and dress the person who is having difficulties, because we know she will manage eventually on her own. It means sometimes taking risks because to be wrapped up in cotton wool is to be deprived of freedom.

Finally, we need to be positive; if we are not, our negative feelings will show and may simply add to the helplessness of the situation. We need to challenge expectations and myths, realising that these can colour events, responses and outcome. Those who use positive approaches, new ideas and have the determination to succeed can create their own special 'miracles'. A realistic optimism and expectation that some change is possible may help to increase elderly persons' self-confidence, and so, in fact, make change more likely to actually occur.

SELECTION OF CLIENTS FOR GROUPS

If interventions are seen not simply as the daily 'therapy' group that 'must' be 'done', but as an integral part of the 24 hour care environment, then the issue of which patients are selected for group work is transformed into which intervention or programme is best suited for each individual. The following principles may prove useful.

Severe impairment. People with a severe level of impairment have in many (but not all) studies proved less responsive to particular interventions. With this type of patient, one-to-one sessions or very small groups are most important; staff need as much information as possible about the person, their life, interests, strengths, needs and specific difficulties, as it will be difficult to check out these aspects with the person themself. Sensory stimulation, touch, music, basic orientation and simple physical exercise are likely to be the most effective means of establishing communication and building a good relationship. Through such a relationship, a minor miracle can sometimes be achieved as something of the person who has been hidden by the ravages of their condition begins again to emerge, seen in a smile, an interest in what is happening, a rare sentence that can be readily comprehended ...

Moderate impairment. These patients will benefit from a variety of programmes and will respond to a 24 hour atmosphere which maintains their abilities and gives as normal a lifestyle as possible. Particular care needs to be given to finding the appropriate level of activities so that the participants do not become bored or threatened or feel their intelligence is being insulted. For example, a person who was previously very intelligent may suffer from a dementia; despite a significant loss of ability he/she may retain knowledge, cultural levels and experience that may not be matched by other participants, or even some care-givers. Equally, some with lower levels of lifetime attainment and experience may feel uncomfortable in the company of those who appear more able. Such considerations need to guide the choice of activities and the composition of groups.

Patients without dementia. The same consideration applies when patients without dementia are included in a programme. These may be patients who have had a stroke or, in some instances, patients who have been in a psychiatric hospital for a number of years. Where disorientation is not evident then the basic approach should aim to draw out from the patient what is happening in their surroundings—both in the immediate vicinity and more generally in the world. Consideration should be given to activity sessions at a higher level than conventional groups.

Deafness. Severely deaf patients, where the hearing loss cannot be corrected, often do not fit well in any sort of group because of their hearing impairment, and may require more individual orientation work. It is worth remembering that hearing aid systems are continually being improved, and some models specially designed for use in groups, using a microphone and earphones, are available.

Poor sight. Patients with very poor eyesight may have difficulty with a number of tasks often included in a group session. Again, individual work is indicated, or a group specifically aimed at utilising the other senses.

Restlessness. Patients who are extremely restless and cannot sit in a chair for a few minutes are not suited to a group approach in view of the disruption they cause. A care programme may have to be done literally on the move: around the lounge, down the corridor ... ! If a person can concentrate for a few minutes, it is better to use those minutes intensively with them, perhaps several times a day, aiming to gradually increase their span till they are settled enough to remain in a group session.

Speech difficulties. Patients with speech problems need careful help. Those whose major difficulty is in expressing themselves may not find the group situation too stressful, whereas those who have particular difficulty in understanding the meaning of what is said may well find the group session a threatening experience; they are then best helped on an individual basis.

Previous experiences. In introducing reminiscence work, it is advisable to first ascertain whether the person enjoys reminiscing; as mentioned in Chapter 8, some older people do not find it as pleasurable as most of their contemporaries do. Staff should be aware of any traumatic experiences in the person's life which might lead to a catastrophic reaction in the group.

Group composition. Group membership should not be constantly changing. If in the early stages, a member appears to be unsuitable, a closer investigation is advisable. Problems may concern behaviour or a specific disability, but the person may just be slow to respond. If essential, exclusion should be made, but individual aid should be considered.

In summary then, positive approaches should be flexible enough to be used with a wide range of elderly patients. If only a proportion of patients can be accommodated in structured group sessions, a good rule of thumb is to work with the most restless and disturbed patients on an individual basis, to encourage the least impaired to initiate their own activities (providing materials and interest) and to work with the other patients in the group session, i.e. those who are moderately impaired. Often these are a comparatively neglected group, needing less physical care than the severely disturbed group and being less able to interact with the care-staff than the mildly impaired group.

Application to community residents

Most of the aspects outlined so far—and indeed virtually all the research that has been carried out on RO, reminiscence, etc—has been primarily concerned with patients in hospital or residents in residential care and nursing homes. Yet only around 5% of all elderly people reside in such institutions (Craig 1983), and even when considering those suffering from some form of dementing condition, a large majority live in the community, alone or with supporting relatives. The reasons for the primary development of such programmes within institutional settings are clear and include the greater impact of people with dementia grouped together in a ward or home as compared with those scattered in the community, the greater ease of carrying out and evaluating intensive treatment programmes consistently and the availability there of more experienced, less emotionally involved care-staff.

Current thinking, rightly in our view, stresses the importance of maintaining elderly persons in their own surroundings, if this is their wish, providing the necessary assistance, and, especially important, support and relief for those such as relatives involved in their care. What part have positive approaches to play in this endeavour?

Day-centres

Work by Greene and his colleagues in Glasgow (Greene et al 1979, 1983) has shown that some impact can be made on the person's orientation and awareness by RO sessions 2 or 3 days a week in a psychogeriatric day unit. In the latter study, improvements in the supporting relative's mood were noted during the RO phase of the study. This is encouraging in suggesting

that work carried out at a day-hospital or day-centre may have some carry-over to the person's situation at home. A number of day-centres and clubs catering for elderly people with dementia on a long-term basis have been established. Applying positive approaches in these settings is a feasible and valuable endeavour. Close links between the day-centre and relatives and other community supports are essential, in order to work towards a consistent approach to the individual person.

RO and reminiscence sessions can certainly be set up in such centres. Mildly impaired people will show benefit even from a fairly infrequent attendance; ideally more impaired people would need to attend three or more times a week for gains to be maintained. Volunteer helpers could well lead sessions in day-centres and clubs, with suitable training and support.

Care at home

For the elderly person living alone the situation is more complex. Regular visitors to the person's home—home help, neighbours, meals-on-wheels attendant, volunteer visitor, etc—can be given some guidance as to the appropriate approach, but some memory aid is needed for the times when the person is alone. Many elderly people have a newspaper delivered regularly and keep the current one available as a reminder of the date; others leave notes in strategic places. Some have a large diary to refer to; in one case the home help assisted in keeping this up-to-date and the elderly person learned to consult it whenever something arose about which she was uncertain. A large electric clock, perhaps with an automatic calendar, might also prove useful. Basically, of course, these are memory aids that most people use at one time or another. When people have memory deficits, the problem is how to teach them to make use of these aids, and it is here that much useful work can be done in the person's own home. The person might, for instance, usefully make a list for shopping but needs to learn where to keep it so it can be easily consulted in the shops. They may well continually 'lose' a purse or handbag and need to be taught to keep these sort of items in particular places. A brightly coloured tag on a key-ring or a reflective strip on a purse may assist in finding frequently lost items. Thus, a retraining session can actually be carried out in the person's home, with the emphasis being on developing and using memory aids and reminders.

Community care

One of a number of community-care schemes is that described by Lodge & McReynolds (1983) in Leicestershire, where volunteers are recruited specifically to work with elderly people with dementia. They provide two forms of help; first, practical help to compensate for the person's loss of skill and, secondly, memory cues and monitoring people with dementia throughout the day. These volunteers are trained and supported in their work, which helps to structure the elderly person's day and ensures that important appointments are kept, day-centre attendance is kept up and meals, drinks and medications are taken regularly.

This is one of a number of schemes that are being developed throughout the UK. It is rare in that its explicit focus is on the particular problems associated with dementing conditions. Probably the most thoroughly evaluated of all these schemes is the Kent Community Care Scheme (Challis & Davies 1985), which aimed to support older people at home, whatever their disability. In the final report of the evaluation project, Challis & Davies (1985) made it clear that a number of people with dementia were included in the research project and highlighted four particular issues which were encountered in supporting people with dementia at home.

In the first place, gaining access was often difficult. Some elderly people might well believe that they have no need of help; so it was vital to establish good relationships initially. This meant offering to meet the needs that the client perceived rather than the more obvious ones they did not see. Support could be built up once this pattern had been accepted.

Secondly, 'process risks' were identified. This refers to areas of increasing decline relating to self-neglect and loss of coping skills, leading to a gradual increase of danger to the person, rather than an immediate crisis. Care was organised (often using local people, neighbours and friends as paid helpers) to provide supervision of food, medicines, etc, and regular stimulation, using RO techniques.

'Event risks'—the danger of a gas explosion, wandering off and getting lost, etc—were dealt with by practical solutions (turning off the gas supply!) and by establishing routines with close supervision.

Fourthly, a clear and regular pattern of care was established, based upon the person's positive, retained abilities. A structured timetable was built around the person's own daily routine, to be meaningful and relevant to the person. Again, RO techniques were emphasised to enhance communication and reinforce the structure being created.

Perhaps most important of all, the scheme offered an individualised approach to developing a package of care for the person with dementia, rather than offering a standard set of services. Assessment is required, which takes a biographical view of the person's situation. This involves making a real effort to understand the person's needs in the context of their skills, preferences, culture, beliefs, resources and difficulties over a lifetime. Without this, the package of care that is devised will not be appropriate to the individual as a whole person, nor sensitive to the subtleties of their individual needs.

The continued development of community care will require those providing care to gain a deeper knowledge and understanding of dementia and its effects and to have access to training, help and advice from other professionals in ways of assessing and working with people with dementia and their families. Inevitably, greater numbers of people with dementia are going to be at home in the future rather than in residential settings; for this to be feasible it is essential that everything possible is done to reduce excess deficits and maximise the person's abilities through a sensitive, creative, realistic and individual approach. People with dementia are numerically the largest and, in many ways, present the most challenging problems of all those who require community care; skilled input and back-up will be needed to achieve a good standard of care.

Support for carers

The community care schemes also, successfully, offer support to carers looking after people with dementia at home (e.g. Challis et al 1988). Indeed, one of the groups for whom the Kent scheme proved most cost-effective consisted of extremely dependent elderly people with both dementia and physical problems being cared for at home by a relative. There is some scope for giving relatives guidance about the techniques of RO and related approaches. Indeed, a number of booklets are now readily available (see Appendix 3) that provide this sort of guidance alongside information about dementia, coping with the emotions that accompany caring and so on. A note of caution must however be sounded. Living with a person with dementia is often very difficult for a relative and, in many cases, however caring the relative is and however good the relationship has been, there may well be some tension, anger and resentment in the relationship. Occasionally, particularly when the relative receives no relief or support, rejection of the elderly person occurs. We would reiterate the importance of attitudes and responses which reinforce the person's dignity, individuality, self-respect, choice and adulthood. Where there are difficulties in the relationship between relatives and the elderly person, some opportunity is necessary to allow the relative to air these negative feelings and the possible resultant guilt. It may then be possible for the relative— with continued support—to allow the elderly person dignity, adulthood, etc, where previously the difficulties in the relationship precluded these attitudes. If it is not possible for this change to occur—perhaps the tensions, resentment and bitterness are too entrenched—then we would not recommend teaching the relative to use a specific programme.

Be this as it may, there is no doubt that any procedure of this kind is more difficult for a relative to carry out than for a care-worker, because of the long-standing emotional attachments and expectations that have built up over the years. However, the relatives do have certain advantages in using RO, reminiscence, etc. They are much more aware of the person's previous interests; they see the elderly person in familiar surroundings; there is ready access to family photographs, souvenirs, etc, from the past right up to the present time; they can work with one individual only; and they can involve the elderly person in tasks around the home. They are particularly well placed, of course, to be involved in drawing up a life-history book with the person, and to help those coming from outside the family to assist in care-giving rapidly to get to know the person in the context of their whole life.

There have been surprisingly few studies of the use of these approaches by relatives. A rare exception is a report by Davies (1981) of a wife who was able to improve her communication with her severely disabled husband using reminiscence. Generally, an effective way of working with relatives is to work through relatives' support groups, preferably made up of people living close by each other. In this setting, relatives may well be able to help each other through such a group by sharing experiences, difficulties, problems and solutions, and might be able to help each other in practical ways, e.g. providing relief for an afternoon or evening on a reciprocal basis.

A number of descriptions of relatives' groups have been published and Woods & Britton (1985) provide a full review of the issues involved. There have been a number of reports of such groups being used to train and educate care-givers, to increase their knowledge regarding dementia, to enhance their coping skills and to teach them ways of managing their feelings of strain (e.g. Morris et al 1992). Brodaty (1992) reviews the evidence on the effects of such interventions, which suggests there is a need for further development of these approaches if a significant impact on the strain experienced by family care-givers is to be achieved. Care-givers differ greatly in their needs: some appreciate a group, expressing surprise at times that they are not alone in their task, and finding it helpful to meet others who are going, or have been, through similar difficulties. Others prefer an individual approach, finding it difficult to listen to others' problems when their own are so pressing. Some relatives are actively seeking information as to how best to communicate with the person with dementia; at present they often feel helpless in the face of the seemingly inevitable deterioration. Procedures like RO and reminiscence may help these carers find some purpose in their interaction with the elderly person and to draw from them their maximal level of functioning.

Some relatives are able to participate regularly in a self-help group (such as those organised by the Alzheimer's Disease Society), and grow in confidence and knowledge together. Often such groups begin to act as a pressure group, calling for better facilities and more resources for older people with dementing conditions. Such groups are valuable in raising awareness of the needs of carers and of their vital role in supporting the majority of elderly people with dementia. Their pressure is vital to maintain and improve the quality and quantity of support services available.

INITIATING CHANGE AND SETTING UP PROGRAMMES

It is well known that the more things change the more they stay the same! The difficulties of promoting and maintaining change have a long history. New laws or policies have been introduced, and even torture and execution have not led to the acceptance of some of them! The new broom works hard and causes a stir for a while; new governments make new policies, only to have them turned around by a succeeding one; committees organise all sorts of new schemes and when their time is up their notes get lost!

We often make more progress when we make changes in our lifestyle and only have ourselves to consider. The influence of family, friends and loved ones complicates decision-making. When it comes to implementing a new system in an institutional setting, the problems multiply.

All the evidence that has accumulated over the years in various fields—with people with learning difficulties, children, psychiatric patients with long-term disabilities, etc—indicates that it can be extremely difficult to establish any positive psychological programme in an institution and that once established these endeavours are liable to encounter obstacles of various kinds, often to the extent of the programme being discontinued or simply drifting into disuse. This process, it should be emphasised, may occur independently of the demonstrated effectiveness of the therapeutic intervention. It seems to be related to the well-documented effects of institutions of any kind, where the needs of the institution are given greater importance than those of the patients they are intended to serve, and where change seems to be resisted and blocked.

Accounts have been written of failure resulting from apparently trivial matters. The problem is consistently raised at meetings and seminars: 'I agree, I want to do this, but how can *I* influence change?' Senior officers are too set in their ways, junior staff are resentful, there is no money, no time, no staff—the excuses and concerns are legion. We cannot offer the perfect answer, but it must be noted that the 1980s have shown remarkable changes in interest in programmes such as RO and reminiscence in hospital and residential settings. The wind of change has already blown far afield.

Where there is a climate for change, there is a chance of moving forward. It is impossible to provide a blueprint to guarantee success, but we can provide some suggestions and describe some general issues that can be adapted to meet the differing needs experienced in practice.

The wrong way

The first question to be raised is from where does the initiative and impetus for the establishment of a particular intervention come? Does it emanate from an 'outsider', e.g. a psychologist wanting to set up reminiscence in a residential home; from someone in a position of authority in the hierarchy of the institution, e.g. a senior nurse, a manager or a consultant; from someone in authority within the ward or residential home unit, e.g. a sister on a ward or an officer-in-charge of a residential home; or from 'shop-floor' level, e.g. a care-worker or ward nurse.

Clearly, there may be different reactions to each of these initiators. However, no matter who initiates change, no matter how inspired that person might be, no matter how interesting or well proven an intervention might be, it is fatal to start today, or even tomorrow! Change takes time.

Unquestionably, the first stumbling block will be provided by other people. Saboteurs are many in number and are often the least expected antagonists.

Junior staff may feel that they are being imposed upon, asked to do more than they are able or need to do, or that this is yet another of the charge-nurse's or matron's crack-pot ideas.

Staff at the same level may feel that the innovator is acting above him or herself as the initiator, is attempting to become ingratiated with senior staff, and is too 'pushy' and ambitious.

Senior staff could resent ideas from lower levels, seeing them as personal criticism or as examples of junior staff interfering and over-stepping their responsibility.

Managerial staff could resent not being consulted, believing other programmes have priority. They may feel concerned about implications for financial resources, about job descriptions possibly being changed without consultation, about paying wages for one sort of job and being supplied with another, and in some places they may well have concerns about the reactions of trade unions.

All staff may feel threatened if the initiator comes from 'outside' the institution, e.g. a community psychiatric nurse in a residential home, or a psychologist in a day-centre. They may feel the very suggestion of change in the pattern of care must constitute a criticism of current standards and procedures. There may be a feeling that the 'outsider' cannot really know the clients in the way the staff do.

Any of these reactions could stifle an idea at birth. Even if the instigator persists and continues to work in the chosen way, responses could be so antagonistic that the person could be forced to leave and the new system, with so much promise, would die unceremoniously with his or her departure.

To start immediately indicates that planning has been overlooked. Many aspects must be considered. For example, where is this going to take place; is there enough room? What about equipment; if needed it takes time to gather it together. What about timing? To run a group session on a ward at the same time as a ward round will hardly win friends! Policies of the institution require consideration in planning, or the whole project will fail.

Preparation is vital. To commence a new scheme without first reading the relevant literature and gathering as much information as possible is to guarantee that mistakes will occur. Clients are not going to happily sit and wait while a therapist races off to read notes before proceeding! Measures of change also need consideration. No one starts a diet without first checking his weight so that any loss can be measured!

The methods to be used must be clearly stated from the beginning so that the programme is not changing constantly with ideas being introduced too late in the day to be useful. Staff resources must be evaluated. Illness, time off, new or different staff must all be catered for or else there will be no back-up system or continuity. If the instigator is the sole leader or therapist, an absence or departure will guarantee that the programme will stop abruptly.

There are some people who do naturally plan well, can 'sell' ideas to other staff and possess the charisma to inspire and convince, but they are very few in number. The 'hero-innovator' who rushes in without preparation and careful thought will indeed, as Georgiades & Phillimore (1975) suggest, be eaten for breakfast by the institutional dragon! Far from saving anyone, or improving anything, this individual creates havoc. A little patience and a great deal of work and thought might prove more effective and indicate possible strategies for a would-be innovator.

Strategies for change

A clear set of strategies can be suggested that will improve the chances of success:

1. Find some allies.
2. Clearly identify what you want to do.
3. Employ salesmanship, consider how to promote change painlessly.
4. Lay the foundations for the new programme.
5. Provide relevant training.
6. Consider the problem of time (and lack of it!).
7. Ensure the assessment and monitoring system is prepared.
8. Consider how to maintain the programme.

1. Find some allies

Identify a group of people with similar ideas to your own, with a shared vision of what might be achieved in the future. The process of change can be stressful and demanding; without the support of like-minded people the going could get very tough. Include in the group people with particular influence or flexibility in their role who could be a particular asset in the process. They too will need continued encouragement and support in facing the obstacles that inevitably other people will place in their paths. Meet regularly to reinforce each other's efforts, to plan a joint strategy and to coordinate a concerted attack on the forces of resistance in the institution.

2. What you want to do

What form are the changes to take? Read, discuss, visit relevant centres and people and attend relevant courses. Be sure the subject is fully understood. Begin to plan the programme. What will happen during it, what will it contain, what are the essential aims, how long will it run and how will it end, or what will replace it? What equipment, space or adaptations will be required? Present policies must be studied. In order to accommodate the programme, do any need to be changed or modified? Who will this effect and how can their cooperation be obtained? All the difficulties that might arise should be covered: illness, staff changes, support systems and people, holidays, rotas and regular meetings or ward rounds.

Involve management. Find out how your scheme can be included and if there are other priorities in the institution. Ask for help: they may have access to equipment, space and other resources of which you were unaware.

Are you going to assess any changes occurring in the clients (or in the staff)? What measures would be appropriate? Does the programme involve selecting particular clients? How will this be carried out? What steps will be taken to consult with the clients before introducing any changes affecting them? Check carefully that any goals set for the programme are appropriate, relevant and realistic.

Is the change being carried out in the form of a research programme? In some instances, approval from the appropriate Ethical Committee will be needed. If groups of clients are to be compared, ensure they are matched on all the relevant attributes (age, sex, level of impairment, etc).

3. Salesmanship

At one time, this word was frowned upon in the NHS and Social Services in the UK—but the market-place culture has changed all that! Another heading for this section might be Machinations, Manipulations and Manoeuvring!

It is not so much a massive public relations drive that is required as a willingness to listen to the needs, fears, reservations, hopes and anxieties of those whose support and permission are required for the changes to happen. Then it will be possible, in many instances, to answer or find a way around their particular problems and worries concerning the programme.

In Table 10.1 we present some common situations and possible response strategies that might be adapted according to the specific circumstances. The aim should be to make people think for themselves, identify areas that could change, either convince them that the proposed idea is a good one or accept another positive approach that they feel is important. *Thinking It Through* (Holden 1984c) could be

Table 10.1 Overcoming obstacles to change

Possible situation/problem	Possible strategy in response
Medical or senior staff opposed to the proposed approach or change	Do not persist with that particular unit. Try to set up the change programme in an adjoining unit where staff initially invited to give support can observe successful changes there. This could encourage them to take a second look
The person 'in charge' is unconvinced or disinterested	Make influential friends—particularly more senior staff. Explain and try to convince them. Enlist enthusiastic support from junior staff. Present a united front
A common response to a new idea is: 'It 's not my/their job to do this'	Again, enlist the help of others. Talk freely at meetings, encourage open discussion. If in a position to do so, offer training, or even demonstrate approach/change in some way. It is important that *all* staff should know that employing authorities include working *with* the elderly as part of the job
Other comments include: a. 'The elderly need total care' b. 'I've been running the unit this way for years' c. 'The elderly are used to their routine'	a and b. As above, example and training with open discussion help. Listing advantages of change, solving staff's problems and meeting *their* needs often opens doors. c. Offering a choice is more acceptable than enforcing a routine which may be boring and meaningless
Excuses include: 'I'd love to, but—no time' 'I'd love to but—no staff'	If staff are convinced that *they* want change, then change will happen. Tempt interest by the use of videos, courses, visiting speakers, arranging visits to active units. Ask staff what *they* need. Examine time—ask staff to look at their way of working: are there ways or things which would improve matters? Use their suggestions. Encourage open discussion. Work to involve staff in planning and expressing ideas and feelings
'I don't know what to do, or where to start'	Confidence is increased by knowledge and practice. All the information from lectures, seminars, articles, etc, plus training and action research projects can lead to more confidence and certainty in ability to cope with change

useful here, as a basis for discussing some of the important issues involved in care for older people.

It is important to identify sources of power and money. Those who control policies and finances will not support new ideas unless they see a call for them. To initiate change, their support is needed. With a good plan, backing *can* be found. It is useful to locate a senior manager who will advise and help to overcome obstacles. Most authorities are, in fact, anxious to promote good, high-quality practice. Junior staff are often unaware of this drive for quality or even that the ideas envisaged are the very ones the authority concerned wishes to see in operation. At any level, constant and public 'nagging' can prove very effective, providing the

argument is logical and well thought out. It might take time to identify supportive people or areas, but it is time well spent. Immovable objects can be circumnavigated and outdated methods can be challenged by more efficient and satisfying ones.

Management can be convinced by demonstrations, good planning and knowledge, considerations of cost and the use of time. Equally valuable is a plea of 'Have you seen what *they* are doing, surely we're just as capable?' Competitiveness is a useful tool!

4. Laying foundations

Appropriate training is the best foundation of all. However, before specific training is started other enticements to think again might be required.

Good speakers at interesting seminars can help. Relevant films, TV programmes and interesting literature or aids all play their part. Competitiveness is found at all levels, so visits or awareness of exciting things happening elsewhere can prove inspiring. Organise regular meetings so that everyone becomes accustomed to open discussion and the exchange of ideas, opinions and concerns. This also provides the opportunity for feedback and encouragement. Always include the night staff, even if it means working overnight to meet them and explain.

A search for the hidden leaders in the unit, and an awareness of those less popular, can indicate where further work is needed. Identify potential leaders or therapists. They will need training, confidence and support. A small pilot study of, for instance, formal RO or reminiscence might prove an inducement. Many staff are afraid of making mistakes, of encountering unexpected problems. Training helps, but the experience of seeing a change in a client as a result of a simple project, with support, has the greatest impact on confidence and will convince staff better than any outside encouragement.

Make sure that your plan includes early and regular submission of reports to whoever might require one. It is much more satisfactory and establishes better confidence if such reports are sent without first being requested. It is preferable to report in your own words rather than to be forced to answer questions which prove to be totally irrelevant or for which answers are not yet available.

5. Providing relevant training

Crucial to the success of any programme is adequate training, so that the staff feel confident in what they are doing and so that their uncertainty is minimised. It must be on-going so that new staff can be familiar with the way others are working, and continuity is protected. Refresher courses are valuable to everyone, so this must be considered in order to avoid boredom and staff becoming stale and running out of ideas. The possible forms that training can take are discussed in more detail on pages 185–187.

6. Time

There are 24 hours in the day; not all should be spent at work! No one can extend the day, nor lengthen a minute. If time is the problem then only the individual can reorganise his or her priorities to fit something else in. To say 'It *must* be done' is to no purpose; only the person concerned can effectively reorganise things to meet the demand. The desire to change must be present in order to achieve anything. When staff are determined to find a way they will voluntarily examine their routines, consider the merits of methods, and look for more useful relevant equipment, policies and systems. Given support for their good ideas, they will identify time-savers for themselves. One home's care-staff discovered that if beds required changing they had to walk all the way downstairs to the linen store (and on the way were delayed by other events and meeting people); every evening they turned back bedclothes as in a hotel; every time something was soiled it was taken to the cleaners by one of the staff; they realised that their need to be seen to be 'working' was such that at mealtimes all staff were on hand, removing each plate as it was finished with. Accordingly, they arranged for linen to be on each floor, for a van to pay a weekly visit for dry-cleaning items, left the bed turning to the residents and found a keen-to-help resident to sit at each of the dining tables to collect together the dirty dishes. Suddenly, they had enough time to run a group each day! Furthermore, at mealtimes all their planned reorganisation became redundant as even the presence of one staff member became barely necessary as the residents took over clearing up without being asked!

If staff can communicate, feel that their ideas are respected and used and if regular meetings occur, many outdated routines will be replaced by more streamlined ones and time will be made available to encourage a more satisfying and stimulating atmosphere for all concerned. It is not always easy to find time for new approaches, but it is always worth trying!

7. Baseline assessments and monitoring

Much of this has been covered in detail in Chapter 6. A written record should be kept of all progress, programmes or sessions. It should list, as appropriate, all present, the subjects discussed, how each elderly person responded, any particular successes made and difficulties encountered. This is of great use when different staff lead sessions each day, so they can ensure variety and can build on previous successes and avoid previously discovered pitfalls. Senior staff can also use the record to monitor progress made by the elderly person in the sessions and to help staff over any difficult issues that arise. If programmes do not appear to be progressing according to the relevant measures in use, then it is advisable to discuss and examine the situation in order to find the problem.

At some stage, ideas may need to be revised or a fresh approach might be indicated. Staff could be proceeding too fast or too slowly, illness may have affected the clients' response, or new staff may not be conversant with the methods. Goals may have been set unrealistically high. Boredom and lack of inspiration in the methods in use may make the staff regard it all as yet another routine. Our section on the misuse of interventions (pp. 188–189) indicates some of the unwelcome developments that can occur if monitoring and supervision of the programme are inadequate. Whatever the problem it should be isolated and efforts made to overcome it.

8. Maintenance

The cautions mentioned above are equally applicable here. Everything possible should be done to ease the staff's taxing task of seeking to communicate with the elderly person. To help the staff member who comes to a group session having had a busy morning with no time to plan what should happen, a number of cards should be provided, each giving a different possible programme for use with the group. Equipment should be readily available for the appropriate activities; the physical setting should be as attractive and comfortable as possible; cards giving details of the elderly person's background—age, number and name of children, occupation, interests, etc—should be available so the staff member can respond appropriately in conversation.

Other aids should be readily available for whatever activity programme is being used. A variety of aids are already available (see Appendix 3). Staff, relatives and volunteers can use imagination and ingenuity in making and finding their own. Quite often active residents or patients can contribute further ideas.

If a programme is to be continued once implemented, it needs to become part of the routine of the ward not an optional extra to be carried out when all other chores are completed. It may be necessary to establish a rota of staff to carry out group sessions or other programmes, to avoid every staff member leaving it to everyone else to lead a group on any particular day. This also ensures that as many staff as possible are involved in the programme, which helps to give the staff intensive practice in the basic approach. Perhaps the testing time for a new programme is when the first staff shortage occurs; what priority will it be awarded then? There will of course be times when it is extremely difficult to carry out the programme. An example of this is a home where there was an outbreak of gastroenteritis among residents and staff; other situations occur that are also difficult to legislate for! However, it is important to plan what will happen during the more predictable staff shortage periods: at weekends, in winter when staff sickness reaches its peak, in summer when many staff will be enjoying a well-earned holiday, in March, when perhaps many staff are on leave to complete their holiday entitlement for the year. If the programme grinds to a halt at times like these, then only a small portion of the year will remain when it will be fully operational.

What is needed is, of course, an emphasis on a 24-hour approach, which takes relatively little additional staff time together, perhaps, with a manageable number of patients involved in daily sessions. It is better to restrict sessions to a small number of patients rather than include a large number involving more staff resources than can always be available.

It may be tempting to include more patients by having a larger group in a session at any one time. Our view is that the group size should be no larger than the staff leading the group can keep fully occupied whilst maintaining attention. Depending on severity of deterioration, this usually precludes a group size larger than four to six. If it is desired to include eight patients, it might be advantageous to split the time available between two groups of four rather than struggle to maintain the concentration of eight confused patients together.

Consideration should be given to the use of volunteers to help lead sessions, given suitable training, support and supervision, of course. Having a structure like RO or reminiscence to work within can help a volunteer worker a great deal to contribute something useful to the care of the elderly person with dementia, and can help reduce the uncertainty and feelings of uselessness that lead to many a voluntary worker only coming to the ward or home once or twice and not returning.

Other resources may also be explored, and it should be emphasised that the task of leading sessions does not have to always fall on the care-staff: occupational therapy staff, or speech therapists, psychologists, etc, may also be willing to be involved in this way. However, when several groups of workers are involved, exactly how the duties are to be shared should be made explicit. It is often said that if a structured programme is stopped the clients will deteriorate quite quickly. As stated earlier, the regression could be caused by replacing a positive, active environment with a negative or unnatural one. If a 24-hour approach or philosophy is operating, then simply to end a series of group sessions will not lead to a definite deterioration. If there is no obvious reason for a deterioration after a regular involvement in a programme, then the environment should be carefully examined for negative, dehumanising factors.

Even when a programme is in full swing, certain events can have a damaging effect: illnesses, staff changes, absences, or the loss of a popular member of the group, staff or other well-known person. Other possibilities are boredom and staleness. Updating will help, another training session or course, an outsider who provides feedback on being impressed by the work being done, or even new equipment or books. Our daily lives are full of ups and downs; we try to find a fresh amusement or interest; so it should be with a ward or home. A short rest from doing things in a particular way, thoughts on other ideas and alternative ways can put new life into a sagging system. Flexibility is desirable. Searching for another way can prove to be a challenge which in itself livens up proceedings.

Approaches to training

What form should the training take? This depends very much on the individual situation, but we have found the following components of training particularly valuable.

Lectures

These should be informal and provide plenty of opportunity for discussion throughout, thus helping the 'lecturer' to ensure real understanding. Some discussion of general attitudes and an understanding of important factors, for instance the basic psychology of ageing, is worth including. It can help staff to consider the behaviour, needs and external influences affecting older people. Specific training will depend on the programme being implemented. Aspects to highlight might include:

- the rationale underlying the approach/ methods being adopted
- the general principles of a 24-hour approach
- examples of the use of the proposed intervention
- environmental factors
- communicating with the person with dementia
- general guidelines on group work
- goals and limitations of the intervention

- how the approach can be applied in a particular setting.

Audio-visual aids

However interesting the lecture, there is no doubt that carefully chosen audio-visual aids are extremely useful in bringing the subject matter to life.

Slides are useful in illustrating what happens in a group session or in demonstrating helpful facilities to be incorporated into the physical environment. They can be used in conjunction with snippets of audiotape from an actual session to show what staff can do to draw the patients out and how they can respond appropriately. This can be especially useful in illustrating how to respond to a given situation using resolution or validation methods.

A tape–slide programme providing a recorded talk illustrated by a set of slides can also be useful. The same talk can be repeated on several occasions, providing an opportunity for all staff on different shifts to see it, and also it can be used with new staff to introduce them to the approach being used. Staff can work through the programme at their own pace. A set of questions to accompany the tape–slide programme is useful to direct the staff member's attention to key points.

Videotapes can also aid training and provide illustrations of the approach to be employed. Careful editing is required to ensure that salient points are made; it can be difficult to assimilate all the information while watching the tape of an entire session of reminiscence or RO as the pace is somewhat slower than TV programmes to which staff are accustomed! A commentary directing attention to particular principles and methods is advisable.

Some audio-visual aids available for sale or hire are listed in Appendix 3.

Hand-outs

The use of hand-outs for staff to keep, peruse at their leisure and refer to when necessary is very important to reinforce the lectures and talks given. They should cover briefly the main points made in the lecture, giving examples as well as guidelines.

Demonstration

A practical demonstration of the approach will make the principles stand out more clearly. A visit to a centre where the approach is already being applied will prove valuable. Or, a person with prior experience could lead a small group with other staff members observing, or someone could lead a session with some other staff role-playing the parts of the patients and others observing. It is in this demonstration that staff observe how the principles are actually put into practice, how the staff member can be encouraging rather than patronising, how even the person with the most severe impairment can be helped to succeed rather than having their failure reinforced yet again. After each demonstration plenty of time should be allowed for comments and discussion of what took place. This should then be followed by role play and involvement.

Role play and involvement

Training group members enjoy remembering their first impressions of age, listing their expectations of ageing and attempting definitions and explanations. The aim should be to help achieve an understanding of older people by referring to everyone's own, personal experience. Staff in training take the role of group leader whilst other staff play the 'confused' elderly patients once more, and other staff observe. This is valuable not only in giving the leaders a gradual exposure to employing a particular system or running a specific type of group, but is also helpful for those playing the role of an elderly person, as it offers an insight into the person's feelings and expectations. The role-played group sessions should be interrupted frequently for observers to make suggestions to leaders or patients and for leaders to ask for help if uncertain how to respond to a patient or how to involve them in the group. This then leads on to feedback.

Feedback

Feedback has a valuable place both in training sessions and in the continuous on-the-job training that should occur. In the role-play sessions, other staff (including those who played the patients) can tell the group leaders in the role play what they thought helpful about what they did and said and about their attitude that came across, and of course what seemed to be less helpful. Giving feedback is never easy, particularly if it is negative. It is important that these training sessions are relaxed and open and that it is remembered that the different approaches all involve certain skills which can only be learned properly if we are able to have our performance monitored—just as when we are, for example, learning to drive a car. If access to video-recording equipment is available, this provides a way in which staff members can see their performance for themselves and, in a sense, provide their own feedback in addition to that of others.

From feedback, the training session may lead on to further demonstrations, more role play and more feedback. For example, in one training session, in a role play, one staff member tended to interrogate the 'patients', pressurising them with questions they were unable to answer, leaving an uncomfortable pause in which the 'patient' seemed likely to become acutely aware of having failed. Feedback was given on this point and a further demonstration showed how the same areas of information could be covered without making the 'patient' feel threatened. The staff member then repeated the role play and was able to be much less interrogative, helping the 'patients' to find the answers for themselves. Feedback was then given by the other staff on how much better this second role play now was, on the noticeable change there had been and how the 'patients' responded much better to this more gentle approach.

Feedback should not be confined to training sessions, and it can be helpful in preventing staff from slipping into bad habits once they have been employing a particular type of intervention for some time (again the analogy with driving a car applies!), and in encouraging them as they find innovative ways to deal with the variety of situations that arise. Feedback should be mutual, not just given by senior staff! What is needed is a continued willingness to learn and to improve skills, not to become over-confident and above all to continue to be sensitive to older people, their needs and what *they* can teach us.

Action research

It is valuable when running courses to encourage staff to use some of the skills that they have encountered during the training session. The best way to do this is to encourage them to form groups and agree on a mini project that they can attempt on their own unit. When the 'action research' has been decided upon, the groups are invited to report back to a follow-up session, in, say, 8 weeks. Support and contact is offered for those who might run into difficulties or need advice. Many ideas, new policies and new problems can be highlighted by this method. Staff learn from it and confidence grows. The skills learned in the training session are then much more likely to actually be applied!

Appendix 3 lists a number of training materials that will be useful for organising training on RO and related approaches and provide a number of ideas for particular activities that can be used within this framework.

Negative effects of positive approaches

Can interventions change patients for the worse and perhaps be harmful to them? Woods & Britton (1977) reviewed reports of negative trends occurring generally in psychological programmes with the elderly. They concluded that some reports indicated a change in the patient from being non-complaining, uncritical and acquiescent to becoming more critical, demanding and challenging as a result of improvements in general functioning and a better awareness of reality.

The change, perhaps, is from being an 'ideal' patient, presenting no nursing problems, to a person becoming aware of a reality which is often by any standards unsatisfactory, who seeks to bring about change by being more complaining and critical. This type of 'negative' change can be seen as, in fact, healthy and adaptive.

Some negative effects specifically related to RO have been identified. Zepelin et al (1981) report deterioration on a number of behavioural measures, particularly social responsiveness, compared with residents in a home where RO was not applied. These results may have emerged in part from difficulties in matching residents adequately and from differences between raters in the two settings in the use of the rating scales. Baines et al (1987) report lower levels of life satisfaction following RO sessions, compared with reminiscence sessions. They suggest this related to RO helping residents appraise more realistically the limitations of their existence. In RO groups, both negative and positive feelings were expressed. The ability of residents to express anger and sadness initially alarmed staff, before they realised these issues deserved careful discussion with the residents.

Possible harmful effects of any approach incorrectly carried out will be considered in the next section. It must be emphasised here, however, that even if properly executed these interventions do not always make patients happy, because reality itself is never all roses. However tactfully we discuss the death—even some years ago—of a patient's spouse or discuss events during the World Wars, these cannot be dismissed with a joke. Reality covers the whole range of emotions, however tempting it is to only look at one side of life. Respect for the patient's dignity may sometimes mean staff facing up to issues that they also find painful to talk about and so would rather avoid. We do need to be aware of negative reactions, however, and, instead of blaming the approach for them, be prepared to work through them with the elderly person, providing warmth in our support of them as they come to terms with what is happening, helping them where possible to express their feelings—which their mental state may make it extremely difficult for them to do unaided.

A further word of warning when beginning work with new patients; it is important to take note of their previous environment. If they have been sitting quietly, withdrawn and non-responsive on a psychogeriatric back-ward for some years, it is not sensible to rush in and stimulate them too quickly, and a gradual approach is more likely to succeed. Change presents difficulties for most people, and in a ward generally, gradual changes will be much less anxiety-provoking—for staff as well as patients!

MISUSE OF INTERVENTIONS

We have become increasingly concerned that a 'little knowledge' of a given technique can lead to it being misapplied, often inadvertently through lack of adequate training or from a misunderstanding of its complexities when, on the surface, it appears so simple.

In the case of RO, several writers have pointed out some of the errors that have been made. For example, the article by Gubrium & Ksander (1975), mentioned in Chapter 5, describes an inflexible, unthinking, mechanical approach to RO. We feel Gubrium & Ksander are right to ask what is the 'reality' of RO in these circumstances. The staff member has learned to go through the RO board, helping the patients to recite the information there. What he has not learned to do is to try to understand the elderly person's viewpoint, to look for what the person is seeking to say and go beyond the rigidly structured session to a situation where real communication can take place. This mechanical type of RO can occur when it is applied without warmth.

Buckholdt & Gubrium (1983) provide further examples of how RO can become an unhelpful approach. They show how in one home's RO-training programme staff are taught to label certain behaviours as 'confused', rather than to seek explanations for the problems or to gain an understanding of what is happening to the person. In care-planning meetings, they observed the use of this label 'confused' or 'disorientated' as an 'explanation' of problems' (leading inevitably to RO being prescribed!), again without a search for alternative ways of looking at the person and their behaviour in a more individualised fashion. Finally, they show how the RO board's 'correct answer' dominated RO sessions at the home to the detriment of real communication and interaction. When staff fail to try to understand the individual person as a whole person—despite the difficulties in communication—then this sort of abuse of RO and other approaches can arise.

More recently, Dietch et al (1989) also criticise the use of RO in practice, arguing that it can prove positively dangerous if the humanistic context is ignored. They provide three examples of a similar nature to those supplied by Feil (1982) as situations where RO can be seen as damaging; for instance, insisting on bringing a person 'up-to-date' regarding the age of a son or the death of parents in such a manner as to provoke a severe emotional reaction. In our opinion, this is not the fault of the techniques, but rather relates to problems of attitudes, inaccurate knowledge and inadequate training. Whatever the approach, what is required is the sensitivity to appreciate what the person is trying to say. This needs thought, time and insight into the feelings being expressed.

RO is not alone in being open to misuse, although its wide application has perhaps helped to generate more examples. Reminiscence work can, at times, run the risk of being too intrusive; it may feel to the elderly person that they are being asked to discuss their personal affairs in front of a group of strangers. As with RO, there is the risk of becoming over interrogative; rather than allowing the person to talk only about those topics they feel comfortable in sharing, the leader persistently asks questions about more personal matters, driving the elderly person into a corner, with possibly harmful consequences. Similarly, where the leader brings up traumatic events the person has experienced in a group setting, considerable distress may be caused that cannot readily be worked through in that setting; such topics may be more appropriate for a one-to-one session, but still the onus is on the worker to be sensitive and to ensure the person really does feel comfortable and secure enough to share such painful memories. Our (often morbid) curiosity must never be the justification for exposing such wounds. Validation work can also become misguided at times; for example, its emphasis on the person resolving past conflicts may obscure real issues in the present. Thus, a frail elderly lady who looks fearful every time a particular male resident walks into the dayroom and starts screaming 'Get away! Get away!' might be viewed as expressing anger at a strict and punitive father; however, discussion with staff might show that the male resident has in fact pushed her over several times and that she is acting on a reality-based current fear. As with other approaches, a sensitive approach is required.

Behavioural approaches have also been subject to possible misuse, particularly where punishment or deprivation of reinforcement has been used, or where social 'reinforcement' has been given in a mechanical or patronising way; even activity programmes may be misused, where attendance is compulsory and no choice is given regarding participation.

A common error is to apply an approach at the wrong level for the individuals concerned, so that it goes over their heads at one extreme, or is demeaning and insulting at the other; flexibility of approach is all-important—a readiness to adjust the activities to the particular group or individual.

To summarise the various misuses of positive approaches, it is fair to say that it is the application of the underlying attitudes, values and principles that must have priority, rather than a rigid adherence to techniques and methods. We need to continually examine our use of these methods in the light of these attitudes. If the person's individuality, dignity and adulthood are respected sensitively, then we have more chance of avoiding some of the pitfalls described here.

MULTICULTURAL ISSUES

Dementing conditions occur worldwide. As the proportion of older people rises dramatically in developing countries such as China, or even Spain and Italy, it is almost certain that the numbers of people with a dementia will increase correspondingly. As numbers increase, the traditional reverence and respect for elders and the imperative given to family care will come under increasing pressure, as is already the case in Japan.

Our whole emphasis on the person with dementia as a whole person with a lifetime of experience that shapes the way they now present makes it clear that any positive approach must be adapted to the person's cultural background and beliefs. However, it must be acknowledged that this is a complex and challenging task, with no easy solutions.

Language barriers in particular may render communication very difficult indeed. Often it seems that the person reverts to their first language, with languages learned subsequently being more severely impaired earlier. Thus a Hungarian man, who had lived in England for many years and spoke perfect English, began to speak more and more in Hungarian, often switching in mid-sentence, unaware that he was not being understood. His English wife found communication very difficult; she had never needed to learn Hungarian in the past as his English had been so good. In countries such as Singapore, where many dialects and languages are in use, the problem becomes even more acute, with patients on a ward being unable to converse with each other, and communication with staff depending on whether there is a staff member with a command of that specific language.

Interpreters are increasingly available in areas of the UK where language barriers arise particularly often, but are an expensive resource and need to be used carefully, to help the staff get to know the person and his/her needs as much as possible and to leave key words and phrases which will assist in the person's day-to-day care. Family members may also be able to assist, but it is wise at some point in the assessment of the person to involve an independent interpreter, so that the person has an opportunity to speak outside the family context.

Even with an interpreter, communication problems may not be resolved, as the dementia may be affecting the person's original language also. Other channels of communication also need to be explored: non-verbal, through gestures and mime, and the use of picture boards depicting common everyday activities, e.g. eating, washing, going to bed and so on, reinforced with a few simple words in the person's own language are worth trying.

It is vital to realise the multiplicity of cultures and not to make assumptions about an individual's beliefs, diet, interests, musical tastes and so on from minimal information. The person's religion may be recorded as Jewish, but this will have quite different implications for different individuals, according to the degree of orthodoxy and sect. Two people may both be recorded as having been born in India, but may well have different languages, religions, food preferences and in fact little in common. The key issue is to ensure the range of choices available extends to allow the person to follow their specific dietary and other requirements. Check out with the person's family the lifestyle the person would follow at home; check out with the person's religious advisor what observances the person was accustomed to follow; as far as possible check out with the individual their own preferences. Where this would clash with ward or home 'policy', query the policy; can a way be found around the problem?

The family have an important role to play, and the difficulties are multiplied where there are no relatives on hand. They can help greatly as already mentioned with language barriers, and to assist in building up a picture of the person's lifestyle. They can help too with the person's life story, which will be of even greater value than usual to staff who do not have the usual background knowledge to flesh out the person's own account. This will be of great use in individual reminiscence work with the person. Staff need to be especially aware of the family's position; they will have their own views of the person's condition and of how care should be provided; staff need to listen carefully to and respect these views, opening up discussion of them as trust develops, offering alternative views for consideration where this seems appropriate and helpful.

What is being described here is not a different approach to older people from cultures other than the most prevalent, but a plea to pursue an individualised, flexible approach to the extent that it is sensitive to the vast individual differences in people, between and within cultures. In working with older people from other cultures, as many care-workers do, we need to recognise and value the differences that exist; to seek to place ourselves in the position of a learner regarding the other's culture; not to expect them to conform to our way but to adapt our approach and the environment so that the person can continue to use their familiar, over-learned skills and abilities, bound up in their culture; to learn and respect their body language and non-verbal communication, which may have important differences from our own; a good way of learning is to celebrate together—to have events in the style of a particular person or group's culture, and to invite others to share in this.

We must avoid dealing in racial or cultural or religious stereotypes; however, we have to recognise that the person with dementia's cognitive impairment may lead them at times to function in this manner, perhaps as a way of simplifying the complex world around them. This can feel hurtful and rejecting at times, particularly if the person makes racist comments, when they seem unable to see the person in us, despite our efforts to work with them as a person. When facing such challenges, we need other staff or a supervisor to talk through our hurt and to acknowledge the reasons behind what has happened; we need to continue working on the relationship, recognising that change is slow, but that as they get to know us better as a person, we might move in their eyes beyond the superficial stereotype.

Concluding remarks

Although research has extended knowledge about older people and the conditions causing dementia, we recognise the continuing difficulties experienced by those working with people suffering from degenerative disorders. Despite the promising research findings, indicating the responsiveness of people with dementia to the environment in which they live, and the expectation that answers may soon be found to some of the disease processes, progressive deterioration remains so often the norm in dementia care. In this context, goals must reflect the knowledge that a relatively small improvement may be a major achievement. Indeed, to maintain a person at a particular level of functioning without further loss is actually a measure of success for the intervention.

Various studies have shown that positive approaches are having an impact in maintaining a better quality of life for people with dementia. Improvements in staff morale and job satisfaction have also been demonstrated. The value of these interventions is that they provide a structure for staff to work within, and a means to train new staff members in order to ensure a consistency of approach and the involvement and understanding of all staff.

In previous years there was little available to help staff solve particular problems, or to provide methods which could be used to improve the environment or to seek to improve the person's abilities. Today there is a much greater choice of methods and approaches, and detailed information and guidelines are readily available. There are now far fewer care-staff who are unaware of approaches such as RO, reminiscence, the importance of environmental influences and the need for activity and stimulation. There is no doubt scope for improvement in the practice of these approaches, but there are now sources of advice and assistance. This book aims to be one such resource but, of course, cannot provide all the answers; whilst we have attempted to cover most of the common interventions, readers will need to follow up references and other resources for greater detail on the implementation of some of these.

Although we have concentrated on older people with dementia, many of the approaches would have a wider applicability, e.g. to functional and neurological conditions. We have stressed the need to clarify behavioural problems, which may be related to 'normal' reactions to unpleasant events or to environmental influences, and specific brain-function problems where other functions are retained and there is a need to avoid mis-interpreting behaviour. There is particular interest in the use of reminiscence in depression (see Garland 1994) and the application of RO principles in areas such as rehabilitation following head injury (Corrigan et al 1985) as well as with elderly people with lifelong mental handicap. As always, the emphasis needs to be on an individualised approach based on the person's strengths and needs.

With elderly people whose decision-making capacity is impaired for one reason or another, it is important to make explicit the ethical issues involved as they form such a vulnerable group, perhaps unable to assert their rights and needs in a conventional manner. We are often asked if these approaches could be harmful (see Ch. 10). Does RO, for instance, treat patients like children, taking them back to 'school'? Should the person who is 'happily demented' be 'disturbed' by being brought back from their withdrawal? Would it not be kinder to leave such people in their twilight world and not expose them to the reality of old age, infirmity, an unsatisfactory environment and so forth?

These and similar questions raise the important issue of the ethics of employing a given approach. Often these issues arouse a great deal of emotion,

perhaps as those working with the elderly imagine themselves in the position of the person with dementia, a fantasy that most people would find threatening and disturbing. Some people favour a passive approach, providing for physical needs until death occurs, keeping the person 'happy' by ensuring a 'no demand' situation. Others opt for a more positive, active approach encouraging awareness and independence. The ethical issues are complex. In some areas of behavioural intervention, it is possible to arrive at an agreed treatment contract with the client, acceptable to both parties. This is extremely difficult—if not impossible—with the person with a severe degree of impairment arising from a dementia. Therefore, there is a need for those working with this group to be clear about their own ethical position as a dementing person may not be capable of making a fully informed decision about treatment.

We will try to make clear the assumptions that we make as we outline the reasons for our preference for the positive approach.

First, it must be emphasised that whether we adopt a positive approach or not we are inter-vening in some way. Not doing anything with a patient still represents some kind of programme, ill-defined as it may be. The advantage of positive approaches is that they make explicit what is being attempted and make it more difficult to shirk responsibility and avoid ethical problems. This is of added importance as those with dementia are a particularly vulnerable group who are less likely to be able to use con-ventional means of self-protection.

Secondly, we see patients with dementia as people, with basic human needs, both physical and emotional. In our view, attempts to meet both sorts of needs are the responsibility of those in the caring role. Emotional needs are more difficult to meet but should not be ignored on this account. Therefore, elderly people who are experiencing decline need to feel cared for and permitted to have opportunities to express care for others. We recognise that these needs may find expression in more restricted ways than seen in the person without dementia, of course. In so far as these approaches aid communication and encourage self-respect, then we would see them as helping in the satisfaction of these emotional needs.

Thirdly, we would draw a parallel with other disabilities, where increasingly the principle of 'normalisation' is being applied. This approach seeks to help a person lead as normal and as valued a life as possible, given the disability that is present (see Ch. 7). We would argue that these positive approaches can be used to help people with dementia experience and achieve much more that is valued than approaches which deny the full range of needs of the person with dementia.

To return to the original question of the 'happily' dementing person, it is difficult to judge to what extent this state does represent a high quality of life; this could be yet another assumption on the part of the onlooker as the people concerned are not capable of expressing their feelings and attitudes coherently. Indeed, the situation may be a means of coping with the failures and difficulties of the dementing process. There may even be a sense in which, by withdrawing in this fashion, the person is missing out to some degree. What we would advocate is to provide opportunities to re-engage, but also to provide a choice. To force the issue is not acceptable, but to nurture and encourage still leaves the options open. In the final analysis, elderly people will shut off the stimulation or will respond to it. Unfortunately, they are not given the choice often enough and it is assumed that they would rather remain withdrawn. We have tried to make it clear that our approach is tactful, flexible and warm rather than pressurised and aggressive. There are dangers with RO and like approaches with the wrong attitudes; there is a need for discussion of ethical issues and monitoring of programmes by those outside the institution as well as those actively involved. Regrettably, advocates for the rights of people with dementia and their supporters are rare; discussion often centres on placement rather than on management and treatment. Working with the supporter and the nurse, the care-attendant or relative should also be considered. Here the ethical situation is simpler; staff members and relatives can make an informed decision

about what they find helpful in caring for and communicating with the elderly person.

A large component of these programmes is in changing the environment rather than necessarily inducing change in the individual. Again, some sort of environment has to be provided: the issue is what the nature of this should be. The environment described in Chapter 7, with its emphasis on basic humanitarian values of respect, dignity and interaction, is an improvement—psychologically—over many current settings. The techniques for facilitating communication also increase the person's quality of life by improving interaction with the staff.

Is it worth adopting a positive approach when the person is to be transferred to a setting where only basic care is given? Again a quality of life consideration applies; if this can be increased in the present then it can be seen as valuable, whatever might or might not happen in the future. There are now fewer and fewer places where some thought is not being given to these approaches. The example of one ward or home can inspire many others. Contact over a particular patient who has benefited from an individualised approach helps to spread the positive attitudes that are needed for real progress to be achieved. These attitudes ensure that there is an ethical, humanitarian basis to these approaches. Abuses are possible (see Ch. 10), but where the approaches are used explicitly and the home or ward is open to external monitoring and scrutiny these can be guarded against.

There is a need for staff supporting people in their own homes to be aware of the major impact their presence will have. They could be welcomed or they could be seen as intruders; they could be perceived as supportive or viewed as interfering. It may seem easier to take over and make decisions, changing things 'for the best' for the person with dementia, who may be accepting of a dependent role. Much work needs to be done to learn ways to use positive approaches appropriately in the community. It is desirable for a person to remain in their own home for as long as possible, but independence must be maintained. The personal touch remains vital, but the means of ensuring that a person retains skills and has a good quality of life is of major importance. Monitoring care given in the person's home is more difficult than in a residential home or hospital ward, but is essential if care in the community is to achieve a higher quality of care than that offered in institutional settings. This is not guaranteed simply because the person is at home; staff involved will require good training, support and supervision systems and adequate resources.

Though research is presently underway concerning the nature of psychological functioning in the conditions which cause dementia, there is still some way to go before there is a flow of information aiding in the development and refining of positive approaches. We are far from being able to consider differences in the general approach to individuals with different underlying conditions, for example. There needs also to be a continued effort to evaluate the effectiveness of positive approaches on a broad front, and to examine in more detail the component parts, to enable further progress in this area.

Approaches like RO and reminiscence and physical exercise may appear simple in concept; others, like validation, seem much more complicated. In practice there are many difficulties and obstacles to the successful implementation of them all. Although answers have been found to some of the concerns over the years, there are always new ones and others which arise again and again for which the answers appear elusive. The vast majority of staff working with older people are enthusiastic and keen to put positive approaches into practice, but they need support. These programmes are hard work and very demanding; they require considerable imagination and often the courage to keep things going, an ability to forget about oneself, to plan, to remember, and even a willingness to make a fool of oneself if it achieves the aim! Yet many staff who have used positive approaches find them extremely satisfying as, at last, they communicate and make personal contact with the elderly person who has appeared so confused, disorientated and inaccessible.

Appendices

APPENDIX 1: Test of verbal orientation and personal and current information

Instructions for use

Ask questions conversationally, varying the exact words used as appropriate to ensure the person understands what is being asked; scoring may be lenient, but no help in giving answers may be offered.

1 What is your name?	0 1
2 How old are you?	0 1
3 When were you born? All correct	0 1
Date correct	0 1
Month correct	0 1
Year correct	0 1
4 Where were you born?	0 1
5 What school did you attend?	0 1
6 What was your occupation (or spouse's)?	0 1
7 Where did you (or spouse) work—which town?	0 1
8 Name of employers for whom you worked?	0 1
9 Name of spouse or sibling?	0 1
10 What is the name of this place?	0 1
11 What type of place is it, i.e. hospital, old people's home, etc?	0 1
12 What is the address of this place, i.e. approximate location?	0 1
13 What is the name of this town/city?	0 1
14 What time of day is it now—morning, afternoon, evening, etc?	0 1
15 What time is it now? (Accept answer if within 30 minutes of actual time.)	0 1
16 What day of the week is it today?	0 1
17 What season is it now—spring, summer, autumn, winter?	0 1
18 What month is it now?	0 1
19 What day of the month is it now?	0 1
20 What year is it now?	0 1
21 Recognition of persons (cleaner, doctor, staff member, resident, relative—any two available), 1 point for each person.	0 1
22 Who is the prime minister at present?	0 1
23 Who was the prime minister immediately before this one?	0 1
24 Who is the president of the USA at present?	0 1
25 Who is on the throne at present? 1 point for name	0 1 2
26 Who was on the throne immediately before her? 1 point for number	0 1 2
27 What are the colours of the Union Jack?	0 1
28 When did the First World War begin, and end? 1 point for each (allow 2 years' error).	0 1 2
29 When did the Second World War begin, and end?	0 1 2
30 Repeat this name and address after me: Mr John/Brown/	0 1 2
42/West Street/Gateshead	3 4 5

   Ask for recall after 5 minutes; score
   1 point for each segment recalled correctly.
   Modify address to suit locality!

Total score   (42 maximum)

As used in Woods' (1979) study.

APPENDIX 2: Holden Communication Scale

Score	0	1	2	3	4
Conversation					
1. Response	Initiates conversation deeply involved with anyone	Good for those familiar to person	Fair response to those close by; no initiation of conversation	Rather confused; poor comprehension	Rarely or never converses
2. Interest in past events	Long, full account of past events	Fairly good description	Short description; a little confused	Confused or disinterested	No response
3. Pleasure	Shows real pleasure in situation/ achievement	Smiles and shows interest	Variable response; slight smile; vague	Rarely shows even a smile	No response or just weeps
4. Humour	Creates situation or tells funny story on own initiative	Enjoys comic situations or stories	Needs an explanation and encouragement to respond	Vague smile; simply copies others	No response or negativistic
Awareness and Knowledge					
5. Names	Knows most people's names on ward	Knows a few names	Needs a constant reminder	Knows own name only	Forgotten even own name
6. General orientation	Knows day, month, weather and whereabouts	Can forget one or two items	Usually gets two right but tries	Vague; may guess one	Very confused
7. General knowledge	Good on current events; generally able	Outstanding events only; fair on general knowledge	No current knowledge; poor general information	Confused about many things; gets anxious and upset	Confused about everything; does not respond
8. Ability to join in games, etc	Joins in games and activities with ease	Requires careful instructions but joins in	Can only join in simple activities	Becomes anxious and upset	Cannot or will not join in
Communication					
9. Speech	No known difficulty	Slight hesitation or odd wording	Very few words; mainly automatic phrases	Inappropriate words; odd sounds; nodding	Little or no verbalisation
10. Attempts at communication	Communicates with ease	Tries hard to speak clearly	Tries to draw; gesticulates needs, etc	Euphoric laughter; weeping; aggressive	No attempt
11. Interest and response to objects	Responds with interest and comment	Despite difficulties shows interest	Shows some interest, but rather vague	Weeps; rejects objects; shows aggression	No response; no comprehension
12. Success in communication	Clearly understood	Uses gestures and sounds effectively	Understanding restricted to a few people	Becomes frustrated and angry	Makes no attempt

APPENDIX 3: Training aids, sources of materials, practical manuals, orientation aids

We recommend that the reader obtains current brochures from the two major suppliers of these aids, for a complete listing of their products and prices:

Winslow Press,
Telford Road,
Bicester, Oxfordshire OX6 OTS
Telephone: 01869 244733

Nottingham Rehab Ltd,
17 Ludlow Hill Road,
West Bridgford,
Nottingham NG2 1BR

Videotapes

1. Black and white tape showing group work at basic and standard RO levels and showing a group over a 6-week period, including pre- and post-group assessments. Details of availability from Una Holden.
2. Videotapes on validation and to assist in reminiscence are available from Winslow Press.

Tape–slide programmes

1. Covers basic attitudes and 24 hour RO (reference number 81–61), 30 minutes.
2. Covers RO sessions (reference number 81–62), 30 minutes. Both prepared by Bob Woods, and are based on Chapters 7 and 8 of this book, respectively. Available for sale or hire from:

Graves Medical Audio-visual Library,
Concord Video & Film Council,
201 Felixstowe Road,
Ipswich IP3 9BJ
Telephone: 01473 726012 / 715754

Training manuals

1. *Reality Orientation—Principles and Practice*, Lorna Rimmer. Available from Winslow Press.
2. *Looking at Confusion*, Una Holden. Winslow Press.
3. *Day into Night*, Una Holden. A handbook for 24 hour care. Winslow Press.
4. *Goal planning with Elderly People; Making Plans To Meet Individual Needs: A Manual of Instruction*, Christine Barrowclough & Ian Fleming, 1986. Manchester University Press, Manchester. ISBN: 0 7190 1802 1.
5. *Reminiscence with Elderly People*, Andrew Norris. Winslow Press.
6. *Group Work with the Elderly*, Mike Bender, Andrew Norris & Paulette Bauckham. Winslow Press.

7. *Wandering*, Graham Stokes. Winslow Press.
8. *Shouting and Screaming*, Graham Stokes. Winslow Press.
9. *Aggression*, Graham Stokes. Winslow Press.
10. *Incontinence and Inappropriate Urinating*, Graham Stokes. Winslow Press.
11. *Working with Dementia*, Graham Stokes & Fiona Goudie (eds). Winslow Press.
12. *The Care Assistant's Guide to Working with Elderly Mentally Infirm People*, Sue Benson & Patrick Carr (eds). Care Concern, 13 Park House, 140 Battersea Park Road, London SW11 4NB.
13. *Making Residential Care Feel Like Home*, Jeff Garland. Winslow Press.

Orientation aids

1. Memory boards, calendars and signposts available from Winslow Press and Nottingham Rehab.
2. *Conversing with Memory Impaired Individuals Using Memory Aids*, Michelle Bourgeois. Winslow Press. A memory aid workbook.
3. *Orientation*, Mike Markey. Winslow Press. An RO board game.

Reminiscence aids

1. Books, pictures, posters, memorabilia, etc, available from Age Exchange, The Reminiscence Centre, 11 Blackheath Village, London SE3 9LA. Telephone: 0181 318 9105.
2. Memory diary; autobiographical scrap-book, for writing and recording life events. Winslow Press.
3. Numerous sets of reminiscence aids available from Winslow Press.

Training packages

1. *Quality Lifestyles for Older People with Dementia*, Hilary Brown & Sue Benson. Pavilion Publishing (Brighton) Ltd, 8 St George's Place, Brighton, East Sussex BN1 4ZZ.
2. The following organisations produce and have lists of relevant training materials:

Age Concern England, Training Department,
Astral House, 1268 London Road, London SW16 4ER
Telephone: 0181 679 8000

Alzheimer's Disease Society,
Gordon House, 10 Greencoat Place, London SW1P 1PH
Telephone: 0171 306 0606

The Dementia Services Development Centre,
University of Stirling,
Stirling, Scotland FK9 4LA
Telephone: 01786 467740

Guides for carers

1. *Failure-free Activities for the Alzheimer's Patient*, Carmel Sheridan, 1992. Macmillan, Basingstoke. ISBN 0 333 55455 8.

2. *Person to Person: A Guide to the Care of Those With Failing Mental Powers*, Tom Kitwood & Kathleen Bredin, 1992. Gale Centre Publications, Whitakers Way, Loughton, Essex IG10 1SQ.

3. *Caring for the Person With Dementia: A Guide for Families and Other Carers*, Bob Woods & Chris Lay; 3rd edn, 1994. Published by and available from the Alzheimer's Disease Society (address above).

4. In addition, numerous books are available for carers: the Alzheimer's Disease Society (address above) can provide lists.

Notes

1. Many of the organisations referred to produce brochures or lists of their publications.

2. Most suppliers will forward their publications outside the UK, but please check availability, conditions and charges.

3. Some of the materials, e.g. some of the reminiscence aids, are not relevant outside the UK.

References

Adelson R, Nasti A, Spratkin J N, Marinelli R, Primnavera L H, Gorman B S 1982 Behavioral ratings of health professionals' interactions with the geriatric patient. Gerontologist 22: 277–281

Ager A 1990 Life experiences checklist. NFER-Nelson, Windsor

Albert M L, Sparks R W, Helm N 1973 Melodic intonation therapy for aphasia. Archives of Neurology 29: 130–131

Albyn-Davis A 1983 A survey of adult aphasia. Prentice Hall, London

Ankus M, Quarrington B 1972 Operant behaviour in the memory disordered. Journal of Gerontology 27: 500–510

Annerstedt L, Gustafson L, Nilsson K 1993 Medical outcome of psychosocial intervention in demented patients: one-year clinical follow-up after relocation into group living units. International Journal of Geriatric Psychiatry 8: 833–841

Applegate W B, Blass J P, Williams T F 1990 Instruments for the functional assessment of older patients. New England Journal of Medicine 322: 1207–1214

Babins L 1988 Conceptual analysis of validation therapy. International Journal of Aging and Human Development 26: 161–168

Backman L 1992 Memory training and memory improvement in Alzheimer's disease: rules and exceptions. Acta Neurologia Scandinavica, suppl 139: 84–89

Bailey E A, Brown S, Goble R E A, Holden U P 1986 24 hour reality orientation: changes for staff and patients. Journal of Advanced Nursing 11: 141–151

Baines S, Saxby P, Ehlert K 1987 Reality orientation and reminiscence therapy: a controlled cross-over study of elderly confused people. British Journal of Psychiatry 151: 222–231

Baltes M M 1988 The etiology and maintenance of dependence in the elderly: three phases of operant research. Behavior Therapy 19: 301–319

Baltes M M, Lascomb S L 1975 Creating a healthy institutional environment: the nurse as a change agent. International Journal of Nursing Studies 12: 5–12

Barrowclough C, Fleming I 1986a Goal planning with elderly people. Manchester University Press, Manchester

Barrowclough C, Fleming I 1986b Training direct care staff in goal-planning with elderly people. Behavioural Psychotherapy 14: 192–209

Bassey E J 1985 Benefits of exercise in the elderly. In: Isaacs B (ed) Recent advances in geriatric medicine—3. Churchill Livingstone, Edinburgh

Beech J R, Harding L (eds) 1990 Assessment of the elderly. NFER-Nelson, Windsor

Beecham J, Cambridge P, Hallam A, Knapp M 1993 The costs of domus care.. International Journal of Geriatric Psychiatry 8: 827–831

Bender M 1994 An interesting confusion: what can we do with reminiscence groupwork? In: Bornat J (ed) Reminiscence reviewed: evaluations, achievements, perspectives. Open University Press, Buckingham, p 32–45

Bender M, Norris A 1987 An introduction to group work with the elderly. Winslow Press, London

Benjamin L C, Spector J 1990 Environments for the dementing. International Journal of Geriatric Psychiatry 5: 15–24

Benson S 1994 Sniff and doze therapy Journal of Dementia Care 2(1): 12–14

Bergert L, Jacobsson E 1976 Training of reality orientation with a group of patients with senile dementia. Scandinavian Journal of Behaviour Therapy 5: 191–200

Bergmann K, Foster E M, Justice A W, Matthews V 1978 Management of the demented elderly patient in the community. British Journal of Psychiatry 132: 441–449

Birchmore T, Clague S 1983 A behavioural approach to reduce shouting. Nursing Times 79(16): 37–39

Birren J E, Schaie K W (eds) 1990 Handbook of the Psychology of Aging, 3rd edn. Academic Press, San Diego

Bleathman C, Morton I 1992 Validation therapy: extracts from 20 groups with dementia sufferers. Journal of Advanced Nursing 17: 658–666

Blessed G, Tomlinson B E, Roth M 1968 The association between quantitative measures of dementia and of senile change in the cerebral grey matter of elderly subjects. British Journal of Psychiatry 114: 797–811

Blumenthal J A, Emery C F, Madden J D, George L, Coleman R E, Riddle M W, McKee D C, Reasoner J, Williams R S 1989 Cardiovascular and behavioral effects of aerobic exercise training in healthy older men and women. Journal of Gerontology 44: M147–157

Booth T, Phillips D 1987 Group living in homes for the elderly: a comparative study of the outcomes of care. British Journal of Social Work 17: 1–20

Bornat J (ed) 1994 Reminiscence reviewed: perspectives, evaluations, achievements. Open University Press, Buckingham

Bourgeois M S 1990 Enhancing conversation skills in patients with Alzheimer's disease using a prosthetic memory aid. Journal of Applied Behavior Analysis 23: 29–42

Bowie P, Mountain G 1993a Life on a long-stay ward: extracts from the diary of an observing researcher. International Journal of Geriatric Psychiatry 8: 1001–1007

Bowie P, Mountain G 1993b Using direct observation to record the behaviour of long-stay patients with dementia. International Journal of Geriatric Psychiatry 8: 857–864

Bowie P, Mountain G, Clayden D 1992 Assessing the environmental quality of long-stay wards for the confused elderly. International Journal of Geriatric Psychiatry 7: 95–104

Bowlby M C 1991 Reality orientation thirty years later: are we still confused? Canadian Journal of Occupational Therapy 58: 114–122

Bracey R 1989 Time for talk. Nursing Times 85(10): 40–42

Brane G, Karlsson I, Kihlgren M, Norberg A 1989 Integrity-promoting care of demented nursing home patients: psychological and biochemical changes. International Journal of Geriatric Psychiatry 4: 165–172

Breuil V, de Rotrou J, Forette F, Tortrat D, Ganansia-Ganem A, Frambourt A, Moulin F, Boller F 1994 Cognitive stimulation of patients with dementia: preliminary results. International Journal of Geriatric Psychiatry 9: 211–217

Bright R 1992 Music therapy in the management of dementia. In: Jones G, Miesen B M L (eds) Care-giving in dementia. Routledge, London, p 162–180

Brodaty H 1992 Carers: training informal carers. In: Arie T (ed) Recent advances in psychogeriatrics - 2. Churchill Livingstone, Edinburgh, p 163–171

Brody E M, Kleban M H, Lawton M P, Silverman H A 1971 Excess disabilities of mentally impaired aged: impact of individualized treatment. Gerontologist 11: 124–133

Brody E M, Kleban M H, Lawton M P, Moss M 1974 A longitudinal look at excess disabilities in the mentally impaired aged. Journal of Gerontology 29: 79–84

Bromley D B 1978 Approaches to the study of personality changes in adult life and old age. In: Isaacs A D, Post F (eds) Studies in geriatric psychiatry. Wiley, Chichester

Brook P, Degun G, Mather M 1975 Reality orientation, a therapy for psychogeriatric patients: a controlled study. British Journal of Psychiatry 127: 42–45

Brooker D J R, Sturmey P, Gatherer A J H, Summerbell C 1993 The Behavioural assessment scale of later life (BASOLL): a description, factor analysis, scale development, validity and reliability data for a new scale for older adults. International Journal of Geriatric Psychiatry 8: 747–754

Brotchie J, Brennan J, Wyke M 1985 Temporal orientation in the presenium and old age. British Journal of Psychiatry 147: 692–695

Buckholdt D R, Gubrium J F 1983 Therapeutic pretence in reality orientation. International Journal of Aging and Human Development 16: 167–181

Burgess I S, Wearden J H, Cox T, Rae M 1992 Operant conditioning with subjects suffering from dementia. Behavioural Psychotherapy 20: 219–237

Burgio L D, Burgio K L, Engel B T, Tice L M 1986 Increasing distance and independence of ambulation in elderly nursing home residents. Journal of Applied Behavior Analysis 19: 357–366

Burgio L, Engel B T, McCormick K, Hawkins A, Scheve A 1988 Behavioral treatment for urinary incontinence in elderly inpatients: initial attempts to modify prompting and toileting procedures. Behavior Therapy 19: 345–357

Burns A (ed) 1993 Ageing and dementia: a methodological approach. Edward Arnold, London

Burns A, Lewis G 1993 Survival in dementia. In: Burns A (ed) Ageing and dementia: a methodological approach. Edward Arnold, London

Burton M 1980 Evaluation and change in a psychogeriatric ward through direct observation and feedback, British Journal of Psychiatry 137: 566–571

Burton M 1982 Reality orientation for the elderly: a critique. Journal of Advanced Nursing 7: 427–433

Butler R N 1963 The life review: an interpretation of reminiscence in the aged. Psychiatry 26: 65–76

Byrne E J 1987 Reversible dementia. International Journal of Geriatric Psychiatry 2: 73–81

Cameron D E 1941 Studies in senile nocturnal delirium. Psychiatric Quarterly 15: 47–53

Caplin B (ed) 1987 Rehabilitative psychology: desk reference. Aspen Publications, Chicago

Carr J S, Marshall M 1993 Innovations in long-stay care for people with dementia. Reviews in Clinical Gerontology 3: 157–167

Carroll K, Gray K 1981 Memory development: an approach to the mentally impaired elderly in the long-term care setting. International Journal of Aging and Human Development 13: 15–35

Carstensen L L 1988 The emerging field of behavioral gerontology. Behavior Therapy 19: 259–281

Carstensen I L, Erickson R J 1986 Enhancing the social environments of elderly nursing home residents: are high rates of interaction enough? Journal of Applied Behavior Analysis 19: 349–355

Cautela J R 1966 Behaviour therapy and geriatrics. Journal of Genetic Psychology 108: 9–17

Cautela J R 1969 A classical conditioning approach to the development and modification of behaviour in the aged. Gerontologist 9: 109–113

Chafetz P K 1990 Two-dimensional grid is ineffective against demented patients' exiting through glass doors. Psychology and Aging 5: 146–147

Challis D, Davies B 1985 Long-term care for the elderly: the community care scheme. British Journal of Social Work 15: 563–580

Challis D, Davies B 1986 Case management in community care. Gower, Aldershot

Challis D, Chessum R, Chesterman J, Luckett R, Woods R 1988 Community care for the frail elderly: an urban experiment. British Journal of Social Work 18 (suppl): 13–42

Christensen A L 1975 Luria's neuropsychological investigation. Munksgaard, Copenhagen

Citrin R S, Dixon D N 1977 Reality orientation: a milieu therapy used in an institution for the aged. Gerontologist 17: 39–43

Cohen D, Kennedy G, Eisdorfer C 1984 Phases of change in the patient with Alzheimer's dementia. Journal of American Geriatrics Society 32: 11–15

Coleman P 1986 Issues in the therapeutic use of reminiscence with elderly people. In: Hanley I, Gilhooly M (eds) Psychological therapies for the elderly. Croom Helm, London

Cornbleth T, Cornbleth C 1977 Reality orientation for the elderly. Journal Supplement Abstract Service of the American Psychological Association MS 1539

Corrigan J D, Arnett J A, Houck J A, Jackson R D 1985 Reality orientation for brain injured patients: group treatment and monitoring of recovery. Archives of Physical Medicine and Rehabilitation 66: 626–630

Corso J F 1967 The experimental psychology of sensory behaviour. Holt, Rinehart and Winston, New York

Costa P T, McCrae R R 1978 Age differences in personality structure revisited. Ageing and Human Development 8: 131–142

Craig J 1983 The growth of the elderly population. Population Trends 32: 28–33

Craine J F 1987 Cognitive rehabilitation. In: Trexler L E (ed) Cognitive rehabilitation: conceptualization and intervention. Plenum Press, New York, p 83–98

Cummings J L 1984 Treatable dementias. In: Mayeux R, Rosen W G (eds) Advances in neurology—38: the dementias. Raven Press, New York

Darley F L 1982 Aphasia. Saunders, Philadelphia

Davies A D M 1981 Neither wife nor widow: an intervention with the wife of a chronically handicapped man during hospital visits. Behaviour Research and Therapy 19: 449–451

Davies A D M 1982 Research with elderly people in long-term care: some social and organisational factors affecting psychological interventions. Ageing and Society 2: 285–298

Davies A D M, Snaith P 1980 The social behaviour of geriatric patients at meal-times: an observational and an intervention study. Age and Ageing 9: 93–99

Dean R, Briggs K, Lindesay J 1993a The domus philosophy: a prospective evaluation of two residential units for the elderly mentally ill. International Journal of Geriatric Psychiatry 8: 807–817

Dean R, Proudfoot R, Lindesay J 1993b The quality of interactions schedule (QUIS): development, reliability, and use in the evaluation of two domus units. International Journal of Geriatric Psychiatry 8: 819–826

Dietch J T, Hewett L J, Jones S 1989 Adverse effects of reality orientation. Journal of American Geriatrics Society 37: 974–976

Dimond S 1972 The double brain. Williams and Wilkins, Baltimore

Downes J J 1987 Classroom RO and the enhancement of orientation – a critical note. British Journal of Clinical Psychology 26: 147–148

Drummond L, Kirchoff L, Scarbrough D R 1978 A practical guide to reality orientation: a treatment approach for confusion and disorientation. Gerontologist 18: 568-573

Eagger S, Levy R, Sahakian B J 1991 Tacrine in Alzheimer's disease. Lancet 337: 989–992

Elliott V, Milne D 1991 Patients' best friend? Nursing Times 87(6): 34–35

Feher E P, Larrabee G J, Crook T H 1992 Factors attenuating the validity of the geriatric depression scale in a dementia population. Journal of American Geriatrics Society 40: 906–909

Feil N 1982 Validation: the Feil method. Edward Feil Productions, Cleveland

Feil N 1989 Validation: the Feil method, 2nd edn. Edward Feil Productions/Winslow Press, Cleveland

Feil N 1992 Validation therapy with late-onset dementia populations. In: Jones G , Miesen B (eds) Care-giving in dementia: research and applications. Routledge, London, p 199–218

Feil N 1993 The validation breakthrough: simple techniques for communicating with people with 'Alzheimer's type dementia'. Health Professions Press, Baltimore

Fisher P 1994 Creative movements for older adults. Winslow Press, Bicester

Folstein M F 1991 Rating scales for use in the elderly. Current Opinion in Psychiatry 4: 591–595

Folstein M F, Folstein S E, McHugh P R 1975 'Mini–mental state': a practical method for grading the cognitive state of patients for the clinician. Journal of Psychiatric Research 12: 189–198

Fussey I, Muir Giles G (eds) 1988 Rehabilitation of the severely brain injured adult: a practical approach. Croom Helm, London

Gaebler H C, Hemsley D R 1991 The assessment and short-term manipulation of affect in the severely demented. Behavioural Psychotherapy 19: 145–156

Garland J 1985 A model for the understanding and behavioural management of excess noise making by old people in residential care. Paper presented at XIIIth International Congress of Gerontology, New York

Garland J 1991 Making residential care feel like home. Winslow, Bicester

Garland J 1994 What splendour, it all coheres: life-review therapy with older people. In: Bornat J (ed) Reminiscence reviewed. Open University Press, Buckingham, p 21–31

Gazzaniga M S 1970 The bisected brain. Appleton Century-Crofts, New York

Georgiades N J, Phillimore L 1975 The myth of the hero-innovator and alternative strategies for organisational change. In: Kiernan C C, Woodford F P (eds) Behaviour modification with the severely retarded. Associated Scientific Publishers, New York, p 313–319

Gibson F 1994 What can reminiscence contribute to people with dementia? In: Bornat J (ed) Reminiscence reviewed: evaluations, achievements, perspectives. Open University Press, Buckingham, p 46–60

Gilhooly M 1984 The social dimensions of senile dementia. In: Hanley I, Hodge J (eds) Psychological approaches to the care of the elderly. Croom Helm, London, p 88–135

Gilleard C J 1984a Assessment of cognitive impairment in the elderly. In: Hanley I, Hodge J (eds) Psychological approaches to the care of the elderly. Croom Helm, London

Gilleard C J 1984b Assessment of behavioural impairment in the elderly: a review. In: Hanley I, Hodge J (eds) Psychological approaches to the care of the elderly. Croom Helm, London

Gilleard C J 1984c Living with dementia. Croom Helm, London

Gilleard C J 1992 Carers: recent research findings. In: Arie T (ed) Recent advances in psychogeriatrics—2. Churchill Livingstone, Edinburgh, p 137–152

Gilleard C J, Mitchell R G, Riordan J 1981 Ward orientation training with psychogeriatric patients. Journal of Advanced Nursing 6: 95–98

Godlove C, Dunn G, Wright H 1980 Caring for old people in New York and London: the 'nurses' aide' interviews. Journal of the Royal Society of Medicine 73: 713–723

Golding E 1989 Middlesex elderly assessment of mental state. Thames Valley Test Company, Titchfield

Goldstein G, Turner S M, Holzman A, Kanagy M, Elmore S, Barry K 1982 An evaluation of reality orientation therapy. Journal of Behavioural Assessment 4: 165–178

Goldwasser A N, Auerbach S M, Harkins S W 1987 Cognitive, affective and behavioral effects of reminiscence group therapy on demented elderly. International Journal of Aging and Human Development 25: 209–222

Gray P, Stevenson J S 1980 Changes in verbal interaction among members of resocialisation groups. Journal of Gerontological Nursing 6: 86–90

Green G R, Linsk N L, Pinkston E M 1986 Modification of verbal behaviour of the mentally impaired elderly by their spouses. Journal of Applied Behavior Analysis 19: 329–336

Greene J G, Nicol R, Jamieson H 1979 Reality orientation with psychogeriatric patients. Behaviour Research and Therapy 17: 615–617

Greene J G, Smith R, Gardiner M, Timbury G C 1982 Measuring behavioural disturbance of elderly demented patients in the community and its effects on relatives: a factor-analytic study. Age and Ageing 11: 121–126

Greene J G, Timbury G C, Smith R, Gardiner M 1983 Reality orientation with elderly patients in the community: an empirical evaluation. Age and Ageing 12: 38–43

Gubrium J F, Ksander M 1975 On multiple realities and reality orientation. Gerontologist 15: 142–145

Haight B 1992 The structured life-review process: a community approach to the ageing client. In: Jones G M M, Miesen B M L (eds) Care-giving in dementia. Routledge, London, p 272–292

Haight B K, Burnside I 1992 Reminiscence and life review: conducting the process. Journal of Gerontological Nursing 18: 39–42

Haight B K, Burnside I 1993 Reminiscence and life review: explaining the differences. Archives of Psychiatric Nursing 7: 91–98

Hall J N 1980 Ward rating scales for long-stay patients: a review. Psychological Medicine 10: 277–288

Hallberg I R, Edberg A K, Nordmark A, Johnsson K 1993 Daytime vocal activity in institutionalized severely demented patients identified as vocally disruptive by nurses. International Journal of Geriatric Psychiatry 8: 155–164

Hanley I G 1981 The use of signposts and active training to modify ward disorientation in elderly patients. Journal of Behaviour Therapy and Experimental Psychiatry 12: 241–247

Hanley I G 1982 A manual for the modification of confused behaviour. Lothian Regional Council Department of Social Work, Edinburgh

Hanley I G 1984 Theoretical and practical considerations in reality orientation therapy with the elderly. In: Hanley I, Hodge J (eds) Psychological approaches to the care of the elderly. Croom Helm, London

Hanley I G 1986 Reality orientation in the care of the elderly person with dementia – three case studies. In: Hanley I, Gilhooly M (eds) Psychological therapies for the elderly. Croom Helm, London

Hanley I G 1988 Individualised reality orientation: creative therapy with confused elderly people. Winslow Press, Bicester

Hanley I G, Lusty K 1984 Memory aids in reality orientation: a single-case study. Behaviour Research and Therapy 22: 709–712

Hanley I G, McGuire R J, Boyd W D 1981b Reality orientation and dementia: a controlled trial of two approaches. British Journal of Psychiatry 138: 10–14

Harris C S, Ivory P B C B 1976 An outcome evaluation of reality orientation therapy with geriatric patients in a state mental hospital. Gerontologist 16: 496–503

Hart J, Fleming R 1985 An experimental evaluation of a modified reality orientation therapy. Clinical Gerontologist 3(4): 35–44

Haugen P K 1985 Dementia in old age – treatment approaches. Report 5/85, Norsk Gerontologisk Institutt, Oslo

Haughie E, Milne D, Elliott V 1992 An evaluation of companion dogs with elderly psychiatric patients. Behavioural Psychotherapy 20: 367–372

Hausman C 1992 Dynamic psychotherapy with elderly demented patients. In: Jones G, Miesen B M L (eds) Care-giving in dementia: research and applications. Routledge, London, p 181–198

Head D, Portnoy S, Woods R T 1990 The impact of reminiscence groups in two different settings. International Journal of Geriatric Psychiatry 5: 295–302

Hecaen H, Albert M L 1978 Human neuropsychology. Wiley, New York

Hecaen H, Assal G 1970 A comparison of construction deficits following right and left hemisphere lesions. Neuropsychologia 8: 289–304

Help the Aged 1981 Recall – a handbook. Help the Aged Education Department, London

Hinchliffe A C, Hyman I, Blizard B, Livingston G 1992 The impact on carers of behavioural difficulties in dementia: a pilot study on management. International Journal of Geriatric Psychiatry 7: 579–583

Hodge J 1984 Towards a behavioural analysis of dementia. In: Hanley I, Hodge J (eds) Psychological approaches to the care of the elderly. Croom Helm, London

Hofman A, Rocca W A, Brayne C et al 1991 The prevalence of dementia in Europe: a collaborative study of the 1980–1990 findings. International Journal of Epidemiology 20: 736–748

Hogstel M O 1979 Use of reality orientation with ageing confused patients. Nursing Research 28: 161–165

Holden U P 1984a Assessment of dementia: the case against standard test batteries. Clinical Gerontologist 3(2): 48–52

Holden U P 1984b Reality orientation reminders. Winslow Press, London

Holden U P 1984c Thinking it through. Winslow Press, London

Holden U P 1988 Neuropsychology and ageing: definitions, explanations and practical approaches. Croom Helm, London

Holden U P 1991 Day into night. Winslow Press, Bicester

Holden U P, Sinebruchow A 1978 Reality orientation therapy: a study investigating the value of this therapy in the rehabilitation of elderly people. Age and Ageing 7: 83–90

Holden U P, Woods R T 1988 Reality orientation: psychological approaches to the 'confused' elderly, 2nd edn. Churchill Livingstone, Edinburgh

Holland C A, Rabbitt P 1991 The course and causes of cognitive change with advancing age. Reviews in Clinical Gerontology 1: 81–96

Hong C S 1989 Doubly disadvantaged. Nursing Times 85: 69–70

Hope R A, Fairburn C G 1990 The nature of wandering in dementia: a community-based study. International Journal of Geriatric Psychiatry 5: 239–245

Huppert F A 1988 Age related changes. In: Boller F, Grafman A (eds) Handbook of neuropsychology. Elsevier, Oxford

Hussian R A 1981 Geriatric psychology: a behavioural perspective. Van Nostrand Reinhold, New York

Hussian R A 1984 Behavioral geriatrics. Progress in Behaviour Modification 16: 159–183

Hussian R A, Brown D C 1987 Use of two-dimensional grid patterns to limit hazardous ambulation in demented patients. Journal of Gerontology 42: 558–560

Hutt S J, Hutt C 1970 Direct observation and measurement of behaviour. Thomas, Springfield

Ingstad P J, Gotestam K G 1987 Staff attitude changes after environmental changes on a ward for psychogeriatric patients. International Journal of Social Psychiatry 33: 237–244

Jagger C, Lindesay J 1993 The epidemiology of senile dementia. In: Burns A (ed) Ageing and dementia. Edward Arnold, London

Jenkins J, Felce D, Lunt B, Powell E 1977 Increasing engagement in activity of residents in old people's homes by providing recreational materials. Behaviour Research and Therapy 15: 429–434

Johnson C M, McLaren S M, McPherson F M 1981 The comparative effectiveness of three versions of 'classroom' reality orientation. Age and Ageing 10: 33–35

Jones G 1985 Validation therapy: a companion to reality orientation. Canadian Nurse (March): 20–23

Jones G M, Clark P 1984 The use of memory 'recall' on a psychogeriatric ward. British Journal of Occupational Therapy 47: 315–316

Josephsson S, Backman L, Borell L, Bernspang B, Nygard L, Ronnberg L 1993 Supporting everyday activities in dementia: an intervention study. International Journal of Geriatric Psychiatry 8: 395–400

Katona C L E, Aldridge C R 1985 The dexamethasone suppression test and depressive signs in dementia. Journal of Affective Disorders 8: 83–89

Keen J 1989 Interiors: architecture in the lives of people with dementia. International Journal of Geriatric Psychiatry 4: 255–272

King's Fund 1986 Living well into old age: applying principles of good practice to services for elderly people with severe mental disabilities. King's Fund, London

Kitwood T 1990 The dialectics of dementia: with particular reference to Alzheimer's disease. Ageing & Society 10: 177–196

Kitwood T 1992a How valid is validation therapy. Geriatric Medicine (April): 23

Kitwood T 1992b Quality assurance in dementia care. Geriatric Medicine (Sept): 34–38

Kitwood T 1993 Towards a theory of dementia care: the interpersonal process. Ageing and Society 13: 51–67

Kitwood T, Bredin K 1992 Towards a theory of dementia care: personhood and well-being. Ageing and Society 12: 269–287

Koh K, Ray R, Lee J, Nair A, Ho T, Ang P C 1994 Dementia in elderly patients: can the 3R mental stimulation programme improve mental status? Age and Ageing 23: 195–199

Kuriansky J, Gurland B 1976 The performance test of activities of daily living. International Journal of Aging and Human Development 7: 343–352

Kuriansky J, Gurland B, Cowan D 1976 The usefulness of a psychological test battery. International Journal of Aging and Human Development 7: 331–342

Lam D H, Woods R T 1986 Ward orientation training in dementia: a single case study. International Journal of Geriatric Psychiatry 1: 145–147

Langford S 1993 A shared vision. Nursing Times 89(44): 66–69

Lemke S, Moos R H 1980 Assessing the institutional policies of sheltered care settings. Journal of Gerontology 35: 96–107

Lemke S, Moos R 1986 Quality of residential settings for elderly adults. Journal of Gerontology 41: 268–276

Lincoln N B 1989 Management of memory problems in a hospital setting. In: Poon L W, Rubin D C, Wilson B A (eds) Everyday cognition in adulthood and late life. Cambridge University Press, Cambridge, p 639–658

Lindesay J, Briggs K, Lawes M, Macdonald A, Herzberg J 1991 The domus philosophy: a comparative evaluation of a new approach to residential care for the demented elderly. International Journal of Geriatric Psychiatry B: 727–736

Lindsley O R 1964 Geriatric behavioural prosthetics. In: Kastenbaum R (ed) New thoughts on old age. Springer, New York

Little A G, Levy R, Chuaqui–Kidd P, Hand D 1985 A double-blind, placebo controlled trial of high dose lecithin in Alzheimer's disease. Journal of Neurology, Neurosurgery and Psychiatry 48: 736–742

Little A G, Volans P J, Hemsley D R, Levy R 1986 The retention of new information in senile dementia. British Journal of Clinical Psychology 25: 71–72

Livingston G, Hinchliffe A C 1993 The epidemiology of psychiatric disorders in the elderly. International Review of Psychiatry 5: 317–326

Lodge B, McReynolds S 1983 Quadruple support for dementia. Age Concern Leicestershire, Leicester

Loewenstein D A, Amigo E, Duara R, Guterman A, Hurwitz D, Berkowitz N, Wilkie F, Weinberg G, Black B, Gittelman B, Eisdorfer C 1989 A new scale for the assessment of functional status in Alzheimer's disease and related disorders. Journal of Gerontology 44: 114–121

Lord T R, Garner J E 1993 Effects of music on Alzheimer patients. Perceptual and Motor Skills 76: 451–455

Luria A R 1963 Restoration of function after brain injury. Pergamon Press, Oxford

McCormack D, Whitehead A 1981 The effect of providing recreational activities on the engagement level of long-stay geriatric patients. Age and Ageing 10: 287–291

Macdonald A J D, Craig T K J, Warner L A R 1985 The development of a short observational method for the study of the activity and contacts of old people in residential settings. Psychological Medicine 15: 167–172

MacDonald M L, Settin J M 1978 Reality orientation vs sheltered workshops as treatment for the institutionalized aging. Journal of Gerontology 33: 416–421

McFadyen M 1984 The measurement of engagement in the institutionalised elderly. In: Hanley I, Hodge J (eds) Psychological approaches to the care of the elderly. Croom Helm, London

McFadyen M, Prior T, Kindness K 1980 Engagement: an important variable in institutional care of the elderly. Paper presented at British Psychological Society Annual Conference, Aberdeen

Mahurin R K, DeBettignies B H, Pirozzolo F J 1991 Structured assessment of independent living skills: preliminary report of a performance measure of functional abilities in dementia. Journal of Gerontology 46: 58–66

Malmberg B, Zarit S H 1993 Group homes for people with dementia: a Swedish example. Gerontologist 33: 682–686

Manser M 1991 Design of environments. In: Jacoby R, Oppenheimer C (eds) Psychiatry in the elderly. Oxford University Press, Oxford, p 550–570

Mayer R, Darby S 1991 Does a mirror deter wandering in demented older people? International Journal of Geriatric Psychiatry 6: 607–609

Meir H J, Benton A L, Diller L 1986 Neuropsychological rehabilitation. Churchill Livingstone, Edinburgh

Melin L, Gotestam K G 1981 The effects of rearranging ward routines on communication and eating behaviours of psychogeriatric patients. Journal of Applied Behavioural Analysis 14: 47–51

Merchant M, Saxby P 1981 Reality orientation: a way forward. Nursing Times 77(33): 1442–1445

Merriam S 1980 The concept and function of reminiscence: a review of the research. Gerontologist 20: 604–608

Miesen B M L 1992 Attachment theory and dementia. In: Jones G, Miesen B M L (eds) Care-giving in dementia. Routledge, London, p 38–56

Miesen B M L 1993 Alzheimer's disease, the phenomenon of parent fixation and Bowlby's attachment theory. International Journal of Geriatric Psychiatry 8: 147–153

Miller A 1985 A study of the dependency of elderly patients in wards using different methods of nursing care. Age and Ageing 14: 132–138

Miller E 1977 The management of dementia: a review of some possibilities. British Journal of Social and Clinical Psychology 16: 77–83

Miller E 1984 Recovery and management of neuropsychological impairments. Wiley, Chichester

Miller E 1987 Reality orientation with psychiatric patients: the limitations. Clinical Rehabilitation 1: 231–233

Miller E, Morris R 1993 The psychology of dementia. Wiley, Chichester

Milne D 1985 An observational evaluation of the effects of nurse training in behaviour therapy on unstructured ward activities and interactions. British Journal of Clinical Psychology 24: 149–158

Mintzer J E, Lewis L, Pennypaker L, Simpson W, Bachman D, Wohlreich G, Meeks A, Hunt S, Sampson R 1993 Behavioral intensive care unit (BICU): a new concept in the management of acute agitated behavior in elderly demented patients. Gerontologist 33: 801–806

Moffat N J 1989 Home-based cognitive rehabilitation with the elderly. In: Poon L W, Rubin D C, Wilson B A (eds) Everyday cognition in adulthood and late life. Cambridge University Press, Cambridge, p 659–680

Molloy D W, Richardson L D, Crilly R G 1988 The effects of a three-month exercise programme on neuropsychological function in elderly institutionalized women: a randomized controlled trial. Age and Ageing 17: 303–310

Moore V, Wyke M 1984 Drawing disability in patients with senile dementia. Psychological Medicine 14: 97–105

Moos R H, Lemke S 1980 Assessing the physical and architectural features of sheltered care settings. Journal of Gerontology 35: 571–583

Morgan K 1987 Sleep and ageing. Croom Helm, London

Morgan K 1991 Trial and error: evaluating the psychological benefits of physical activity. International Journal of Geriatric Psychiatry 4: 125–127

Morgan K, Gledhill K 1991 Managing sleep and insomnia in the older person. Winslow Press, Bicester

Moriarty J, Levin E 1993 Interventions to assist caregivers. Reviews in Clinical Gerontology 3: 301–308

Morris R G 1987 Matching and oddity learning in moderate to severe dementia. Quarterly Journal of Experimental Psychology 39: 215–227

Morris R G, Morris L W 1993 Psychosocial aspects of caring for people with dementia: conceptual and methodological issues. In: Burns A (ed) Ageing and dementia. Edward Arnold, London

Morris R, Wheatley J, Britton P G 1983 Retrieval from long term memory in senile dementia – cued recall revisited. British Journal of Clinical Psychology 22: 141–142

Morris R G, Morris L W, Britton P G 1988 Factors affecting the emotional well-being of the caregivers of dementia sufferers. British Journal of Psychiatry 153: 147–156

Morris R G, Woods R T, Davies K S, Berry J, Morris L W 1992 The use of a coping strategy focused support group for carers of dementia sufferers. Counselling Psychology Quarterly 5: 337–348

Morton I, Bleathman C 1991 The effectiveness of validation therapy in dementia: a pilot study. International Journal of Geriatric Psychiatry 6: 327–330

Mountain G, Bowie P 1992 The possessions owned by long-stay psychogeriatric patients. International Journal of Geriatric Psychiatry 7: 285–290

Murphy G, Goodall E 1980 Measurement error in direct observations: a comparison of common recording methods. Behaviour Research and Therapy 18: 147–150

Naylor G, Harwood E 1975 Old dogs, new tricks: age and ability. Psychology Today 1: 29–33

Nelson H E, Willison J 1991 National adult reading test: test manual. NFER-Nelson, Windsor

Netten A 1989 Environment, orientation and behaviour; the effect of the design of residential homes in creating dependency among confused elderly residents. International Journal of Geriatric Psychiatry 4: 143–152

Netten A 1993 A positive environment? Physical and social influences on people with senile dementia in residential care. Ashgate, Aldershot

Norberg A, Melin E, Asplund K 1986 Reactions to music, touch and object presentation in the final stage of dementia: an exploratory study. International Journal of Nursing Studies 23: 315–323

Norman A 1987 Severe dementia: The provision of long-stay care. Centre for Policy on Ageing, London

Norris A 1986 Reminiscence. Winslow Press, London

Oberleder M 1962 An attitude scale to determine adjustment in institutions for the aged. Journal of Chronic Diseases 15: 915–923

Orrell M, Howard R, Payne A, Bergmann K, Woods R, Everitt B S, Levy R 1992 Differentiation between organic and functional psychiatric illness in the elderly: an evaluation of four cognitive tests. International Journal of Geriatric Psychiatry 7: 263–275

Parmelee P A, Lawton M P 1990 The design of special environments for the aged. In: Birren J E, Schaie K W (eds) Handbook of the psychology of aging. Academic Press, San Diego, p 464–488

Patel V, Hope R A 1992 A rating scale for aggressive behaviour in the elderly. Psychological Medicine 22: 211–221

Patterson R L 1982 Overcoming deficits of aging: a behavioural approach. Plenum Press, New York

Pattie A H 1988 Measuring levels of disability – the Clifton assessment procedures for the elderly. In: Wattis J P, Hindmarch I (eds) Psychological assessment of the elderly. Churchill Livingstone, Edinburgh, p 61–80

Pattie A H, Gilleard C J 1979 Manual of the Clifton assessment procedures for the elderly (CAPE). Hodder and Stoughton Educational, Sevenoaks

Peisah C, Sachdev P, Brodaty H 1993 Vascular dementia. International Review of Psychiatry 5: 381–395

Perry E K, Perry R H 1993 Neurochemical pathology and therapeutic strategies in degenerative dementia. International Review of Psychiatry 5: 363–380

Perry R H, Irving D, Blessed G, Fairbairn A F, Perry E K 1990 Senile dementia of the Lewy body type: a clinically distinct form of Lewy body dementia in the elderly. Journal of Neurological Science 95: 119–139

Pinkston E M, Linsk N L 1984 Care of the elderly: a family approach. Pergamon, New York

Portalska R Z, Bernstein M 1988 The differentiation of depression from senile dementia in the elderly. International Journal of Geriatric Psychiatry 3: 137–144

Powell-Proctor L, Miller E 1982 Reality orientation: a critical appraisal. British Journal of Psychiatry 140: 457–463

Praderas K, MacDonald M L 1986 Telephone conversational skills training with socially isolated, impaired nursing home residents. Journal of Applied Behavior Analysis 19: 337–348

Quattrochi–Tubin S, Jones J W, Breedlove V 1982 The burnout syndrome in geriatric counsellors and service workers. Activities, Adaptation and Ageing 3: 65–76

Rabbitt P 1988 Social psychology, neurosciences and cognitive psychology need each other (and gerontology needs all three of them). Psychologist 12: 500–506

Reeve W, Ivison D 1985 Use of environmental manipulation and classroom and modified informal reality orientation with institutionalized, confused elderly patients. Age and Ageing 14: 119–121

Regnier V, Pynoos J 1992 Environmental intervention for cognitively impaired older persons. In: Birren J E, Sloane R B, Cohen G D (eds) Handbook of mental health and aging. Academic Press, San Diego, p 763–792

Riegler J 1980 Comparison of a reality orientation programme for geriatric patients with and without music. Journal of Music Therapy 17: 26–33

Rimmer L 1982 Reality orientation: principles and practice. Winslow Press, London

Rinke C L, Williams J J, Lloyd K E, Smith-Scott W 1978 The effects of prompting and reinforcement on self-bathing by elderly residents of a nursing home. Behavior Therapy 9: 873–881

Ritchie K, Colvez A, Ankri J, Ledesert B, Gardent H, Fontaine A 1992 The evaluation of long-term care for the dementing elderly: a comparative study of hospital and collective non-medical care in France. International Journal of Geriatric Psychiatry 7: 549–557

Rona D, Bellwood S, Wylie B 1984 Assessment of a behavioural programme to treat incontinent patients in psychogeriatric wards. British Journal of Clinical Psychology 23: 273–280

Rona D, Wylie B, Bellwood S 1986 Behaviour treatment of daytime incontinence in elderly male and female patients. Behavioural Psychotherapy 14: 13–20

Roth M, Tym E, Mountjoy C Q, Huppert F, Hendrie H, Verma S, Goddard R 1986 CAMDEX – a standardised instrument for the diagnosis of mental disorders in the elderly with special reference to the early detection of dementia. British Journal of Psychiatry 149: 698–709

Roth M, Huppert F A, Tym E, Mountjoy C Q 1988 CAMDEX – Cambridge examination for mental disorders of the elderly. Cambridge University Press, Cambridge

Rothi L J, Horner J 1983 Restitution and substitution: two theories of recovery with application to neurobehavioural treatment. Journal of Clinical Neuropsychology 5: 73–81

Rothwell N, Britton P G, Woods R T 1983 The effects of group living in a residential home for the elderly. British Journal of Social Work 13: 639–643

Ryan D H 1994 Misdiagnosis in dementia: comparisons of diagnostic error rate and range of hospital investigation according to medical specialty. International Journal of Geriatric Psychiatry 9: 141–147

Rybash J M, Hoyer W J, Roodin P A 1986 Adult cognition and aging: developmental changes in processing, knowing and thinking. Pergamon, New York

Sahakian B J 1991 Depressive pseudodementia in the elderly. International Journal of Geriatric Psychiatry 6: 453–458

Sanavio E 1981 Toilet retraining psychogeriatric residents. Behavior Modification 5: 417–427

Sandman C A 1993 Memory rehabilitation in Alzheimer's disease: preliminary findings. Clinical Gerontologist 13: 19–33

Saxby P, Jeffery D 1983 In a strange land. Social Work Today 15 (Sept 6): 16–17

Scarbrough D R, Drummond L, Kirchhoff L 1978 Letter to the editor. Journal of Gerontology 33: 588

Schaie K W 1990 Intellectual development in adulthood. In: Birren J E, Schaie K W (eds) Handbook of the psychology of aging. Academic Press, San Diego, p 291–309

Schaie K W, Willis S L 1986 Can intellectual decline in the elderly be reversed? Developmental Psychology 22: 223–232

Schnelle J F, Traughber B, Morgan D B, Embry J E, Binion A F, Coleman A 1983 Management of geriatric incontinence in nursing homes. Journal of Applied Behavior Analysis 16: 235–241

Schnelle J F, Traughber B, Sowell V A, Newman D R, Petrilli C O, Ory M 1989 Prompted voiding treatment of urinary incontinence in nursing home patients: a behavior management approach for nursing home staff. Journal of American Geriatrics Society 37: 1051–1057

Schnelle J F, Newman D, White M, Abbey J, Wallston K A, Fogarty T, Ory M G 1993 Maintaining continence in nursing home residents through the application of industrial quality control. Gerontologist 33: 114–121

Schwenk M A 1981 Reality orientation for the institutionalized aged: does it help? Gerontologist 19: 373–377

Scogin F, McElreath L 1994 Efficacy of psychosocial treatments for geriatric depression: a quantitative review. Journal of Consulting and Clinical Psychology 62: 69–74

Seligman M 1975 Helplessness: on depression, development and death. W. H. Freeman, San Francisco

Sinason V 1992 The man who was losing his brain. In: Sinason V (ed) Mental handicap and the human condition: new approaches from the Tavistock. Free Association Books, London, p 87–110

Sixsmith A, Hawley C, Stilwell J, Copeland J 1993a Delivering 'positive care' in nursing homes. International Journal of Geriatric Psychiatry 8: 407–412

Sixsmith A, Stilwell J, Copeland J 1993b Rementia: challenging the limits of dementia care. International Journal of Geriatric Psychiatry 8: 993–1000

Skurla E, Rogers J C, Sunderland T 1988 Direct assessment of activities of daily living in Alzheimer's disease: a controlled study. Journal of the American Geriatrics Society 36: 97–103

Smith P, Smith L 1986 Continence and incontinence: psychological approaches to development and treatment. Croom Helm, London

Snyder L H, Rupprecht P, Pyrek J, Brekhus S, Moss T 1978 Wandering. Gerontologist 18: 272–280

Sofroniew M V 1993 Cellular recovery. In: Greenwood R, Barnes M P, McMillan T M, Ward C D (eds) Neurological rehabilitation. Churchill Livingstone, Edinburgh, p 67–84

Sparks R, Helm N, Albert M L 1974 Aphasia rehabilitation resulting from melodic intonation therapy. Cortex 10: 303–316

Stephens L P (ed) 1969 Reality orientation: a technique to rehabilitate elderly and brain-damaged patients with a moderate to severe degree of disorientation. American Psychiatric Association Hospital and Community Psychiatric Service, Washington DC

Stockwell F 1985 The nursing process in psychiatric nursing. Croom Helm, London

Stokes G 1986a Wandering. Winslow Press, London

Stokes G 1986b Screaming and shouting. Winslow Press, London

Stokes G 1987 Aggression. Winslow Press, Bicester

Stokes G 1989 Managing aggression in dementia: the do's and don't's. Geriatric Medicine (April): 35–40

Stokes G 1992 On being old: The psychology of later life. Falmer Press, London

Stokes G, Goudie F (eds) 1990 Working with dementia. Winslow Press, Bicester

Strickland R, Hill P 1992 Gentle exercises for the elderly. Winslow Press, Bicester

Stuart-Hamilton I 1994 The Psychology of ageing: an introduction, 2nd edn. Jessica Kingsley, London

Tarrier N, Larner S 1983 The effects of manipulation of social reinforcement on toilet requests on a geriatric ward. Age & Ageing 12: 234–239

Taulbee L R, Folsom J C 1966 Reality orientation for geriatric patients. Hospital and Community Psychiatry 17: 133–135

Thompson L W, Wagner B, Zeiss A, Gallagher D 1990 Cognitive/behavioural therapy with early stage Alzheimer's patients: an exploratory view of the utility of this approach. In: Light E, Lebowitz B D (eds) Alzheimer's disease: treatment and family stress. Hemisphere, New York, p 383–397

Thornton S, Brotchie J 1987 Reminiscence: a critical review of the empirical literature. British Journal of Clinical Psychology 26: 93–111

Ulatowska H K (ed) 1985 The aging brain: communication in the elderly. Taylor and Francis, London

Voelkel D 1978 A study of reality orientation and resocialization groups with confused elderly. Journal of Gerontological Nursing 4: 3–18

Wallis G G, Baldwin M, Higginbotham P 1983 Reality orientation therapy: a controlled trial. British Journal of Medical Psychology 56: 271–278

Walsh K W 1987 Neuropsychology: a clinical approach, 2nd edn. Churchill Livingstone, Edinburgh

Ward T, Murphy E, Procter A 1991 Functional assessment in severely demented patients. Age and Ageing 20: 212–216

Ward T, Murphy E, Procter A, Weinman J 1992 An observational study of two long-stay psychogeriatric wards. International Journal of Geriatric Psychiatry 7: 211–217

Ward T, Dawe B, Procter A, Murphy E, Weinman J 1993 Assessment in severe dementia: the Guy's advanced dementia schedule. Age and Ageing 22: 183–189

Ware C J G, Fairburn C G, Hope R A 1990 A community based study of aggressive behaviour in dementia. International Journal of Geriatric Psychiatry 5: 337–342

Warrington E K, James M, Kinsbourne M 1966 Drawing disability in relation to laterality of lesion. Brain 89: 53–82

Wattis J P, Church M 1986 Practical psychiatry of old age. Croom Helm, London

Welden S, Yesavage J A 1982 Behavioral improvement with relaxation training in senile dementia. Clinical Gerontologist 1: 45–49

West B, Brockman S 1994 The calming power of aromatherapy. Journal of Dementia Care 2(2): 20–22

Wilcock G 1984 Dementia. In: Dawson A M, Compston N, Besser G M (eds) Recent advances in medicine 19. Churchill Livingstone, Edinburgh

Wilcock G, Esiri M M 1982 Plaques, tangles and dementia: a quantitative study. Journal of the Neurological Sciences 56: 343–356

Wilkinson A M 1993 Dementia care mapping: a pilot study of its implementation in a psychogeriatric service.

International Journal of Geriatric Psychiatry 8: 1027–1029

Willcocks D M, Peace S M, Kellaher L A 1987 Private lives in public places. Tavistock, London

Williams R, Reeve W, Ivison D, Kavanagh D 1987 Use of environmental manipulation and modified informal reality orientation with institutionalized confused elderly subjects: a replication. Age and Ageing 16: 315–318

Willmott M 1986 The effect of a vinyl floor surface and a carpeted floor surface upon walking in elderly hospital in-patients. Age and Ageing 15: 119–120

Wilson B A, Moffat N 1984 Running a memory group. In: Wilson B A, Moffat N (eds) Clinical management of memory problems. Croom Helm, Beckenham, p 171–198

Wimo A, Wallin J O, Lundgren K, Ronnback E, Asplund K, Mattsson B, Krakau I 1991 Group living, an alternative for dementia patients: a cost analysis. International Journal of Geriatric Psychiatry 6: 21–29

Wisocki P 1984 Behavioral approaches to gerontology. Progress in Behavior Modification 16: 121–157

Woods R T 1979 Reality orientation and staff attention: a controlled study. British Journal of Psychiatry 134: 502–507

Woods R T 1983 Specificity of learning in reality orientation sessions: a single-case study. Behaviour Research and Therapy 21: 173–175

Woods R T 1987 Psychological management of dementia. In: Pitt B (ed) Dementia. Churchill Livingstone, Edinburgh

Woods R T 1989 Alzheimer's disease: coping with a living death. Souvenir Press, London

Woods R T 1992 What can be learned from studies on reality orientation? In: Jones G, Miesen B (eds) Care-giving in dementia. Routledge, London, p 121–136

Woods R T, Britton P G 1977 Psychological approaches to the treatment of the elderly. Age and Ageing 6: 104–112

Woods R T, Britton P G 1985 Clinical psychology with the elderly. Croom Helm Chapman Hall, London

Woods R T, McKiernan F 1995 Evaluating the impact of reminiscence on older people with dementia. In: Haight B K, Taylor J (eds) The art and science of reminiscing: theory, research, methods and applications. Taylor and Francis, Washington DC

Woods R T, Portnoy S, Head D, Jones G 1992 Reminiscence and life-review with persons with dementia: which way forward? In: Jones G, Miesen B (eds) Care-giving in dementia. Routledge, London, p 137–161

Yesavage J A, Rose T L, Spiegel D 1982 Relaxation training and memory improvement in elderly normals: correlation of anxiety ratings and recall improvement. Experimental Aging Research 8: 195–198

Zanetti O, Bianchetti A, Montini M, Trabocchi M 1993 Reality orientation therapy in demented patients: useful or not? (Abstract) Paper presented at International Congress of Gerontology, Budapest

Zepelin H, Wolfe C S, Kleinplatz F 1981 Evaluation of a year-long reality orientation program. Journal of Gerontology 36: 70–77

Author Index

Subject Index